Semantic Cognition

30.00

Semantic Cognition

A Parallel Distributed Processing Approach

Timothy T. Rogers and James L. McClelland

A Bradford Book
The MIT Press
Cambridge, Massachusetts
London, England

First MIT Press paperback edition, 2006

© 2004 Massachusetts Institute of Technology

This book was set in Melior and Helvetica Condensed by Asco Typesetters, Hong Kong. Printed and bound in the United States of America.

Library of Congress Cataloging-in-Publication Data

Rogers, Timothy T.
Semantic cognition : a parallel distributed processing approach / Timothy T. Rogers and James L. McClelland.
    p.   cm.
Includes bibliographical references and index.
ISBN 978-0-262-18239-3 (hc. : alk. paper)— 978-0-262-68157-5 (pb. : alk. paper)
1. Dementia—Miscellanea. 2. Cognition. 3. Semantics. 4. Dementia. I. McClelland, James L. II. Title.

RC521.R64   2004
153—dc22   2003070600

10 9 8 7 6 5 4 3 2

Contents

Preface

Attempts to understand the basis of human semantic abilities are central to the effort to understand human cognition. Since antiquity, philosophers have considered how we make semantic judgments, and the investigation of semantic processing was a focal point for both experimental and computational investigations in the early phases of the cognitive revolution. Yet the mechanistic basis of semantic cognition remains very much open to question. While explicit computational theories were offered in the 1960s and into the 1970s, the mid-1970s saw the introduction of findings on the gradedness of category membership and on the privileged status of some categories that these theories did not encompass. Eleanor Rosch, who introduced most of these phenomena, eschewed any sort of explicit mechanistic theorizing.

Subsequently a new thrust of research has emerged within a framework that is often called "theory theory." This framework has been very useful as a springboard for powerful experimental demonstrations of the subtlety and sophistication of the semantic judgments that adults and even children can make, but it has left the field without an explicit mechanistic theory of the representation and use of semantic knowledge, since the fundamental tenets of theory theory are general principles whose main use has been to guide the design of ingenious experiments rather than the explicit formulation of computational mechanisms.

The subtlety of the semantic capabilities of human adults and even of rather young children, and the ways these abilities evolve and become elaborated over the course of development, make the prospect of offering any sort of mechanistic framework for understanding semantic cognition daunting. Nevertheless, we find ourselves in the position of offering, if not a full characterization of the mechanistic basis of semantic knowledge, then at least some demonstrations of the properties of a type of mechanism that may suggest the general form such a characterization might take.

When we began our work we had a specific and rather narrow focus: to address the progressive differentiation of conceptual knowledge in development and the progressive deterioration of conceptual knowledge in dementia. As we explored a model that exhibited these properties, we found ourselves thinking of ways our approach might address other findings in the literature as well. While we would not disagree with those who may feel that we are still far from a complete model of human semantic abilities, we nevertheless have come to feel that our modeling work has addressed a sufficient range of basic findings for it to be useful to lay out what we have done in the form of an integrative theoretical statement. Our main goal in presenting our work at this point is to solicit the participation of others in its further development. We hope to gain the benefit of the reactions of others who have considered these matters. We also hope that our progress to date will seem promising enough that some researchers will join us in the further development of our approach.

The framework that we offer is by no means new or original with us. Indeed, the essential theoretical ideas were developed by others, starting twenty years ago, near the beginning of the period when interest in neural network or connectionist models began to reemerge after fifteen years of dormancy following Minsky and Papert's *Perceptrons* (1969). In 1981, Geoffrey Hinton's influential model of semantic memory appeared as a chapter in Hinton and James Anderson's book *Parallel Models of Associative Memory* (1981). This is the earliest source we know of in which the idea of property inheritance was implemented, not through traversal of links in a network of propositions, but through the use of similarity-based generalization within a distributed, connectionist net. Hinton's ideas provide the basic foundation for all our current work. The chief limitation of Hinton's model was that at the time the field lacked a method for discovering useful representations; instead Hinton handcrafted the distributed representations in his network to illustrate how the idea might work. The emergence of the backpropagation learning algorithm in the mid-1980s addressed this fundamental problem, and immediately Hinton demonstrated how it could be used to discover useful representations to facilitate semantic inference, in a paper presented at the Cognitive Science Society meeting in 1986.

Our own work takes as its point of departure a subsequent model developed by David Rumelhart. Rumelhart talked about this model in colloquia during the late 1980s, and it appeared in a book chapter in 1990 and subsequently in an *Attention and Performance* article with Peter Todd in 1993. Rumelhart made some simplifications to the architecture Hinton had introduced, and used it to illustrate how some of the attractive features of Quillian's hierarchical propositional network for representing semantic information could be captured in a connectionist net.

One of the properties that Rumelhart's model exhibited was a progressive differentiation of conceptual representations—a property observed in the development of children's concepts as noted in the work of Frank Keil. This connection with development was not itself a focus of Rumelhart's interests: he and Hinton both offered their models for their general computational properties, as connectionist alternatives to symbolic models of semantic knowledge representation. However, it was the convergence of the progressive differentiation in Rumelhart's model with the corresponding psychological phenomenon observed in the work of Frank Keil that led one of us (James McClelland) to think that distributed connectionist networks might provide a useful starting point for a psychological theory of semantic cognition. In a subsequent paper with McNaughton and O'Reilly, McClelland made use of the Rumelhart model to illustrate the benefits of gradual, interleaved learning for the discovery of structure in a body of information, and to demonstrate the deleterious effects of any attempt to integrate a new item of semantic information rapidly into such a structured knowledge representation. While working with Rumelhart's model in that context, McClelland learned of the work of John Hodges, Karalyn Patterson, and their colleagues, and of the earlier work by Elisabeth Warrington on the progressive disintegration of conceptual knowledge in semantic dementia. At that time the two of us (Rogers and McClelland) began to work together on the extension of the model to address these phenomena. We hoped that Rumelhart would also participate in these investigations. Tragically, this became impossible, since Rumelhart fell victim to this very condition himself. To us this remains a staggering irony, given the extreme rarity of semantic dementia.

As we began our explorations of progressive disintegration of conceptual knowledge in semantic dementia, several additional phenomena came to our attention, and so the scope of our effort gradually expanded. A major issue, frequently confronted in the early stages of the work, was the advisability of continuing with Rumelhart's very simple feed-forward network model. This choice involves some major simplifications, and at times we have been concerned that many readers may find the model oversimplified. However, Rumelhart himself would certainly have urged us to retain this simplicity, and we feel that it has paid off to follow this course. It is of course essential to be clear that the simplifications of the model are adopted for the sake of clarity and tractability, and should not be confused with the properties of the real mechanism that the model imperfectly reflects. We have tried throughout the book to be clear about where we feel the simplifications lie, and how the properties of the simple model relate to those of the more elaborate mechanism we believe actually underlies semantic abilities in the brain.

In addition to its historical roots in the ideas of Hinton and Rumelhart, the approach we take has a vibrant ongoing life of its own in the hands of many other contemporary investigators. We have chosen to focus on a range of phenomena bridging between topics in adult cognition, cognitive development, and cognitive neuropsychology. Many others are pursuing the application of models with similar properties to a broad range of sometimes overlapping phenomena. We consider our efforts and theirs to reflect an ongoing exploratory process that we hope will eventually lead to a fuller understanding of the mechanisms underlying human semantics abilities. Many of the same principles that govern the phenomena exhibited in the model we explore are also at work in the models used by these other investigators.

Our work has been supported by a Program Project Grant MH-47566 from the National Institute of Mental Health, which has also supported a range of closely related efforts by ourselves and several colleagues. The insights and observations that have come out of collaborations and ongoing interactions with John Hodges, Matthew Lambon Ralph, Karalyn Patterson, David Plaut, and Mark Seidenberg have helped to shape the direction of our efforts. The early phases of Rogers's effort were supported by a graduate traineeship from the National Science and Engineering Research Council in Canada, and a version of some of the material in this book appeared as a section in Rogers's Ph.D. dissertation. We are grateful to Robert Siegler and John Anderson for their input during this phase of our work. Subsequently our effort continued during Rogers's time as a postdoctoral researcher with Karalyn Patterson at the MRC Cognition and Brain Sciences Unit in Cambridge, England. We are especially grateful to Karalyn for her supportive collegiality throughout the project. In fall 2001, McClelland benefited greatly from the opportunity to focus on this project while visiting at the Gatsby Computational Neuroscience Unit at University College, London, where he had several helpful discussions with Peter Dayan, Geoffrey Hinton, and Alberto Paccanaro, as well as others in the rich Cognitive Neuroscience environment in and around UCL, including Mark Johnson, Annette Karmiloff-Smith, Denis Mareschal, Timothy Shallice, Michael Thomas, and Gabriella Vigliocco. We have also benefited from discussions and/or comments on various parts of the book from Susan Carey, Clark Glymour, Alison Gopnik, Scott Johnson, Jean Mandler, David Plaut, Kim Plunkett, Paul Quinn, David Rakison, James Russell,

and Lorraine Tyler. The Carnegie Symposium in May 2002, organized by David Rakison and Lisa Gershkoff-Stowe, and a meeting
on semantic processes at the British Academy in June 2002 organized by Lorraine Tyler, provided opportunities for interactions
with these and a number of other important contributors. Gregory
Murphy read the entire draft of the book and provided helpful,
detailed comments and pointers to important work we did not
know about. Finally, we would like to acknowledge Lee Brooks,
who urged us at a formative point in our effort to consider how our
model relates to the phenomena considered by the protagonists of
theory theory.

1 Categories, Hierarchies, and Theories

How do we perform semantic tasks, such as attributing a property to an object? How do we represent the information that we use as the basis for performing such tasks, and how do we acquire this information? We will propose answers to these questions that are quite different from those that have traditionally been offered by philosophers and psychologists. We will suggest that performance in semantic tasks arises through the propagation of graded signals in a system of simple but massively interconnected processing units. We will argue that the representations we use in performing these tasks are distributed, comprising patterns of activation across units in a neural network, and that these patterns are governed by weighted connections among the units. We will further suggest that semantic knowledge is acquired through the gradual adjustment of the strengths of these connections, in the course of processing semantic information in day-to-day experience.

In this chapter we lay the groundwork for our argument by reviewing classical findings and theories in the area of semantic memory. We will begin by considering work conducted primarily in the 1970s and 1980s that was carried out under the (sometimes implicit) assumption that semantic knowledge is represented in stored category representations, linked together in a taxonomically organized processing hierarchy (Collins and Quillian 1969; Collins and Loftus 1975). Processing models developed under this general approach have considerable appeal by virtue of their potential to provide detailed accounts for data from a variety of semantic tasks (e.g., Anderson 1991). However, we will uncover several difficulties with hierarchical, categorization-based models, and we will review several findings that have been used to suggest that categorization-based approaches must be augmented by invoking additional knowledge, often characterized as a naive or informal causal theory, to guide the process of making semantic judgments (e.g., Carey 1985; Gopnik and Wellman 1994; Keil 1991; Murphy and Medin 1985). Many of the ideas expressed by researchers working within this *theory-theory* approach also have obvious appeal, but as yet there has been no mechanistic proposal describing (in processing terms) what a theory is, how theories are represented in memory, and how they operate to constrain learning and processing in semantic tasks.

We suggest that this grounding of the study of semantic task performance in a theory based on categorization and domain theories may not be the optimal approach. Instead, it may be useful to construe performance in semantic tasks as arising within networks of simple processing units that learn by gradually adjusting the strengths of their connections in response to experience. We will demonstrate that within such an approach, many of the functions attributed to categorization-based mechanisms still arise. But we will also see that many of the difficulties such theories encounter can be reduced or eliminated, and several apparent paradoxes they face can be resolved. Moreover, we will suggest that our alternative approach offers a mechanistic means of understanding the phenomena that have motivated the appeal to informal causal theories.

Before we begin, we must be clear about what kinds of tasks count as semantic. We define *semantic tasks* as those that require a person to produce or verify semantic information about an object, a depiction of an object, or a set of objects indicated verbally (e.g., by a word). By *semantic information*, we refer to information that has not previously been associated with the particular stimulus object itself (though it may well have been associated with other objects), and that is not available more or less directly from the perceptual input provided by the object or object depiction. Obviously the boundaries of these conditions are difficult to draw, and may be contentious in some cases. However, there are certainly some cases that are clear enough. For example, verifying that the object shown in a picture is a cat, or that the pictured object can purr, are clear cases of semantic tasks, as long as the required information has not previously been directly associated with the particular picture. Likewise verifying sentences like *cats have fur* is also clearly a semantic task. In contrast, verifying that two cats depicted in color are in fact the same in color is not a semantic task, because the judgment can be made based on the color information in the picture and without reference to semantic information about the objects.

Categorization-Based Models

Semantic task performance is usually thought to depend on a mediating process of categorization. Under such approaches, a representation exists in memory (perhaps a node in a semantic network; perhaps a record in a database) corresponding to each of many concepts or categories, and information about these concepts is either stored in the representation itself, or is otherwise only accessible from it. Within such a model, then, performance on semantic tasks depends on access to the relevant category representations. This idea has a long history in science and philosophy, extending back at least to Aristotle and the invention of the syllogism, which can be viewed as an early categorization-based theory of knowledge storage and retrieval. For example, in the classic example of syllogistic reasoning, Aristotle is able to determine that Socrates is mortal by reasoning that Socrates is a man, and making use of stored knowledge about the category *man*—specifically, that all men are mortal:

1. Socrates is a man.
2. All men are mortal.
3. Therefore, Socrates is mortal.

Categorization-based approaches lie either implicitly or explicitly at the base of a great deal of theorizing about semantic knowledge and its use in semantic tasks. It will be useful, therefore, to

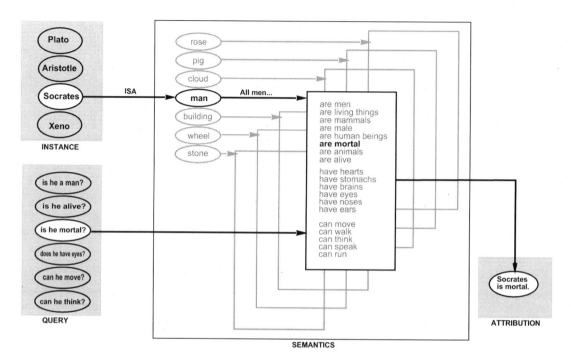

Figure 1.1   Schematic of a simple categorization-based approach to semantic task performance. Individual objects in the environment are represented by ovals in the box labeled *Instance*. Contextual constraints in the box labeled *Query* determine the kind of information to be retrieved. Semantic information is stored in discrete category representations that contain lists of the attributes typically true of the category exemplars. To determine that Socrates is mortal, the system first categorizes Socrates as an instance of the category *man*, and then searches the list of attributes for the property *is mortal*.

consider the strengths and weaknesses of such approaches, and to review some of the empirical findings on which they rest. In figure 1.1 we show what a simple categorization-based model of a semantic task might look like. Unique objects in the environment (such as Socrates) are represented by the ovals in the box labeled *Instance*. The ovals in the box labeled *Query* represent contextual factors constraining the kind of information to be retrieved. In the example given, the context might be a conversation in which Xeno has asked Aristotle whether Socrates is mortal.

The ovals in the middle of the diagram indicate stored representations of various categories. Associated with each is a list of properties that are generally true of the category's exemplars. To decide whether Socrates is mortal, the model categorizes the instance (Socrates) as a *man*. It then accesses the stored list of properties common to all men, and determines whether the property indicated in the query is contained in the list.

Similar models have been used to account for a wealth of empirical data from studies of semantic task performance. In turn, the empirical phenomena have motivated the introduction of increasingly sophisticated processes and constructs to the framework. Many detailed categorization-based models have been put forward in the literature, and it may be impossible to articulate a single characterization of the approach on which everyone will agree. However, across particular instantiations, there are broad commonalities. In this section, we consider three constructs that are frequently invoked in categorization-based theories to explain empirical data: *hierarchical structure*, which directs the sharing of information across related concepts at different levels of abstraction; *privileged categories*, which contain information that is accessed directly, and not by means of spreading activation in the hierarchy; and *category prototypes*, which are the means of computing similarity between individual instances and stored category representations.

Our aim in this review is to suggest that while each of these constructs has some appeal, they offer an incomplete and in some ways paradoxical basis for accounting for the relevant empirical phenomena. In making this point, we will lay out a body of findings that require explanation; these phenomena will be the target of our own subsequent modeling effort.

Hierarchical Structure

For many natural domains, there exist constraints on category membership, such that exemplars of one category must also be

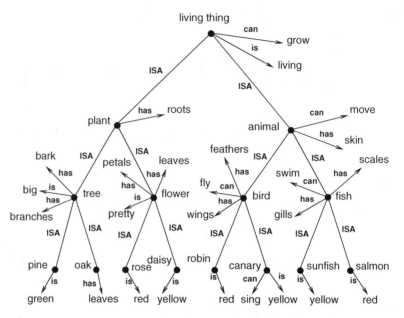

Figure 1.2 A taxonomic hierarchy of the type used by Collins and Quillian in their model of the organization of knowledge in memory. The schematic indicates that living things can grow, that a tree is a plant, and that a plant is a living thing. Therefore it follows that a tree can grow. *Note:* Redrawn with alterations from figure 1.8 of "Learning and connectionist representations" (p. 14), by D. E. Rumelhart and P. M. Todd, in *Attention and Performance XIV: Synergies in Experimental Psychology, Artificial Intelligence, and Cognitive Neuroscience*, edited by D. E. Meyer and S. Kornblum (1993), Cambridge, MA: MIT Press. Copyright 1993 by MIT Press.

members of another. For example, if an object is a kind of cat, it must also be a kind of animal. Often, these class-inclusion constraints can be described by a *taxonomic hierarchy*, such as the one shown in figure 1.2. In an influential early paper, Quillian (1968) pointed out that the taxonomic hierarchy can provide an efficient mechanism for storing and retrieving semantic information. A key aspect of the appeal of Quillian's proposal flows from the observation that category membership at each level entails a number of properties shared by all the members of the more specific included categories. Thus, the properties shared by all animals, say, but not by all living things, could be stored only once, at the concept *animal*. Then, by consulting stored taxonomic relations, a subject could determine that more particular types of animals (e.g., cats) should inherit the properties of animals. To allow for this consultation, Quillian proposed a spreading activation mechanism that permitted the activation of a category representation to spread to taxonomically superordinate concepts. Under this view, when an object is categorized as a cat, activation of the concept *cat* spreads to the related concept *animal*, and properties stored there are attributed to the object. In addition to its economy, this model provided an elegant mechanism for property inheritance and generalization of new knowledge: new facts could be stored with the appropriate category node, and would then automatically be inherited by all subordinate concepts. Similarly, a new subcategory, such as *mahimahi*, could be added as a subordinate of a more general category such as *fish*, and existing knowledge about the properties of fish would automatically generalize to it.

The Quillian model is appealing in many ways, but some of the key predictions derived from it have not held up to experimental tests. Collins and Quillian (1969) assumed that it would take time to traverse the ISA links that form the backbone of the taxonomic hierarchy. Hence, they predicted that propositions stored directly with a concept would be verified the fastest, with verification time increasing with the number of ISA links that would have to be traversed to find the property in question. To test this prediction, the authors devised a speeded property-verification task. Subjects were shown propositions about object properties, and were asked to decide as quickly and accurately as possible whether the propositions were true. Some propositions were about general properties (e.g., "A canary has skin"), while others were about more specific properties (e.g., "A canary can sing"). Data from the initial experiments reported by Collins and Quillian (1969) supported the hierarchical processing model: subjects took longer to verify statements about general properties than about more specific properties, putatively because such properties were stored higher in the tree and thus required a greater number of inferences. However, subsequent work has shown that reaction times in property-verification tasks are influenced by a variety of factors other than the property's putative position in the taxonomic hierarchy. These factors include its typicality (Rips, Shoben, and Smith 1973), its frequency (Conrad 1972), and its pairwise correlation with other properties across objects (McRae, De Sa, and Seidenberg 1997). When such factors are controlled, the predicted advantage of specific over superordinate properties can fail to materialize (McCloskey and Glucksberg 1979; Murphy and Brownell 1985). Furthermore, it has been shown that the time it takes to verify category membership at various levels can often violate the predictions of the taxonomic hierarchy model. For example, Rips and colleagues (1973) found that subjects can more quickly verify that a chicken is an animal than that it is a bird.

In spite of the failure of these predictions, the idea that concepts are stored within a taxonomic processing hierarchy has continued to receive at least qualified endorsement (see, for example, Murphy and Lassaline 1997), partly because such an organization has proven useful for explaining other aspects of data from semantic tasks. In the domain of neuropsychology, Warrington (1975) invoked hierarchical structure to account for patterns of deficits witnessed in cases of progressive fluent aphasia, today better known as *semantic dementia*. Patients with semantic dementia exhibit a progressive deterioration of semantic knowledge, while other cognitive faculties remain relatively spared (Snowden, Goulding, and Neary 1989). Warrington's patients appeared to lose information about specific categories at the bottom of the taxonomy earliest in the progression of the disease. For example, they were often able to provide general names for objects when they had lost more specific labels, and were more accurate at verifying general properties (e.g., *a canary has skin*) than more specific ones (e.g., *a canary can sing*). These observations have more recently been complemented by a series of studies by Hodges, Patterson, and their colleagues (Patterson, Graham, and Hodges 1994a, 1994b;

Patterson and Hodges 1992; Graham and Hodges 1997; Hodges and Patterson 1995; Hodges, Graham, and Patterson 1995), showing that semantic dementia patients exhibit relatively preserved general knowledge in a variety of semantic tasks, including word and picture sorting, word and picture definition, and word-to-picture matching. Warrington suggested that such deficits might arise within Collins and Quillian's framework if category representations at the top of the taxonomy are the first to be activated during retrieval. Under this view, the structure apparent in impaired performance of semantic tasks reveals the organizational structure of concepts in memory: semantic dementia patients first lose the specific representations stored at the bottom of the taxonomy, but retain access to the general knowledge stored in more inclusive categories.

Taxonomic structure has also been invoked to explain patterns of concept differentiation during development. For example, Warrington observed that the deterioration of semantic memory in her patients, progressing as it did from the bottom toward the top of the taxonomic hierarchy, mirrored the progression of conceptual differentiation in children reported by Clark (1973). She suggested that the categories located at the top of the taxonomy are not only the first to be activated during access, but are also the first to be acquired in development. The theory that children first acquire broad, global category representations is consistent with several findings that have emerged since Warrington introduced this suggestion, particularly in the work of Keil (1979) and Mandler (Mandler 1988; Mandler and Bauer 1988; Mandler 1992; Mandler, Bauer, and McDonough 1991; Mandler 1997; Mandler and McDonough 1993; Mandler 2000a).

Keil (1979) asked children of varying ages (kindergarten–grade 6) to judge whether particular propositions and their negations were acceptable. For example, he might ask whether it is silly to say that a pig could be sorry, or that a rock could be an hour long. Based on their responses, Keil constructed a set of *predicability trees*, which described the "ontological distinctions" indicated by

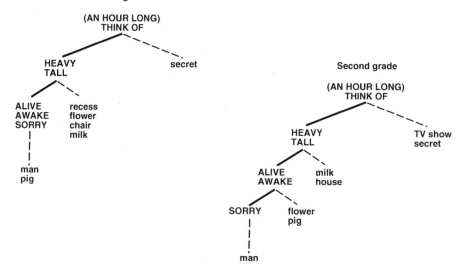

Kindergarten

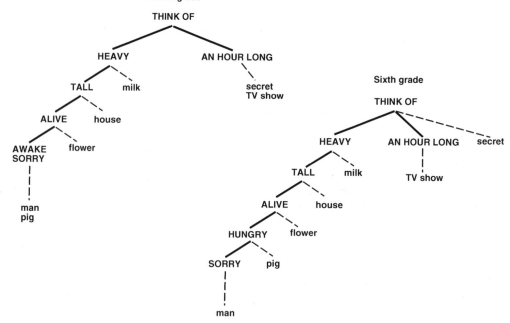

Fourth grade

each child's responses (see figure 1.3). For example, the kindergartner whose tree is shown accepted the predicate *is heavy* (or its negation) as applicable to the concepts *recess, flower, chair,* and *milk,* but not to *secret.* Concepts occupy the same node on the tree if children accept that they can enter into the same set of propositions. As figure 1.3 illustrates, predicability trees become increasingly differentiated over the course of development, suggesting that broader conceptual distinctions are acquired earliest.

The studies of Mandler and her collaborators have investigated infants' abilities to differentiate objects on semantic grounds using a variety of methods, including an object-manipulation analog of the well-known preferential-looking procedure. In this task, there is a familiarization phase, in which the infant is handed a series of toy objects exemplifying a particular semantic category (e.g., *animal*). This phase is followed by a test phase, in which the infant is given one novel item from the same category and one novel item from a different category. Sensitivity to the semantic distinction between the categories is inferred if infants spend longer exploring the test object that does not belong to the category presented during familiarization.

In one such study, Mandler and McDonough (1993) familiarized infants with a series of toy birds by allowing them to examine and manipulate each bird for a period of 15 seconds. They then presented each infant with a tray holding a novel bird and a toy plane. The investigators endeavored to choose the test items in such a way that the novel bird and the novel plane were both perceptually

Figure 1.3 Examples of the predicability trees constructed by Keil (1979), involving four individual children from four different age groups. The trees indicate which of several predicate terms are accepted by the individual children as being applicable to various concepts; concepts accepting the same set of predicates are grouped together at the same branch of the tree. See text for further discussion. *Note:* Redrawn from *Semantic and Conceptual Development: An Ontological Perspective* (A3 from p. 181, A17 from p. 183, A37 from p. 185, and A54 from p. 187), by F. C. Keil 1979, Cambridge, MA: Harvard University Press. Copyright 1979 by Harvard University Press.

similar to the birds used in familiarization. Even so, 9-month-old infants preferred to play with the plane, suggesting a novelty preference for the out-of-category item, in spite of its intended perceptual similarity to the familiarization items. Infants did not show analogous preferences based on more fine-grained conceptual distinctions (such as dogs vs. fish) until 12 months. Similar findings have now been reported independently by Pauen (2002b).

Based on such findings, Mandler (2000a) has proposed that infants are sensitive to broad semantic distinctions as soon as they are testable using her methods (around 7 months), and subsequently exhibit progressive differentiation. These claims have been controversial, largely because of uncertainty about the degree to which the investigators succeeded in ruling out the possibility that the results could reflect greater perceptual similarity within than between categories. However, support for Mandler's view comes from a series of studies by Pauen (2002a) in which the possible role of perceptual similarity of various types was extensively explored in a test for global category versus specific object differentiation in an object-examination task. Among other things, Pauen found global differentiation in 10- and 11-month-olds even with stimuli in which independently rated perceptual similarity was greater between the categories used (furniture versus animals) than within each category—as would be expected if performance was based on conceptual, rather than perceptual, distinctions. A significant effect indicating specific-object differentiation was only found with 11-month-olds. While perceptual factors can often be important in related tasks, these findings do suggest a role for conceptual and not perceptual similarity, at least in Pauen's particular task situation. We provide further discussion of these issues in chapter 4. For present purposes, we take the findings to be consistent with Warrington's (1975) suggestion that infants' semantic representations first honor very general semantic distinctions and only later come to be sensitive to more specific distinctions.

Finally, taxonomic structure may be used to explain the influence of general category membership on the processing of more specific category information. One example of such an influence is that the relevance of a given feature can vary from category to category—for example, color appears to be more important for discriminating among foods than toys. To demonstrate this, Macario (1991) showed wax objects that varied in shape and color to 3- and 4-year-old children. The children were introduced to a toy alligator, and were taught a new fact about one of the wax objects. In one condition, children were told that the toy alligator liked to eat the object; in the other, they were told the alligator liked to play with the object. They were then asked to guess which other nonsense objects the alligator would like to eat or play with. When led to treat the objects as foods, children were more likely to choose the other object of the same color. When led to treat the objects as toys, they were more likely to choose the object of the same shape. Thus children as young as 3 treat the color of an object as more important than its shape if it is a kind of food, but less important if it is a kind of toy (see Jones, Smith, and Landau 1991 for similar findings).

It is easy to see that taxonomic structure can go some way toward explaining this differential weighting of properties across categories. Information stored with more general representations can determine the feature weights for more specific categorizations (Anderson 1991; Anderson and Matessa 1992; Anderson and Fincham 1996). Children in Macario's (1991) experiment are told that the novel object is either something to eat or something to play with, allowing them to categorize it at a general level (e.g., *food* or *toy*). Information stored with the general representation might then constrain the saliency of shape and color in making more specific distinctions (Anderson, personal communication, 1999). As far as we know, no developmental mechanism has yet been proposed to explain how such knowledge is acquired, or to determine where in a hierarchy particular information of this type should be stored. However, a taxonomic hierarchy does provide one mechanism by which, once the knowledge is acquired, differential weights could be assigned to particular properties in different branches of the hierarchy.

A second way general knowledge may influence the processing of more specific information stems from the literature on so-called illusory correlations. Several studies have shown that people are not very good at estimating the frequency with which objects and properties co-occur across a particular set of events (e.g., Chapman 1967; Anderson and Lindsay 1998). Subjects may persist in the belief that particular objects and properties have occurred together frequently, even in the face of empirical evidence to the contrary, and they may discount or ignore the co-occurrence of object-property pairs during learning (Keil 1991; Murphy and Medin 1985). For example, R. Gelman (Gelman 1990; Massey and Gelman 1988) showed preschoolers static pictures of various unfamiliar objects, living and nonliving, and asked them to decide whether each object would be able to move up and down a hill on its own. Some of the nonliving things were shaped like animate objects (e.g., a figurine), whereas some of the living things were extremely atypical animals (e.g., an echidna). The ontological status of each item (i.e., living or nonliving) was not revealed to the child, but had to be inferred from the appearance of the object. After making their decision, the experimenters asked children to explain their choices. As these protocols from Gelman 1990 show, children often referred to properties of objects that were clearly not present in the picture, and ignored the presence of other properties that were not consistent with their decision:

M. B. (3 years 7 months)
Insect-eye figurine
DOWN BY SELF? No.
WHY NOT? Because it's metal and doesn't have any shoes or feet.
ARE THOSE FEET? (E POINTS TO THE FEET.) No.
Echidna
DOWN BY SELF? Yeah.
WHY? It has feet and no shoes.
CAN YOU POINT TO THE FEET? I can't see them.

Although such phenomena have typically been discussed by researchers within the theory-theory approach to semantic cognition, one might turn to a taxonomic processing hierarchy to explain them. If children in Massey and Gelman's (1988) experiment were able to categorize the stimuli at a general level such as *animate* or *inanimate*, they may have simply attributed the typical properties of animate or inanimate items to the unfamiliar stimuli, even though these properties were not visible in the picture. That is, they may have used information stored with a general category representation to make inferences about the individual objects that contradicted their immediate perceptual experience—attributing unseen legs to the echidna and ignoring the feet on the figurine.

In summary, a taxonomic hierarchy is useful for explaining a variety of empirical findings. The key relevant phenomena are summarized in table 1.1. However, there are findings on latency of category- and property-verification responses that are inconsistent with Quillian's initial proposal, and to our knowledge no comprehensive alternative theory has been proposed that encompasses the phenomena listed in the table. In the next section we review some additional findings that such a comprehensive account would need to explain.

Privileged Categories at Intermediate Levels of the Hierarchy

A second major influence on categorization-based theories of semantic task performance stems from studies by Rosch and colleagues regarding what she called the *basic level of categorization* (Rosch et al. 1976; Rosch 1978; Mervis and Rosch 1981). Rosch observed that, of the several categories to which a particular object might belong, some appear to be particularly informative and meaningful. For example, an individual dog might belong to the categories *Rover*, *German shepherd*, *dog*, *animal*, and *living thing*; of these, the category *dog* appears to be especially useful. Rosch dubbed such categories *basic*, and showed that subjects often

Table 1.1   Empirical phenomena consistent with the claim that category representations are organized within a taxonomic hierarchy

PHENOMENON	EXPERIMENTAL PARADIGM	TRADITIONAL ACCOUNT
Children and infants are sensitive to broad semantic distinctions earliest in development.	• Object manipulation • Preferential looking • Predicability trees	Children acquire the broad category representations at the top of the taxonomy first in development. Taxonomic structure guides the subsequent differentiation of concepts.
General information is more robust in semantic dementia.	• Sorting words and pictures • Picture naming • Word-to-picture matching • Feature verification	Category representations at the top of the taxonomy are the first to be accessed during retrieval and the last to be lost in dementia.
Illusory correlations in children and adults show that semantic knowledge can influence the extent to which we perceive or infer the presence of particular object properties.	• Estimates of object-property co-occurrences • Children's explanations of their decisions in reasoning tasks	General category representations are activated whenever specific instances are encountered, influencing the attribution of particular features to the object.
A given property has differential importance for different categories.	• Generalization of a new property to objects described as foods or toys	Categorization at a more general level determines the importance of various features for more specific categories.

perform best in semantic tasks requiring them to identify objects at this level. In general, Rosch et al. (1976) demonstrated that:

1. Subjects are fastest to verify membership at the basic level.
2. They prefer to use the basic label in picture-naming tasks.
3. They are fastest to discriminate objects at the basic level.
4. They show a larger effect of visual priming to the basic label.
5. Children first learn to name objects with their basic-level name.

Rosch suggested that basic-level advantages are observed because the cognitive system exploits representations that correspond to information-rich bundles of co-occurring attributes in the environment. She showed that basic categories tend to have special statistical properties, in that their exemplars share many properties with one another and few with the exemplars of contrasting categories (Rosch et al. 1976). Murphy and Lassaline (1997) have described basic categories as maximizing both *informativeness* and *distinctiveness*. More general categories are not very informative, because their exemplars have little in common—for example, when told that something is a piece of furniture, one cannot infer very many of its properties. More specific categories are informative but not particularly distinctive, because they have few distinguishing characteristics. Thus, wingback chairs have many properties in common with one another, but they share most of these with other kinds of chairs. Objects from the same basic category tend to share many properties with one another, and few with exemplars of contrasting categories, and thus basic categories are considered particularly useful (Rosch 1978; Murphy and Brownell 1985; Murphy and Lassaline 1997).

Rosch et al. (1976) proposed that cognitive faculties develop to take advantage of this structure by "carving the world at its joints" —that is, by forming summary representations of maximally distinct and informative categories of objects. Rosch initially supposed that there might be a single level of abstraction in the taxonomic hierarchy at which such useful categories tend to occur, and early cross-cultural studies of natural-kind concepts provided at least some support for this interpretation (e.g., Berlin 1972). However, from early on in Rosch's research it became apparent that the so-called basic level was not invariant across cultures. In Rosch's own studies, her American undergraduate subjects treated the folk-generic level as basic for many mammals (e.g., horse, dog, pig), but in other cases treated as basic what had previously been thought of as the more general "life-form" level (e.g., bird, fish) (Rosch et al. 1976). It thus appeared from the beginning that what constitutes the basic level may reflect not only similarities and differences among objects themselves, but also differences in experience, with more specific levels being treated as basic in cultures where there is more experience with the relevant objects. It should also be noted that while the so-called basic level has an advantage for typical members of the basic-level category, this is not always the case for less typical members. Thus, it is easier to call a sparrow a "bird" than is is to call it a "sparrow," but it is easier to call a chicken a "chicken" or an "animal" than to call it a "bird" (Rips et al. 1973; Jolicoeur, Gluck, and Kosslyn 1984).

The exact way basic-level structure influenced processing was left to others to work out, since Rosch herself explicitly disavowed any commitment to such issues (Rosch 1978). One hypothesis compatible with categorization-based theories is that basic-level concept representations constitute the entry point into a taxonomic processing hierarchy (Jolicoeur, Gluck, and Kosslyn 1984; Murphy and Brownell 1985). Under this view, a given stimulus directly activates only its basic (or *entry-level*) category representation. Information stored at other levels of abstraction must be retrieved by means of spreading activation in the taxonomy. Such *privileged-access* theories, then, introduce a distinction between semantic information retrieved *directly* by means of categorization, and *indirectly*, through reference to stored class-inclusion links. Access to information stored with concepts superordinate or subordinate to the entry level depends on prior activation of the entry-level representation. Consequently, the system will always be fastest to retrieve information stored with the entry-level concept. According to this view, basic-level phenomena are observed because information stored at more general or specific levels of abstraction is only accessible through the prior activation of basic-level concept representations. Jolicoeur and colleagues (1984) further stipulated that entry-level categories need not reside at the same level of taxonomic specificity for all exemplars, and might be found at a more specific level of the hierarchy for atypical instances. For example, a picture of a sparrow might directly activate the concept *bird*, whereas a picture of an ostrich might first activate the concept *os-*

trich. Consequently, subjects are fastest to verify category membership at the "basic" level for the sparrow, but at a more specific level for the ostrich.

Primacy in Lexical Acquisition and Dementia Basic categories are thought by many to be primal in another sense as well: Rosch et al. (1976) argued that they are the first to be acquired in development, albeit in primitive form (Mervis and Rosch 1981). As evidence for this hypothesis, they turned to studies of sorting and naming with young children. Rosch et al. (1976) purported to demonstrate that children at 3 years could sort toy objects into basic, but not superordinate, categories. However, the basic-level categories the children had to distinguish also contrasted at the superordinate level (Mandler 1997). When Bauer and Mandler (1989) tested children on an unconfounded sorting task, they found that they could sort objects at both levels as early as they were able to understand the instructions. Rosch's (Rosch et al. 1976) studies of children's naming, however, have proven more robust; it is now well accepted that children can name many objects with the correct basic label before being able to name them at more general or specific levels (Brown 1958; Chapman and Mervis 1989). Mervis (Mervis 1984, 1987a) and others (e.g., Anglin 1977) have taken this as evidence that children acquire basic category representations first in development.

Interestingly, semantic dementia patients show a similar preservation of some basic-level names as their disease progresses. For example, in a picture-naming task, patient J. L. showed preservation of the basic-level names "dog," "cat," and "horse" after he had lost such names for other animals, and indeed overextended these labels to other, similar animals, naming many large animals "horse," medium-sized animals "dog," and small animals "cat" (Hodges, Graham, and Patterson 1995). In general, there is a tendency for relatively frequent basic-level labels to be preserved and sometimes overextended, even while the patient appears to have only very general information about many other concepts.

The Influence of Expertise Finally, some studies have found that basic-level advantages can shift with increasing expertise in a domain, suggesting that such effects are at least in part constrained by experience. For example, Tanaka and Taylor (1991) have shown that experts are equally quick to verify category membership at basic and more specific levels, within their domain of expertise (also see Johnson and Mervis 1997). Experts also prefer to name at the subordinate level in their domain of expertise, whereas novices prefer to name at the basic level, even when they know the correct subordinate label (Tanaka and Taylor 1991; Johnson and Mervis 1997).

Explanations of these effects consistent with categorization-based theories have tended to be more descriptive than mechanistic. For example, Johnson and Mervis (1997, 271) write that expertise serves to make subordinate categories "function as basic," but are unclear about exactly how this happens or what it might mean. Tanaka and Taylor (1991) come closer to a mechanistic account when they suggest that expertise serves to make subordinate categories more distinct and informative. There appears to be reliable data supporting this idea. For example, experts can list many more properties unique to subordinate-level concepts than can novices in their domain of expertise (Tanaka and Taylor 1991; Palmer et al. 1989), and fishermen sort pictures of fish into a larger number of groups than do novices (Boster and Johnson 1989). But, to our knowledge, no theory has been offered describing the mechanisms by which expertise serves to make subordinate concepts more distinct and informative, or how such transformations influence the speed with which subordinate information can be accessed. The same may be said of existing accounts of basic-level advantages generally: they offer no explanation of the mechanism by which the statistical properties of basic categories lead them to become privileged in processing.

Moreover, other studies of expertise have shown that experts in a given domain may derive somewhat different conceptions about how items in the domain are similar to one another, depending on the kind of expertise they have acquired (Medin, Lynch, and Coley 1997; Lopex et al. 1997; Coley, Medin, and Atran 1997). For example, Medin and colleagues (1997) performed sorting experiments with three kinds of tree experts: landscapers, biologists, and park maintenance workers. All the experts sorted photographs of trees into groups at various grains. While there was some consistency in the categories formed by different kinds of experts, they were not perfectly consistent. Biologists tended to stick close to the scientific taxonomy, regardless of the surface characteristics of various trees, whereas landscapers and maintenance workers were more likely to deviate from the scientific taxonomy for uncharacteristic trees (such as the ginkgo—according to biological classification a coniferous tree, which shares surface properties with deciduous trees). Landscapers and maintenance workers also consistently grouped together some trees on the basis of their utilitarian properties. That is, they formed a category of "weed" trees, whose members shared no essential or biological characteristics, but were grouped together presumably because they demand similar treatment in the day-to-day tasks of the maintenance workers and landscapers. These results suggest to us that the processes by which we construct semantic representations are sensitive to the details of the experience we have with the categories in question, which itself appears to reflect the different ways individuals from different professions interact with these objects. Again, existing theories have not offered specific mechanisms that account for these experience-dependent effects.

To summarize, the hypothesis that some categories are "privileged" relative to others has been used to explain the order in which names at different levels of specificity are learned in lexical acquisitions, the basic-level advantage in naming and property verification for typical objects, and the absence of such an advantage for atypical objects. The empirical findings supporting these claims are shown in table 1.2. However, a certain puzzle arises at this point. On the one hand, there is support for Warrington's idea that the most general levels of category structure are the most robust, in

Table 1.2 Empirical phenomena consistent with the claim that some categories are privileged

PHENOMENON	EXPERIMENTAL PARADIGM	TRADITIONAL ACCOUNT
Children first learn to name objects with their basic label.	• Speech protocols • Picture naming	Children acquire basic category representations earliest in development.
For typical exemplars, adults are faster at retrieving or verifying basic-level information.	• Category verification • Feature verification • Picture naming	"Entry-level" category representations are the first to be accessed during retrieval. For typical instances, these are basic-level representations residing in the middle of the taxonomy.
For atypical instances, adults are faster at retrieving or verifying subordinate-level information.	• Category verification • Picture naming	"Entry-level" representations are lower on the taxonomy for atypical instances than for typical instances.
In free-naming experiments, adults prefer to name typical objects with their basic name, and atypical objects with their subordinate name.	• Picture naming	"Entry-level" category representations are the first to be accessed during retrieval. These are basic categories for typical objects, and subordinate categories for atypical objects.

that they are the first to be acquired in development and last to be lost in dementia. Yet there is considerable evidence that a level of category structure intermediate between the most specific and the most general has primacy over the most general level, as evidenced by data from normal adults, child language acquisition, and aspects of semantic dementia. No existing theoretical framework has integrated these apparently contrasting bodies of evidence.

Furthermore, studies of expertise suggest that the level of specificity at which the basic-level advantage is observed can vary as a function of experience, and also that experts may come to represent the same set of items differently, depending on the nature of their expertise. These findings, summarized in table 1.3, seem to

Table 1.3 Empirical data from the study of expertise suggesting that basic-level effects are constrained by experience

PHENOMENON	EXPERIMENTAL PARADIGM
Experts use more specific names in their domain of expertise than do novices.	• Picture naming
Experts are equally fast at verifying membership in basic and more specific categories in their domain of expertise.	• Category verification
Experts differentiate objects to a greater extent in their domain of expertise.	• Picture sorting • Attribute listing
Different kinds of experts sort objects differently in their domain of expertise.	• Picture sorting • Word sorting

indicate that basic-level advantages do not derive strictly from fixed structure in the environment, regardless of one's experience, but must be constrained to some degree by the nature of one's interactions with the domain. Again, we are not aware of any mechanistic theory explaining how experience will constrain basic-level advantages.

Category Prototypes

In addition to introducing the privileged status of an intermediate level of concept structure, Rosch (Rosch and Mervis 1975; Rosch 1975) also challenged the classical notion that, in semantic tasks, objects are categorized on the basis of necessary and sufficient criteria (see, for example, Katz 1972). Borrowing from Wittgenstein (1953), she argued that for most natural categories, no such criteria exist. Instead, natural kinds have a tendency to share *family resemblances*. Attributes are not distributed randomly across instances in the world, but have a tendency to occur in clusters. For instance, objects with beaks are also likely to have feathers and wings. Rosch suggested that the cognitive system exploits such discontinuities by forming summary representations of categories that correspond to clusters of correlated attributes in the environment.

In support of this theory, Rosch observed that membership in most natural categories is not all-or-none, as suggested by the classical theory, but is instead graded: some objects are better examples of a category than are others. Subjects make remarkably consistent judgments of category "goodness" for many natural kinds (Rosch, Simpson, and Miller 1976; Rosch 1975), and these judgments correlate strongly with performance on semantic tasks such as category and property verification (Rosch and Mervis 1975; Rips, Shoben, and Smith 1973; Smith, Shoben, and Rips 1974). In general, poor or *atypical* members of a category take longer to verify than do good or *typical* members. These data would seem to have strong implications for processing models of semantic memory, but again Rosch was cool about her commitment to such issues. With her colleague Mervis, she suggested that the semantic system may store summary category representations as a prototypical set of descriptors that are generally, but not necessarily, true of the category's exemplars (Rosch and Mervis 1975). For example, the prototype for *cat* might include the features *has fur*, *can reproduce*, and *ISA pet*,[1] even though some cats do not have fur, cannot reproduce, and are not pets. Rosch showed that time to classify a given instance is inversely proportional to the number of attributes it shares with a prototypical category member (Rosch and Mervis 1975). However, she later recanted any interest in processing models, stating that her use of the word *prototype* was simply meant as a shorthand to describe the empirical fact that typical category members are easier to classify than are atypical members (Rosch 1978).

This reticence has not prevented others from adopting the prototype theory as a processing model, and there have been several proposals about how category prototypes might be employed to store and retrieve semantic information (e.g., Hampton 1993,

1997). Common to these approaches is the idea that natural categories are represented by summary descriptions that are abstracted through exposure to instances in the environment. Novel instances are compared to these stored summary descriptions, and are assigned to the category with the closest match under some measure of similarity. The amount of time taken to perform this assignment depends on the feature overlap (potentially weighted by feature "importance") between the novel instance, the correct category, and the competing categories. Typical instances are categorized quickly, because they are highly similar to the correct category, and are dissimilar to contrasting categories. Atypical instances, which share fewer properties with the category prototype, and which may share more properties with competing prototypes, take longer to categorize.

Mervis (Mervis 1987b; Mervis and Rosch 1981; Mervis, Catlin, and Rosch 1976) extended the prototype theory to account for data from lexical acquisition. She showed that during early word learning, children often restrict their use of a category label to typical members of the category—for example, in denying that a football could be a kind of ball. Similarly, children often inappropriately extend the use of a familiar category name to out-of-category objects that share properties with typical category members—for instance, by calling a round piggy bank a "ball." Mervis (1984) suggested that immature or *child-basic* category prototypes include a small number of properties relative to adult category prototypes. As a consequence, atypical instances that do not share these properties get excluded from the category, whereas out-of-category instances that do share these properties are inappropriately included. One might correspondingly suggest that the tendency of semantic dementia patients to overextend frequent basic-level category names might reflect the loss of some differentiating properties, while still preserving a few more central properties.

Thus, category prototype representations may be used to explain the effect of typicality on reaction times in category- and property-verification tasks in adults, and also to explain the overextension

Table 1.4 Empirical phenomena consistent with the claim that conceptual information is stored in category prototypes

PHENOMENON	EXPERIMENTAL PARADIGM	TRADITIONAL ACCOUNT
Category membership is verified more quickly for typical exemplars than for atypical exemplars.	• Category verification	Typical exemplars are more similar to their category prototype, and less similar to neighboring category prototypes.
Familiar names are overextended to related objects during early language learning.	• Picture naming • Category verification • Speech protocols	Children's impoverished category prototypes are insufficient to correctly differentiate objects.
Familiar names are overextended to similar objects in dementia.	• Picture naming	When unfamiliar category representations degrade, instances are assigned to the closest-matching category remaining in their repertoire.
Children restrict names to typical category instances during early language learning.	• Picture naming • Category verification • Speech protocols	Children's impoverished category prototypes are insufficient to identify atypical exemplars.

of familiar names to inappropriate but related objects in lexical acquisition and dementia, as well as the inappropriate restriction of familiar names to typical objects during early word learning. The empirical findings encompassed by these ideas are listed in table 1.4.

Although category prototypes provide a fairly intuitive way of thinking about effects of typicality on naming and category and property verification, we should note that it is not clear how these ideas might be integrated with the hypothesis that category representations are organized within a taxonomic processing hierarchy. Prototype theory suggests that instances are assigned to categories on the basis of their similarity to stored prototypes, and that categorization latencies (and subsequent retrieval of semantic information) depend on the degree of similarity between the instance and stored category representations. By contrast, spreading activation theories of semantic knowledge representation, and privileged-access accounts of basic-level effects, suggest that the time to retrieve semantic information depends on the distance between concepts in the processing hierarchy, and on which concept constitutes the "entry point" to the system. It is not clear how these different factors will interact in the context of a particular task. If time to categorize depends in part on similarity to stored prototypes, and in part on spreading activation in the taxonomy, how does an item's similarity to a superordinate concept such as *animal* influence the retrieval of superordinate information? Is the item compared simultaneously to superordinate, basic, and more specific concepts, with similarity determining the strength of activation of these nodes? If so, what is the role of spreading activation in the taxonomy? How does similarity to representations at different levels of abstraction influence the way that activation spreads in the taxonomy? In what sense are intermediate representations privileged under this view?

Both constructs—hierarchical processing mechanisms and similarity-based categorization mechanisms—could be exploited to explain some of the data. However, neither construct alone seems sufficient to capture all of it. Similarity-based models of categorization that attempt to do away with taxonomic processing structure will have difficulty explaining how more general category membership can influence categorization and processing at more specific levels, as discussed earlier. On the other hand, hierarchically organized processing models will have difficulty explaining the strong influence of typicality on semantic judgments. One response to the situation is to seek a marriage between the two ideas; however, we are not aware of any processing model that has done so successfully (see Murphy and Lassaline 1997 for a useful discussion of this issue).

The Theory-Theory

In addition to the difficulties we have outlined above, categorization-based theories face further challenges that derive from a different perspective on semantic cognition, namely, the *theory-theory* approach (Murphy and Medin 1985; Carey 1985; Keil 1989; Gopnik and Meltzoff 1997). The basic tenet of the theory-theory is that semantic cognition is constrained to a large extent by the naive domain knowledge—often referred to as a "theory"—that people hold about the causal relations that exist between entities in a domain. It is difficult to characterize just what "naive theories" are in information processing terms, and not all researchers in this tradition always refer to the naive domain knowledge as a theory as such (Murphy 2002). However, some researchers working in this tradition have stressed that a key function of a naive domain theory is to explain and predict observed events in the environment, and that domain theories serve this function with reference to stored knowledge about the causal properties of (and causal relations between) objects (e.g., Gopnik and Meltzoff 1997). According to this view, children and adults make sense of the "blooming, buzzing confusion" that constitutes the environment by employing domain-specific constraints (Gelman 1990) that specify the causal relationships between objects and their essential properties (Keil 1991). For many investigators, there is a strong tendency to assume that some form of constraint or prototheory is available initially to shape children's thinking from birth. Other investigators stress the developmental changes that occur in children's thinking and seek ways of understanding how domain knowledge evolves with experience from its initial state. Regardless of relative emphasis on these points, researchers in this tradition tend to agree that reliance on such domain knowledge constrains semantic knowledge acquisition and semantic task performance (Gopnik and Meltzoff 1997; Gelman and Williams 1998).

Although some researchers are agnostic about the relationship between categorization-based theories and the theory-theory (e.g.,

Carey 1985), most investigators in this tradition seem to view the theory-theory as a complementary approach that can help categorization-based theories overcome some of their limitations (e.g., Murphy and Medin 1985; Keil et al. 1998). From this standpoint, categorization-based theories in and of themselves are thought to provide an inadequate framework for explaining semantic cognition without further constraints to determine which categories and properties are stored in memory, and how these are consulted in particular tasks.

In this section we will review what we consider to be the core issues raised within the theory-theory framework, and the empirical phenomena they encompass. While some of the issues overlap with those discussed above in the context of categorization-based models, others have yet to be addressed. Thus, this review will allow us to identify further difficulties with categorization-based approaches, and to identify additional empirical findings to be addressed in the simulations in later chapters.

Category Coherence

The first issue concerns what Murphy and Medin (1985) have referred to as *category coherence*—that is, the tendency for some groupings of objects to "hang together" in seemingly natural categories, whereas other groupings do not. Murphy and Medin (1985) pointed out that, although categorization-based theories can explain how the semantic system gives rise to a particular behavior once the appropriate category representations have been stored and linked to one another with the requisite processing structure, they lack the crucial explanation of how the "appropriate" representations and processes are settled on in the first place. For example, it seems reasonable to suppose that the semantic system stores a representation of the concept *dog*, and unreasonable to suppose that it stores a representation for the concept *grue* (things that are green before the year 2010, and blue thereafter; see Goodman 1954). But what are the principles by which the semantic system "knows" to create a category for *dog* and not for *grue*?

One possible answer to this question is that proposed by Rosch, and discussed above: perhaps the system forms summary representations for groups of objects that are similar to one another but somewhat different from other items. The problem is that the determination of how similar two objects are to one another itself depends on what kind of things they are (Murphy and Medin 1985). Recall for example that an object's shape may be more important than its color if the object is a toy, but that the reverse might be true if the object is a kind of food. In assessing how similar two novel objects are to one another (and to other items stored in memory), one must consider how their shape and color contribute to the measure of similarity, but the contributions of these properties differ depending on whether the items are toys or foods. Murphy and Medin (1985, 291) put it this way:

Certainly, objects in a category appear similar to one another. But does this similarity explain why the category was formed (instead of some other) or its ease of use? Suppose we follow A. Tversky's (1977) influential theory of similarity, which defines it as a function of common and distinctive features weighted for salience or importance. If similarity is the sole explanation of category structure, then an immediate problem is that the similarity relations among a set of entities depend heavily on the particular weights given to individual features. A barber pole and a zebra would be more similar than a horse and a zebra if the feature *striped* had sufficient weight. Of course, if these feature weights were fixed, then these similarity relations would be constrained, but as Tversky (1977) demonstrated convincingly, the relative weighting of a feature ... varies with the stimulus context and experimental task, so that there is no unique answer to the question of how similar one object is to another. To further complicate matters, Ortony, Vondruska, Jones, and Foss (1985) argue persuasively that the weight of a feature is not independent of the entity in which it inheres. The situation begins to look very much as if there are more free parameters than degrees of freedom, making similarity too flexible to explain conceptual coherence.

The problem identified in this quotation, and emphasized by other theory-theorists (e.g., Gelman and Williams 1998, Keil 1991), is that the relevance of any given property in the performance of a given semantic task depends upon the other attributes that constitute the stimulus description and upon the particular task that is being performed. In some cases, reliance on a superordinate category might be invoked to explain sensitivity to such interdependencies, as we discussed earlier. For example, to explain the fact that children use color to discriminate foods, but not toys, we may suppose that information about how color should be weighted is stored in the superordinate categories *food* and *toy*. However, a closer consideration of this solution suggests that it has limitations. Although some categorization-based theories provide detailed mechanistic accounts of how the category representations themselves are acquired, they do not necessarily explain how the taxonomic processing structure that links these representations is formed. For example, Anderson's (1991) Rational model provides a mechanism for acquisition of category representations, but no specification of how these might be linked into a taxonomic hierarchy so that the correct superordinate can be identified to specify what properties are relevant to a given subordinate category. Furthermore, there is no specification of how the child learns which types of features are important within different superordinate categories.

According to Murphy and Medin (1985), categorization-based theories are somewhat underconstrained without answers to these questions. They may provide detailed and mechanistic accounts of behavior given a particular choice of category representations and feature weightings, but if the motivation for these choices does not extend beyond fitting the data, the theory has in effect assumed what it purports to explain.

Under the theory-theory, the constraints that determine which properties are important for which concepts in which tasks—and hence, which concepts are coherent and which are not—derive from naive theories about the causal forces by which properties inhere in objects. That is, some constellations of properties (and the groupings of objects that share these properties) "hang together" because they are related to one another in a causal theory. For example, wings, hollow bones, feathers, and flight hang together and render *birds* a coherent category, because these properties are related to one another in a causal theory of flight: hollow bones make birds light, feathers and wings provide lots of air resistance, and these properties together allow birds to fly. Knowledge about these causal relationships among properties may render such properties particularly useful, salient, or informative. Keil (1991, 243), initially paraphrasing Boyd (1986), makes the case quite clearly:

Although most properties in the world may be ultimately connectable through an elaborate causal chain to almost all others, these causal links are not distributed in equal density among all properties. On the contrary, they tend to cluster in tight bundles separated by relatively empty spaces. What makes them cluster is a homeostatic mechanism wherein the presence of each of several features tends to support the presence of several others in the same cluster and not so much in other clusters. Thus, the properties tend to mutually support each other in a highly interactive manner. To return to an example used previously, feathers, wings, flight, and light weight don't just co-occur; they all tend to mutually support the presence of each other, and, by doing so, segregate the set of things known as birds into a natural kind.

Boyd's claim is about natural kinds and what they are, not about psychology. At the psychological level, however, we may be especially sensitive to picking up many of these sorts of homeostatic causal clusters such that beliefs about those causal relations provide an especially powerful cognitive "glue," making features cohere and be easier to remember and induce later on.

Thus category coherence would depend crucially on the causal theories that relate different properties, and not solely on independent and objective structure in the environment. That is, in order to know that wings, feathers, and flight are important properties of birds, and that the category *birds* itself is coherent, one must have a causal theory about how wings and feathers give rise to the ability to fly.

The theory-theory offers somewhat different explanations for some of the empirical phenomena we reviewed earlier. Specifically, Murphy and Medin (1985) and Keil (1991) have argued that illusory correlations provide strong evidence that semantic task performance is constrained by causal theories. In this view, children and adults may ignore or downplay the importance of co-occurring properties in the environment, if such co-occurrences do not fit their implicit theories, and may enhance the importance of feature correlations that do fit such theories. In R. Gelman's (1990) experiment described above, children attributed feet to an echidna even though no feet were visibly apparent, but denied that a metal figurine had feet, despite the fact that the figure's feet were evident from the picture. One account of these phenomena consistent with theory-theory is that children hold an implicit belief that feet are necessary for self-initiated movement. Hence, objects that can move must have feet, and objects that cannot move must not.

Similarly, causal theories might be invoked to explain the data from Macario's (1991) experiment, demonstrating that children generalize on the basis of shared color for objects construed as foods, but on the basis of shared shape for objects construed as toys. In this view, color is important for determining category membership for fruits, because the color of a fruit is understood to have arisen from biological processes that are essential to it as a particular type of biological kind. By contrast, color may be unimportant for the particular types of toys, because the color of a toy is understood to be incidental to the causal properties that make it a particular kind of toy. For example, the roundness of a toy ball is causally linked to its ability to roll, but its color is not.

More generally, category-coherence phenomena suggest that a theory of semantic memory should explain why some constellations of properties are, in Keil's words, easier to learn, induce, and remember than others; where constraints on the acquisition of knowledge about object-property correspondences come from; and how these phenomena are influenced by causal knowledge.

Differential Generalization of Different Types of Information

A second challenge posed by the theory-theory stems from the observation that human beings are able to generalize different types of information in different ways. These abilities may be present even in young children. For example, Gelman and Markman (1986) showed that preschoolers use category membership to guide inferences about biological properties, but use perceptual similarity to guide inferences about physical properties. In one study, children were shown a picture of a brontosaurus and a picture of a rhinoceros. They were taught the names of the animals ("dinosaur" and "rhino"), and a new fact about each. Half the children were taught a biological fact (e.g., the dinosaur has cold blood, but the rhino has warm blood), and half were taught a physical property (e.g., the dinosaur weighs ten tons, but the rhino weighs one ton). The children were then shown a picture of a triceratops, which they were told was another kind of dinosaur; however, the triceratops more closely resembled the rhinoceros. Children who learned the biological fact extended it to the triceratops on the basis of category membership—that is, they were more likely to say that the triceratops was cold-blooded like the brontosaurus. By contrast, children who were taught the physical property were less likely to use the category as the basis for generalization: most either guessed that the triceratops was one ton, like the rhino, or were uncertain. A very few overemphasized the importance of category membership, and consistently guessed that the triceratops would weigh ten tons like the brontosaurus.

This pattern of property generalization is difficult to explain within a hierarchical categorization-based model, because it violates the constraints of the taxonomic hierarchy. In order for biological information to generalize from brontosaurus to triceratops, but not to rhino, *brontosaurus* and *triceratops* representations must reside beneath a common node somewhere in the taxonomy, in a branching structure that excludes *rhinoceros*. The generalization of physical properties from rhino to triceratops, but not to brontosaurus, requires that *rhino* and *triceratops* reside beneath a common node that is not superordinate to *brontosaurus*. It is easy to see that these constraints are not compatible with a hierarchical scheme; there are too few degrees of freedom.

Taxanomic organization imposes further unnecessary restrictions on the relationships that can be represented in categorization-based theories. For example, a biological taxonomy of animal concepts has no means of encoding the important similarities that exist among domestic animals, which distinguish these from wild animals. In the biological taxonomy, dogs are more similar to wolves than to cats; however, there are many properties shared by cats and dogs but not by wolves, which are captured by the concept *pet*—for example, they are tame, friendly, companionable, and so on. These properties may be stored separately with each individual concept to which they apply, but such a scheme fails to capture the important regularities shared by all pets. That is, there is no way to represent (in a biological taxonomy) that dogs, cats, and horses are in some respect the same kind of thing. Again, there are too few degrees of freedom.

We might suppose that the semantic system makes use of more than one hierarchical structure—that one taxonomic system is used to govern the generalization of biological properties, and another for physical properties. But such *heterarchies* open themselves up to intractable inheritance conflicts. For example, in Gelman and Markman's (1986) experiment above, suppose children were taught that the rhinoceros eats a small amount of food, while the brontosaurus eats a large amount. Eating is a biological process, but large animals need to eat lots of food. Should the biological taxonomy or the physical taxonomy be used in directing the inference? What criteria should be used to select the appropriate structure? By organizing concepts in a single taxonomy, one may avoid such conflicts, but there appears to be no way of doing so that does justice to the flexibility with which human beings can use their semantic knowledge to reason about objects and their properties.

The alternative offered by the theory-theory is that generalization and induction of semantic information are partially governed by naive theories appropriate to the domain (Carey 1985). For example, children may generalize information about body temperature on the basis of shared category membership, because they adhere to a naive theory of biology in which living things are construed as similar when they have similar names, regardless of their visual appearance. In this case, a theory specific to the domain of biology is appropriate, because body heat is understood to arise from fundamentally biological causal mechanisms, which are appropriate for understanding and explaining certain properties of animals. When making judgments about nonbiological properties of animals, such as their weight, children (and adults) may refer to naive theories specific to an alternative domain—for example, a naive physics—in which animals are construed as similar when they share certain physical characteristics, like size. That is, the flexibility exhibited by children and adults in their induction behavior may arise from their ability to bring different domain theories to bear on different kinds of induction tasks.

Although this idea seems reasonable enough, it is worth pointing out that it raises many of the same questions unanswered by categorization-based models. How does the system know which domain theories are appropriate to which phenomena? Which criteria determine that size and weight are physical phenomena, whereas body heat is biological? Once the appropriate domain is determined, how do the corresponding theories constrain behavior in the task? These are the sorts of questions that any theory of semantic task performance must address.

Conceptual Reorganization

A third challenge posed by the theory-theory stems from studies of developmental change in children's inductive projection of properties of one object to other objects. An influential series of studies by Carey (1985) suggests that children's conceptual knowledge undergoes substantial reorganization over development. In one experiment, children were shown pictures of unusual and presumably unfamiliar animals (such as aardvarks and dodo birds) and were asked to decide whether each had particular biological properties (e.g., Does the aardvark have a heart? Does the dodo bird sleep? See Carey 1985). At age 4, children attributed all the properties probed to each novel animal roughly according to its similarity to people. For example, they were most likely to guess that the aardvark breathes, has bones, and can sleep; were moderately likely to draw the same conclusions for a dodo bird; and were least likely to guess that the stinkoo (a kind of worm) shares these properties. Older children showed a quite different pattern of induction: some properties (such as *breathes* and *eats*) were judged to be true of all animals regardless of their similarity to people; others (such as *has bones*) were attributed with equal likelihood to vertebrates but with very little likelihood to invertebrates; and still others (such as *thinks*) were again attributed to the novel animals on the basis of their similarity to humans (Carey 1985). When taught a new biological property of an object (e.g., that it has a *spleen*), children's willingness to generalize this property to other objects paralleled the pattern of extension of other biological properties.

On the basis of these and many more related data, Carey (1985) has argued that the representations and processes that govern human performance in these kinds of induction tasks undergo a radical reorganization between the ages of 4 and 10. In this view, the different induction profiles shown by 4- and 10-year-olds indicate that profoundly different conceptual structures underlie their judgments. The behavior of the youngest children is marked by a simple proximity rule, in which biological properties are attributed to objects in proportion to their similarity to human beings. The more sophisticated behavior of older children and adults is thought to reflect the emergence of a naive theory of biology, within which human beings are construed as one among many sorts of living things, all sharing certain essential properties. The observation that the older groups will extend some kinds of properties in an all-or-none fashion to all animals (and only to animals) indicates that they have achieved a biological concept of *animal* not available to the younger children.

The conceptual reorganization investigated in Carey's work can involve more than an increasing differentiation of concepts with experience, of the sort documented by Keil (1989) and Mandler (1997). It can also involve the incorporation of many superficially different items within a superordinate concept, as when animals, insects, birds, and plants are subsumed under the general concept *living thing*, as well as the discovery of new concepts that have no obvious progenitor in the earlier system. Conceptual reorganization can also reflect itself in the gradual restructuring of knowledge about different kinds of properties (Gelman and Markman 1986; Gelman and Coley 1990; Gelman and Wellman 1991; Gelman and Kremer 1991). For example, young children attribute various biological properties (such as breathing, having bones, and thinking) to unfamiliar animals in more or less the same way: specifically, in proportion to the animal's proximity to people. Older children, on the other hand, treat different properties differently—attributing some behaviors such as sleeping and breathing to all animals, and restricting others (such as having bones) to narrower categories (i.e., vertebrates).

We have already made the point that taxonomic processing models have not tended to provide very concrete explanations about how the taxonomic processing structure on which they depend is acquired. However, we have suggested that work on the progressive differentiation of concept knowledge in childhood described by Keil (1989) and Mandler (1997) is at least consistent with the notion that concepts are organized within a taxonomic hierarchy. Carey's (1985) work suggests that conceptual change can be somewhat more complex, and further undermines the usefulness of invoking the taxonomic hierarchy to explain the organization of semantic memory. An account of conceptual change consistent with hierarchically organized processing models must explain how the links between nodes stored in the hierarchy change with development, and also how the nodes of the hierarchy themselves differentiate and coalesce into new concepts. It hardly needs saying that this complicates the developmental picture painted by Warrington (1975) considerably. How and why does such dramatic change happen? The shifts in induction behavior that Carey (1985) documents render a mechanistic account of the acquisition of conceptual knowledge the more pressing, and the lack of such an account in hierarchical categorization-based theories the more wanting.

The Importance of Causal Knowledge

Finally, research in the theory-theory framework has led to an increasing appreciation of the important role causal knowledge plays in semantic cognition. By *causal knowledge*, we mean a person's knowledge about the causal relationships that exist between different objects, as well as knowledge about the causal mechanisms by which particular properties inhere in objects. Much of the research encompassed by the theory-theory has focused on documenting the ways that causal knowledge can influence semantic task performance.

For example, influential research described by Keil (e.g., Keil 1989) has shown that knowledge about the causal mechanisms by which properties are understood to have arisen in a particular object provides strong constraints on the inferences the object supports. Keil composed short stories in which a particular object was transformed in some way that altered its appearance. In one example, children were told about a raccoon that was altered to make it look like a skunk. After hearing the story, children were asked whether the object had changed its identity—for instance, whether it had become a skunk as a result of the transformation, or whether it was still "really" a raccoon. Keil found that children's answers varied depending on the particular transformation stories they were told. If the animal was transformed by means of relatively superficial mechanisms (such as dying it black and painting a stripe down its back), older children were much less likely to decide that the object had changed its kind. If the mechanism was more "biological" (for example, if the raccoon had been given an injection that caused it to "grow up into" something that looked like a skunk), children were more likely to accept that it had changed kinds. Moreover, Keil documented a developmental progression in the likelihood that children would accept that the object had changed its kind, with younger children accepting that almost any change in appearance signaled a change in identity. In Keil's view, such developmental change signals the elaboration of increasingly sophisticated intuitive domain theories.

These studies demonstrate that knowledge about the causal forces that give rise to an object's appearance has strong consequences for the inferences that children and adults will make about the object's kind, and hence about many of its properties. That is, causal knowledge about an object seems especially important for determining many of the object's properties, including what "kind" of thing it is (see also Gopnik and Sobel 2000). We have already seen that categorization-based theories may have difficulty explaining why some kinds of properties are more important than others for determining category membership. The discovery that causal knowledge in particular may prove especially important adds a wrinkle to this general dilemma: how is causal knowledge to be represented in a categorization-based framework to begin with, and moreover, why should causal knowledge prove especially important for directing and constraining semantic task performance?

Theory-theorists have also pointed out that categorization-based theories fail to capture another potentially important aspect of semantic cognition: specifically, the ability of children and adults to explain why they made a certain semantic judgment. For example, in R. Gelman's experiment with the echidna, children were not only asked whether the unfamiliar animal could move up and down the hill by itself; they were also asked to explain how they came to their decision. Part of the interest of the experiment lay in the fact that children provided answers to the question that were taken as indicating the presence of an underlying "causal-explanatory" reasoning process, which (it might be argued) partially supported their ultimate decision. Recall for instance that some children stated that they knew the echidna could move "because" it had feet, suggesting that knowledge about a causal relationship between having feet and the ability to move informed the child's decision in the task. Under the theory-theory, such causal-explanatory reasoning lies at the heart of human cognition, and the knowledge that makes this reasoning possible—causal-explanatory domain theories—is reflected both in the patterns of judgments that children and adults make in different semantic tasks, and in the reasons that they explicitly provide for their decisions in these tasks. Categorization-based theories may be able to account for the former—for example, they may explain how children are able to correctly conclude that the echidna can move up and down the hill by itself—but the accounts such theories offer preclude a concurrent understanding of the explicit causal explanations children provide for their own decisions. That is, categorization-based theories may explain a subject's behavior in semantic tasks, but without additional constructs, they cannot explain the causal-explanatory "reasons" subjects give for this behavior.

In summary, the theory-theory raises a number of issues that we believe seriously challenge the sufficiency of categorization-based approaches to semantic cognition. These are listed in table 1.5.

Toward a Mechanistic Model of Semantic Knowledge

We find some of the insights offered by the theory-theory appealing —specifically, its emphasis on the ways existing semantic knowledge can interact with experience to constrain acquisition and processing in particular semantic tasks, and its stipulation that semantic representations and processes must be more flexible than many categorization-based theories suggest. However, the notion of a naive or implicit theory has been somewhat vaguely specified in the literature. The framework has not yet produced a mechanistically explicit account of what a theory is, or how theories work to constrain performance in semantic tasks. Though several studies are consistent with the idea that prior knowledge can influence how children and adults reason about objects (Gelman and Kremer 1991; Carey and Gelman 1991; Springer and Keil 1991; Murphy and Allopenna 1994), and the ease with which they learn new information (Gelman 1990; Gelman and Williams 1998; Tomasello 1999), it is not clear how (or whether) it makes sense to distinguish between knowledge that takes the form of a theory from other kinds of semantic knowledge (Murphy 2002). The strength of categorization-based models and their like resides in the explicitness of the mechanisms they invoke, which allows the models to be tested empirically through studies such as those devised by Collins and Quillian (1969), Rips, Shoben, and Smith (1973), and Rosch et al. (1976). In our view, theory-theorists have convincingly demonstrated that knowledge acquisition is somewhat more constrained, and semantic task performance somewhat more flexible, than suggested by categorization-based theories, but have not yet articulated a comparably explicit account of the mechanisms that underpin these aspects of human cognition. We believe that a theory of semantic task performance should offer an explicit account of the processes that give rise to the empirical phenomena addressed by the researchers working in the theory-theory framework, but none of these researchers has proposed such a theory as yet.

Table 1.5   Empirical phenomena consistent with the theory-theory

PHENOMENON	EXPERIMENTAL PARADIGM	THEORY-THEORY ACCOUNT
Some feature constellations are easier to learn, induce, and remember than others.	• Concept learning tasks	Features that are related to one another in a causal theory are easier to learn, induce, and remember.
Illusory correlations in children and adults suggest that perceptual experience is insufficient to explain knowledge of object-property correspondences.	• Estimates of object-property co-occurrences • Children's explanations of their decisions in reasoning tasks	Children and adults use naive theories to explain, and thereby filter or supplement, their perceptual experience.
A given property has differential importance for different categories.	• Generalization of a new property to objects described as members of different categories	Naive theories determine which properties are important for which categories.
Children's conceptual knowledge undergoes extensive reorganization between the ages of 3 and 10.	• Semantic induction tasks	Children acquire new domain theories, which constrain their conceptual knowledge and hence their induction behavior.
Different kinds of properties generalize across different groups of objects.	• Semantic induction tasks	Children apply different domain theories to different types of properties.
Causal knowledge strongly constrains the inferences children and adults make about an object.	• Transformation studies • Semantic induction tasks	Causal-explanatory theories are especially important for constraining semantic knowledge.
Children and adults can provide explicit causal-explanatory "reasons" for their decisions in semantic tasks.	• Protocols from semantic induction tasks	Causal-explanatory theories and the reasoning processes they support underlie performance of semantic tasks.

One response to this critique might be to develop new models based on categorization that also incorporate aspects of the theory-theory in order to address all of the phenomena outlined above. Indeed, just such an approach has been pursued by several investigators (see Sloman and Rips 1998), and we expect that many theorists will continue to make such an effort. We have chosen to follow a different course, employing a distributed, connectionist framework for the representation and use of semantic information. Here we consider some of the reasons we feel it may be useful to consider such an alternative.

First of all, we adopt the view, inherent in a great deal of earlier work within the PDP framework, that categorization-based models may be too restrictive or constraining to capture the nuances of human knowlege of all sorts of things (Rumelhart et al. 1986c). The boundaries between different categories are not at all clear, and the characteristics of individual category members are sensitive to subtle contextual shading (McClelland, St. John, and Taraban 1989), and to dependencies among the features that make up a stimulus description (e.g., Aha and Goldstone 1990; Anderson and Fincham 1996). As Rumelhart et al. (1986c) pointed out, the adoption of categorization mechanisms to explain semantic memory involves the all-or-none discretization of an essentially graded set of similarity relations—a process that of necessity discards important information about subregularities in the domain. Consider the graded similarities existing among various birds: robins, sparrows, ravens, chickens, penguins. To capture the fact that all of these objects are similar in many respects, we might create a concept such as *bird*, which describes all the properties they are likely to share. To capture the differences among the classes, we might also posit a subordinate category representation for each, all of which are attached to the *bird* representation by a stored class-inclusion link. In this case, we have represented that the various kinds of birds are similar to one another by virtue of attaching to the same superordinate node, but different from one another by virtue of properties stored with the subordinate representations. However, many similarities between robins and sparrows are not captured by this scheme. Properties shared by robins and sparrows, but not by birds generally, must be represented separately in each of the *robin* and *sparrow* concepts respectively. We might suppose that these regularities are themselves captured by an intermediate concept (such as *songbird*) that interposes between *bird* and *robin*, and that captures the similarities between robins and sparrows. However, this choice would fail to capture the similarities between songbirds and, say, ravens—which, though fairly distinct from robins and sparrows, nevertheless share properties with these birds not associated with, say, gulls and terns.

It is easy to see that any particular choice of categories will neglect some of the regularities apparent in the domain. Chickens, ostriches, and turkeys are quite distinct from one another; nevertheless, all are large, flightless birds. The relationship between *large* and *flightless* is not arbitrary; among birds, these properties have a tendency to co-occur together and to predict other properties—for example, large, flightless birds are less likely to build nests, are more likely to be edible, and so on. Such relationships cannot be described by hard-and-fast rules—there are plenty of large birds that can fly, for instance—but are better characterized as graded constraints (Rumelhart et al. 1986c). Attempts to capture them with a set of discrete category distinctions are often forced and artificial.

A related but equally important point is that semantics is a *quasi-regular* domain—that is, a domain that exhibits systematic tendencies, but that also tolerates exceptions that may deviate from these tendencies in some ways, while respecting them in others (McClelland and Seidenberg 1995). Though some perfectly reliable relationships may exist, many other relationships are not perfectly reliable, but are informative nonetheless (e.g., most furry creatures walk, most feathered creatures fly). Exceptional objects that do not perfectly respect the regularities of the domain may still share some of its systematicity. For example, although penguins cannot fly, they do have many of the typical properties of other feathered creatures; they lay eggs, they have beaks, and so on. Thus, items that seem exceptional in some (or even many) respects may also be quite ordinary in others. The semantic system appears to capitalize on such regularities where they exist, while also accommodating exceptional information. This poses a problem for any model that assigns items to equivalence classes. While it is possible to build in overrides for particular properties in categorization-based models, this can lead to further complications. These complications are avoided in connectionist models: their graded, similarity-based generalization properties have proven very useful for capturing quasi-regular structure in several domains.

Based on considerations such as these, Rumelhart et al. (1986c) argued that perhaps the best approach would be to view knowledge of a particular kind of thing not as a prespecified cognitive entity (whether it be called a concept, a category, a schema, or something else), but as an emergent property of an underlyingly connectionist semantic system. This is the approach that will be taken throughout the rest of this book.

Summary

The long history of research into semantic cognition has generated a wealth of data from semantic tasks in the domains of development, adult cognition, and dementia. Many of these findings, summarized in tables 1.1 through 1.5, have been interpreted within a categorization-based approach to understanding semantic task performance. Several powerful constructs have been invoked within this framework, including taxonomic processing hierarchies, category prototypes, and privileged or "basic" category representations. However, we have identified a variety of challenges to categorization-based accounts. First, although each of the constructs invoked in the framework may help to explain a portion of the data, they sometimes appear to conflict with one another. These conflicts are particularly obvious in the apparent primacy of superordinate category knowledge on the one hand and intermediate, basic-level category knowledge on the other; and in the tendency to explain processing latencies sometimes with reference to taxonomic processing structure, and sometimes with reference to similarity-based mechanisms. Second, there are a variety of empirical findings that remain to be fully explained by any existing account. Third, no full developmental theory of the acquisition of conceptual knowledge has been provided, and more specifically, categorization-based models have thus far not described the mechanisms by which the processing structure assumed to link category representations at different levels of specificity is acquired. Hence, the framework offers at best an incomplete account of conceptual development and expertise. Fourth, the flexibility with which children and adults can generalize new knowledge suggests that more than one taxonomy is needed to direct semantic induction, but such heterarchies can result in intractable inheritance conflicts. While the proposals of theory-theorists afford one way to address these difficulties, these proposals have thus far been underspecified. Fifth, human performance in semantic tasks may be sensitive to multiple high-order dependencies among stimulus features; the discrete nature of category representations makes it difficult to explain these dependencies without sacrificing the qualities that make such representations appealing in the first place. Finally, semantics appears to us to be a quasi-regular domain, in which many graded regularities may be observed. The discrete equivalence classes of categorization-based models provide a procrustean bed, insufficient to capture fully the graded structure of semantic relationships.

We believe that these shortcomings warrant the exploration of an alternative to the categorization-based approach—one that addresses the phenomena that have motivated categorization-based models as well as those that have motivated the theory-theory approach. The parallel distributed processing framework appears to provide a promising starting place for such an alternative, because it naturally captures the graded nature of semantic knowledge, its gradual acquisition in development, and its graceful degradation under damage in dementia.

In this chapter we put forward a theory of semantic cognition quite different from the categorization-based theories discussed in chapter 1. Our theory adopts different assumptions about the nature of the representations and processes that subserve semantic memory, namely, those articulated in the parallel distributed processing (PDP) framework (Rumelhart, McClelland, and the PDP Research Group 1986). PDP networks offer a powerful set of tools for characterizing learning and development, generalization and induction, the time course of processing, and the breakdown of cognitive function as a result of neuroanatomic deterioration—phenomena relevant to human cognition generally and to the domain of semantic cognition in particular. Properties of PDP networks that have been useful in understanding other domains of human cognition may also help to explain the phenomena discussed in chapter 1. We refer in particular to the ability of PDP networks to acquire useful representations in quasi-regular domains such as word reading and English past-tense formation (Seidenberg and McClelland 1989; Plaut et al. 1996); their accommodation of context-sensitive representations, which has been explored in schema theory (Rumelhart et al. 1986c) and text comprehension (McClelland, St. John, and Taraban 1989; St. John 1992); and their specification of a general mechanism for cognitive change in learning and development (McClelland 1995; Munakata et al. 1997; Elman et al. 1996).

The application of PDP networks to semantic cognition has its roots in early work conducted by Hinton (1981, 1986). Hinton (1981) outlined a general framework for storing propositional knowledge (of the kind described in a Quillian-like semantic network) in a distributed connectionist network. An illustration of the model is included in figure 2.1. Here, the structure of a simple proposition of the form *Item-Relation-Attribute* is reflected in the architecture of the network: there is a separate bank of units for each part of the proposition. Different fillers for each slot are represented as different patterns of activation across the corresponding units. For example, the representation of the proposition *Clyde color gray* (to use one of Hinton's examples) would correspond to one pattern of activity across each of the three groups of units: one for *Clyde*, one for *color*, and one for *gray*.

All three banks have bidirectional connections to a fourth layer (labeled *Prop* in the illustration), such that a pattern of activity across the three input layers generates a unique pattern across the *Prop* units. These in turn send new signals to the *Item*, *Relation*, and *Attribute* units, which update their states in response. The process iterates until the unit states stop changing, at which point the network is said to have *settled* into a steady state. Hinton demonstrated that individual propositions could be stored in the network by adjusting the weights to make the patterns representing the proposition stable. Each stored proposition would then be represented in the network by a unique pattern of activity across the *Prop* units, which simultaneously activated and received support from the input patterns.

Hinton's network had several interesting properties and implications. First, he showed that the network was capable of completing stored propositions when given two of its terms as inputs. For example, when provided with the inputs *Clyde* and *color*, the network settled into a steady state in which the pattern representing the correct completion of the proposition (*gray*) was observed across the *Attribute* units. Second, several such propositions could be stored in the network, in the same set of weights, and new propositions could be added without requiring additional computational elements. Third, Hinton showed that when appropriate representations were chosen, the network provided a natural

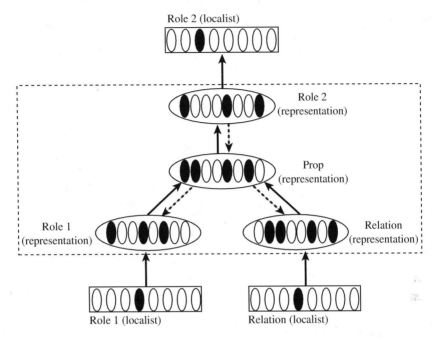

Figure 2.1   Our depiction of Hinton's (1981) model for storing propositional knowledge in a distributed connectionist network (layers and connections within the dotted box), also reflecting the structure of the network used in Hinton (1986; complete model including items within and outside the dotted box). The structure of a simple proposition is reflected in the architecture of the network, with a separate bank of units dedicated to representing *Role 1*, *Relation*, and *Role 2*. In Hinton 1981, the filler for any two of the slots could be directly provided as a pattern of activity, and the task of the network was to fill in the pattern in the remaining slot. The patterns in the three slots interact by means of the units in the *Prop* layer, which contain units that respond to various conjunctions of roles and relations. In the 1981 model, there were bidirectional connections (both solid and dashed arrows), as well as connections from the units in the Prop layer back to themselves (not shown). Specific propositions can be stored in the network by adjusting the connection weights. In later work, Hinton (1986) used the backpropagation algorithm in a feed-forward variant of this model to train the connection weights. For this work, inputs could be presented only to the Role 1 and Relation slots; Role 2 was always used for the output. Only the connections illustrated with solid arrows were used, propagating activation forward via the Role 1 and Relation Representation layers, to the Prop Representation layer, to the Role 2 Representation layer, and finally to the Role 2 localist output. In Hinton (1986), all connection weights were adjusted by the learning procedure so that the representations of the slot fillers and of the overall proposition were all learned.

mechanism for generalization. If related objects (such as different elephants) were represented by similar patterns of activity across the *Item* units, they would contribute similar inputs to the *Prop* units. As a result, the entire network would tend to settle into an appropriate steady state (corresponding to the most similar stored proposition) when given a novel input that overlapped with a familiar stored proposition. For example, if the network had stored the proposition *Clyde color gray*, and was then given the inputs *Elmer color* in the *Item* and *Relation* units, it would settle into a state in which the pattern corresponding to *gray* was observed across *Attribute* units—provided that the representations of *Clyde* and *Elmer* were sufficiently similar. Note that similarity to known items, rather than explicit categorization of *Elmer* as an elephant, provides the basis for generalization in this case.

The properties of pattern completion and similarity-based generalization captured in Hinton's model are key consequences of the use of distributed representations in connectionist networks (Hinton, McClelland, and Rumelhart 1986). Distributed representations, in which a pattern of activity over a set of units is used to represent some object of thought, can be more efficient than local representations, where an individual unit is used to stand for a each possible alternative object. The essential observation is that with N units, one may distinguish only N objects using localist representations, but one may distinguish 2^N using distributed representations. The use of distributed representations brings with it an automatic tendency to generalize: If a network already makes a certain response to one pattern, it will tend to make a similar response to a similar pattern. Generalization is essential for intelligent behavior, since hardly anything ever repeats itself exactly (Marr 1969). Thus the two properties that motivate discrete category representations under other approaches—economy of storage and knowledge generalization—are also captured by distributed representations. The core of our theory is its reliance on distributed representations to provide the basis for intelligent generalization.

Hinton also pointed out that the network was sensitive to inter-dependencies among its inputs. When many propositions are stored in the network, neither the *Item* nor the *Relation* inputs alone are sufficient to uniquely determine a correct pattern of activation in the *Attribute* units. Instead, the conjunction of the *Item* and *Relation* fillers must be taken into account. For example, the completions of *Clyde color*, *Scott color*, and *Clyde size* are quite different if Scott is a human being and Clyde is an elephant. Put another way, the state into which the network settles when given a particular pattern in the *Item* slot depends on the state of the units in the *Relation* slot, and vice versa. Both the *Item* and *Relation* representations provide constraints on the ultimate state the network settles into. These interactions of *Item* and *Relation* information are a specific instance of a general property of connectionist networks: All aspects of the input—in this case, the item and the relation input—impose constraints on the output of the system, so that different conjunctions of inputs can work together to influence the outputs that correspond to overt responses.

The network's ability to produce appropriate responses to given item and relation inputs derives from the particular representations assigned to the different inputs. In his early model, Hinton (1981) directly specified the representations for each of the slots, including the *Prop* slot, and used a simple procedure to set the weights so that particular inputs would work together to support pattern completion. However, this sidestepped the same sticky question of acquisition faced by categorization-based models. Where do useful representations come from? If the internal representations are doing all of the interesting work in the network, the question of their origin is of paramount importance. Must they be separately specified (perhaps by evolution), or can they be acquired as a result of a learning process?

The introduction of the back-propagation learning algorithm (Rumelhart, Hinton, and Williams 1986) provided an important step forward in the pursuit of the idea, certainly favored by Hinton (1981), that useful representations (or more specifically, the connection weights that determine such representations) might be learned. Indeed, Hinton (1986) was the first to use the backpropagation algorithm to address the acquisition of semantic representations. He created a network with an architecture similar to that of the semantic network shown in figure 2.1, and taught it to respond to queries about family relationships. For example, when given the name of an individual *Person1* (e.g., *Colin*) and a *Relation* (*Father*) as input, the network was required to complete the proposition with the name of the correct *Person2* (in this case, Colin's father, *James*). The inputs and outputs were localist in this model—a separate unit was used for each person and each relation in the input, and for each person in the output—but the individual units in each slot had modifiable connections to a pool of units similar to the *Item*, *Relation*, and *Attribute* pools in figure 2.1, and these in turn were connected to a common pool of units corresponding to the *Prop* layer. For simplicity, connections ran in only one direction in Hinton's model, from the input units to the distributed *Person1* and *Relation* pools, to the *Prop* units, to the distributed *Person2* pool, and finally to the output units. Note also that, as in the 1981 model, neither the *Person1* nor the *Relation* fillers, on their own, were sufficient to uniquely determine the correct *Person2*. The network had to learn to respond differently to different conjunctions of person and relation fillers.

Using backpropagation, Hinton trained the network to answer queries about three generations of two families. After learning, the model was able to respond correctly in all cases—demonstrating that the learning process had discovered connection weights that (1) assigned distributed representations to each individual *Person1* and *Relation*, (2) allowed these representations to work together via the *Prop* layer to produce a useful distributed *Person2* representation, and (3) allowed this *Person2* representation to activate the correct local output unit. The particular representations acquired through the learning process captured important and useful regularities across the training examples: analyses of the patterns of activity corresponding to the different people showed that informative aspects of the individual's identity, such as which family and which generation the individual belonged to, were coded along orthogonal dimensions in the network's representation space (McClelland 1995). This structure in turn allowed the model to draw similarity-based inferences about some valid relations that had not been included in the training set.

In summary, the early work by Hinton (1981), bolstered by the backpropagation learning algorithm (Rumelhart et al. 1986a), provides the starting place for our theory of semantic cognition:

- Performance in semantic tasks occurs through the propagation of activation among simple processing units, via weighted connections.
- Connection weights encode the knowledge that determines which distributed representations arise internally, and that governs the joint use of these representations to determine the outcome of the process.
- The connection weights are learned, so that semantic cognitive abilities arise from experience.

In the remainder of this book, we will present the argument that these simple statements actually provide the basis for a useful account of human semantic cognitive abilities and their acquisition. To do so, we will be using networks with the properties listed above to address the empirical phenomena reviewed in the first chapter, and to answer the questions raised in our discussion of categorization-based theories there.

The Rumelhart Feed-Forward Network

In most of the work to be presented in the following chapters, we will work within a simplified connectionist model introduced by Rumelhart (1990; Rumelhart and Todd 1993). This model is a further variant of Hinton's (1986) family-trees model that acquires distributed representations of items by learning about their properties in different relational contexts. The model embodies the

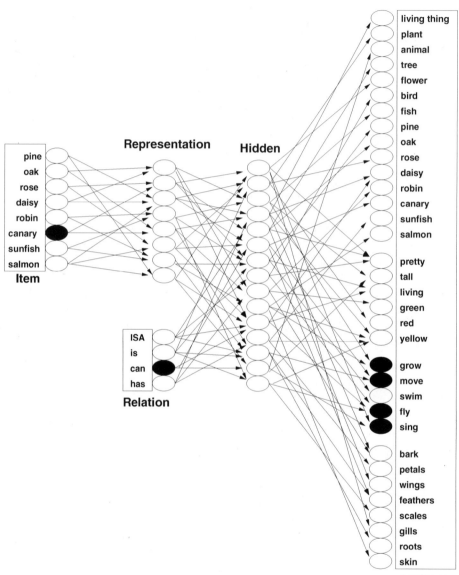

essential properties necessary to address the empirical phenomena raised in chapter 1, and has the added virtues of tractability and simplicity.

Our adaptation of the Rumelhart model is illustrated in figure 2.2. We describe the model and the processing that occurs in it at a level of detail that we hope is sufficient to allow readers not already familiar with such networks to understand the basics of their operation. Additional details of the implementation and of the training patterns are presented in appendixes A and B.

Rumelhart's initial goal was to demonstrate that the propositional content contained in a traditional taxonomic hierarchy could also be captured in the distributed representations acquired by a PDP network trained with backpropagation, and that the network could support the kinds of inferences that can be performed in Quillian's hierarchical propositional network. Rumelhart used individual nodes (or *localist units*) in the network's input and output layers to correspond to the constituents of the propositions—the items or concepts that occupy the first (*subject*) slot in each proposition, the relation terms that occupy the second (*relation*) slot, and the attribute values that occupy the third slot. Each item is represented by an individual input unit in the layer labeled *Item*, different relations are represented by individual units in the layer labeled *Relation*, and the various possible completions of three-element propositions are represented by individual units in the

Figure 2.2   Our depiction of the connectionist model of semantic memory used in the simulations in chapter 3, adapted from Rumelhart (1990; Rumelhart and Todd 1993). The entire set of units used in the network is shown. Input units are shown on the left, and activation propagates from left to right. Where connections are indicated, every unit in the pool on the left is connected to every unit in the pool on the right. Each unit in the *Item* layer corresponds to an individual item in the environment. Each unit in the *Relation* layer represents contextual constraints on the kind of information to be retrieved. Thus, the input pair *canary can* corresponds to a situation in which the network is shown a picture of a canary and asked what it can do. The network is trained to turn on all the units that represent correct completions of the input query, and to turn off all other units. In the example shown, the correct units to activate are *grow*, *move*, *fly*, and *sing*.

layer labeled *Attribute*. When presented with a particular *Item* and *Relation* pair in the input, the network's task is to turn on the attribute units in the output that correspond to valid completions of the proposition. For example, when the units corresponding to *canary* and *can* are activated in the input, the network must learn to activate the output units *move*, *grow*, *fly*, and *sing*. The particular items, relations, and attributes are based on the information contained in figure 1.2. When the network has learned to correctly complete all of the propositions, it has encoded the same information stored in the propositional hierarchy.

We have adapted Rumelhart's model a little to suit our own purposes. We treat the network as a simplified model of experience with objects in the world and of spoken statements about these objects. The *Item* layer is construed as providing a simplified proxy for an input representation of an object as encountered in experience; the units stand for the occurrence of the actual items themselves, not for their names, and in our work they always correspond to the items at the bottom level of the taxonomic hierarchy in figure 1.2. The relation layer is viewed as a simplified specification of the context in which the item is encountered. The attribute layer is thought of as representing the predicted consequences or sequelae following from the occurrence of the object in the given context. The completion of a simple three-term proposition about the object is an example of what we have in mind: given *canary can* _____, the possible sequelae include *grow*, *move*, *fly*, and *sing*. In this approach, the four propositional relations from Quillian's hierarchy are viewed as distinct contexts. The *ISA* relation corresponds to a naming or explicit categorization context, in which the object's name or category label is of relevance, as these might be indicated verbally (e.g., by a sentence such as "This is a bird" or "This is a canary"). The *can* relation corresponds to a context in which the behaviors of the object might be observed, the *is* relation corresponds to a context in which its appearance properties are highlighted, and the *has* relation corresponds to a context in which its parts are highlighted.

The network consists of a series of nonlinear processing units, organized into layers, and connected in a feed-forward manner as shown in figure 2.2. Patterns are presented by activating one unit in each of the *Item* and *Relation* layers (i.e., these activations are set to 1 and activations of all other input units are set to 0). Activation then feeds forward through the network, modulated by the connection weights. Activations are updated sequentially, layer by layer, so that first the representation layer is updated, then the hidden layer, then the attribute layer. To update the activation of a unit, first its net input is calculated: the sum, over each of the unit's incoming connections, of the activity of the unit sending its activation through the connection, multiplied by the value of the connection weight. The net input is then transformed into an activation according to the logistic activation function shown in figure 2.3.

Initially, the connection weights in the network have small random values, so that the activations produced by a given input are weak and random in relation to the target output values. To perform correctly, the network must find a configuration of weights that will produce the correct target state across the output units for a given item-relation input. Each target state consists of a pattern of 1s and 0s like the one shown for the input *canary can* in figure 2.2—the target values for the black units are 1 and for all other units are 0.

To find an appropriate set of weights, the model is trained with the backpropagation algorithm already mentioned (Rumelhart et al. 1986a). Backpropagation is an inherently gradual learning process, which depends on the presentation of many training examples. When the environment is characterized (as in this case) by a relatively small and finite set of training examples, each example is presented multiple times, interleaved with presentations of the other examples. Training consists of a set of epochs, each encompassing the presentation of every item in the training set. There are several possible variants of the general training method. The approach we have used involves presenting each example once per

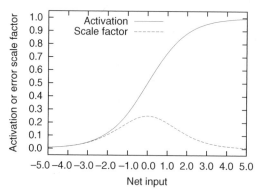

Figure 2.3 Activation function (solid curve) and error-derivative scale factor (dashed curve) used in the model. The activation function is used to convert the net input to each unit into its activation on the forward activation sweep through the network after presentation of an input. Learning depends on the differences between the target and obtained activation of the output units. Adjustments to the weights are made to reduce the error E, the sum of the squares of the differences. The change to a particular weight is the product of (a) the effect of changing the weight on the input to the receiving unit, and (b) the effect of changing the input to the receiving unit on E. Factor (a) depends on the activation of the sending unit; if the activation is 0, changing the weight does nothing. Factor (b), called δ ("delta"), is the product of (c) the effect of changing the unit's input on its activation and (d) the effect of changing its activation on E. Factor (c) is the scale factor shown in the figure. This varies with the net input to the unit that was calculated on the forward activation sweep, as indicated in the figure. For an output unit, factor (d) is the difference between the target and the current activation. For a hidden unit, changing its activation will affect the error at each output unit, via the unit's forward connections. The effect at each output unit is the product of the weight from the hidden unit to the output unit times the effect of changing the output unit's net input on E, the output unit's δ term. Accordingly, the δ terms are computed in a backward pass through the network. First the δ terms for each output unit are computed, then these are passed back to the hidden units. For each hidden unit the back-propagated δ terms are multiplied by the weight from the hidden unit to the output unit, then summed and scaled by factor (c) to obtain the hidden unit's δ term. Once δ has been computed for all the hidden units, it can be propagated back to the representation layer, where it can be used to calculate δ terms for each of the representation units. The eventual change to a connection weight is the product of (a) the activation of the sending unit and (b) the δ term of the receiving unit, scaled by the learning-rate constant ε.

epoch, in random order, and adjusting the weights after every training example. We use this *online* connection-weight adjustment procedure because we imagine that the brain uses a similar procedure: small connection-weight adjustments are made after every experience, and these gradually accumulate to form the basis of semantic knowledge and representation.

For each presentation of a training example, the process works as follows. First, the item and relation are presented to the network as inputs, and activation is propagated forward to the output units as described above. The observed output states are then compared to the target values, and the difference is treated as a measure of error at each output unit. Small adjustments to the connection weights throughout the network are made to reduce the error. A brief description of the procedure is given in the caption to figure 2.3; fuller discussions including derivation of the algorithm are available in Rumelhart et al. 1986a and Hertz, Krogh, and Palmer 1991. What is important conceptually about the procedure is that it involves the propagation of the error information at the output backward through the (forward-projecting) connection weights in the network, so that the changes to each weight—including those from the input units to the representation layer—are dictated by the effect that they will ultimately have on the error at the output. The weight adjustments are scaled by a constant ε, which must be small to ensure progress (McClelland, McNaughton, and O'Reilly 1995). Some adjustments cumulate across examples, while others cancel out. Overall the weights adapt slowly, yielding gradual evolution of the patterns of activation at each level of the network, and gradual reduction of error.

Although the model's inputs are localist (one unit for each item), each individual *Item* unit projects to all of the units in the layer labeled *Representation*. The activation of a single item in the model's input, then, generates a distributed pattern of activity across these units. The weights connecting the *Item* and *Representation* units evolve during learning, so the pattern of activity generated across the *Representation* units for a given item is a *learned internal representation* of the item. Though the model's input and target states are constrained to locally represent particular items, attributes, and relations, the learning process allows it to derive distributed internal representations governed by the structure of the domain.

For reasons we will discuss in the next chapter, the learned representations in the Rumelhart network gradually come to capture the semantic similarity relations that exist among the items in the training environment. Indeed, as Rumelhart (1990; Rumelhart and Todd 1993) showed, the hierarchy explicitly represented by the *ISA* links in Quillian's network come to be represented in a latent form, in the similarity relations among the patterns the network gradually learns to assign to each of the items. Because each item is represented locally in the input, the model has no initial information about how the objects in its virtual world are related to one another. For example, the *pine* and *oak* inputs are no more similar to one another than each is to the *salmon* input. Due to the small, random values of the weights from these units to the *Representation* units, the patterns initially all have very similar internal representations, with only sight random differences. However, as the model learns to complete particular propositions, these representations gradually change, and as we will see later, items that differ on many attributes come to be differentiated, while items that share many attributes continue to be represented by similar patterns of activity across the *Representation* units. Thus, the connections that link *Item* and *Representation* units in the network can be viewed as encoding a set of semantic similarity relationships among a set of otherwise arbitrary markers. The connections in the rest of the network then reflect the learned mappings between these internal representations, in combination with input from the relation context, and the explicit properties coded in the output.

An important departure from other representational schemes (including those used in some other connectionist approaches) is that the internal representations acquired by the Rumelhart network are not lists of semantic features—in no way are they directly interpretable semantically. Individual units in the model's *Representation* layer do not encode the presence or absence of explicit, intuitive object properties. Rather, the representations are abstracted from the featural decomposition of objects represented in the output layer. The network's representations capture the similarities existing among different kinds of objects, not the actual semantic properties themselves. The individual semantic properties can only be recovered through the combined effects of the units in the distributed representation, working in concert with units in other parts of the network.

Interpretation and Storage of New Information

A key aspect of our theory of conceptual knowledge acquisition, captured in the Rumelhart model, is the idea that it occurs through the very gradual adaptation of the connection weights that underlie the processing and representation of semantic content, driven by the overall structure of experience. We have argued elsewhere (McClelland et al. 1995) that slow, interleaved learning is essential for the discovery of the underlying structure of a domain of information through the use of an online learning procedure. A corollary of this aspect of our theory is that the gradual learning process is not the basis for learning in a situation where a person is given some new information and is subsequently asked to recall the information or otherwise make use of it.

According to our theory, the ability to interpret and make use of new information depends on knowledge that has previously accumulated in the semantic network through gradual learning; but neither the information nor its interpretation is stored immediately in the network's connection weights. To make this discussion concrete, imagine that a child who has heretofore experienced the small world encompassed by the Rumelhart network encounters a new item, such as a sparrow, and is told, "This is a bird." From this information, we assume the child can assign an internal representation to the sparrow using the knowledge he or she has previously acquired from encounters with other items in the environment, without any additional learning required. In the Rumelhart model, this assignment of a new representation based on acquired knowledge is accomplished using a variant of a technique introduced by Miikkulainen and Dyer (1987), which we will call *backpropagation-to-representation*.

The technique works as follows. A neutral pattern of activation is imposed on the representation units (all of their inputs are set to zero), and the appropriate relation input unit is activated. In this case, the appropriate relation unit is the *ISA* unit, because the child has been told that the sparrow "is a bird." Activation is fed forward to the output units, and compared to the correct activation of the appropriate output unit only (in this case, the output unit corresponding to the name *bird*). The difference between the activation produced by the network and the target activation generates an error signal that is backpropagated through the network to the representation units, without changing any of the weights. At each of these units, the error signal (d in the caption to figure 2.3) corresponds to the partial derivative of the error with respect to the activation state of the unit. This signal is then used to make a slight change in the unit's activation to reduce the error at the output.[1] The resulting pattern of activation is then fed forward to the output units, a new error is calculated, and this in turn is backpropagated, resulting in a new value of the partial derivative, which again is used to adjust the unit states. The process is iterated several times, until the error on the relevant output unit stops changing (regardless of how much total error has been removed). The resulting pattern of activity across representation units is taken to correspond to the network's interpretation of the sparrow based on the verbally provided information that it "is a bird," and this pattern is assigned to the sparrow as its internal representation (see appendix A for implementational details).

Note that no weight changes are applied to the network during this process—only unit activation states are adjusted. The network must find a pattern of activity across the representation units that, given the existing weights, comes as near as possible to activating the target unit (corresponding to the name *bird* in this case). In this sense, it uses the knowledge already stored in its weights to find an appropriate representation for the novel item, given the explicit information that it is called a "bird." The backpropagation-to-representation process can be generalized so that the representation reflects several items of information about an object. The basic idea is that the different items of information are presented in interleaved fashion, so that the resulting representation incorporates all of the specified properties. For example, the two propositions *sparrow ISA bird* and *sparrow is small* could be used to assign a representation of a small bird. We would accomplish this by first presenting one proposition and doing one step of the iterative adjustment process, then presenting the other proposition and doing another step. The process would then cycle repeatedly as before, until the error on the output units corresponding to "small" and "bird" stops changing.

Once the representation of a novel item is assigned, how is it stored? In our theory, a single learning episode with the sparrow does produce small changes in the connection weights in the semantic network itself, but these adjustments are too small to support retrieval of the new information after one or even a few presentations. Instead, we assume that the new information, and the ability to reinstate the newly assigned representation, is stored in the connections among neurons in a separate, fast-learning system. This fast-learning system encompasses the hippocampus and related structures, whereas the slower-learning semantic system that is the main focus of our analysis is thought to reside in the temporal neocortices, and in connections from these to other neocortical regions. Bidirectional connections between the neocortex and the hippocampus mediate the communication between these complementary learning systems.

These proposals, and the empirical and thoretical basis for them, were developed in McClelland, McNaughton, and O'Reilly 1995, drawing on related earlier proposals by Marr (1969) and several others (Squire, Cohen, and Nadel 1984; McNaughton and Morris 1987; Rolls 1990; see also Alvarez and Squire 1994). The key ideas motivating this account are as follows. First, the discovery of structure in the environment depends on gradual learning, so that changes in connection weights result from whole ensembles of experiences rather than the single most recent experience. Second, the large changes that would be needed to add new information into the neocortical network quickly would produce "catastrophic interference" (McCloskey and Cohen 1989) with information previously acquired. Hence, memory systems with different computational properties are necessary to satisfy different cognitive demands: for rapid learning of new episodes, a system that minimizes overlap of representations is needed, to avoid interference. By contrast, the extraction of common structure across many different experiences—crucial to the semantic knowledge system —requires the deployment of shared and overlapping representations, but learning in such a system must proceed slowly and gradually.

The complementary learning-systems account accords with a large body of evidence on the effects of damage to the hippocampus and related structures. Of most relevance here, individuals with such damage appear have intact semantic knowledge, but lack the ability to learn new semantic information quickly (Squire 1992). Very gradual acquisition of new semantic information does appear to be possible, even after the most complete hippocampal lesions (Bailey and Squire 2002). By contrast, patients with generalized semantic impairment resulting from atrophy of the temporal neocortex can retain the ability to rapidly store new nonsemantic information, while exhibiting profound deficits in semantic task performance (e.g., Graham and Hodges 1997; Graham et al. 2000).

Inferences Based on New Semantic Information

The internal representations derived from the presentation of information about a novel item can be used to make new inferences about the item. For example, once the network has assigned a representation to the sparrow based on the information that it is a bird, it is possible to ask the network to complete other propositions about the sparrow, such as "sparrow can _____," "sparrow is _____," and "sparrow has _____." This is accomplished by applying the assigned pattern for sparrow to the representation units, activating the appropriate relation unit, and propagating activation forward to the output units. The resulting patterns of activation over the output units then indicate the network's inferences based on the given information.

Rumelhart (1990; Rumelhart and Todd 1993) used essentially the technique we have just described to demonstrate that his network could correctly infer the properties of a sparrow, given the information that it is a bird. Once the representation had been established using the backprop-to-representation process, the network was queried in each of the four relation contexts. Although the network had derived its internal representation solely from the information that the sparrow is a bird, it strongly activated all the properties shared by the two known birds (the robin and the canary): *has wings*, *has feathers*, *can grow*, *can fly*, *ISA animal*, and so on. Properties characteristic of specific known birds (such as *is red* or *can sing*) were partially activated. This generalization arises from the fact that the internal representation assigned to the *sparrow* by the backprop-to-representation process is similar to the previously established representations of the *robin* and *canary*. This similarity led the model to attribute to the *sparrow* the properties shared by the *robin* and *canary*, and to partially activate their idiosyncratic properties (with a larger set of known examples, the activation of idiosyncratic properties would further diminish). Thus, Rumelhart's simple model illustrates the property of similarity-based generalization that provided the basis of semantic inferences in Hinton's 1981 model; the difference is that the semantic representations have been learned in this case.

It is worth noting the differences between inference in these connectionist networks and inference in categorization-based models. In the connectionist models, the inferences flow directly from the pattern of activity assigned to represent an item, based on whatever information has been provided about the item. There is no explicit act of categorization at the time the inference is made, only the instantiation of the assigned pattern across representation units. We think this corresponds to the situation that holds for many of the everyday, natural "inferences" humans beings draw, more or less automatically, in day-to-day behavior. To know intuitively that Socrates will die if he drinks the hemlock, we do not need to explicitly call to mind the fact that Socrates is a man and that all men are mortal—"mortality" is implicit in our representation of Socrates, which is shaped by prior experiences that lead us to assign to him a representation like that assigned to other individual human beings.

A related difference between our approach and categorization-based approaches is that it does not require explicit search of the taxonomic propositional hierarchy to retrieve item-relevant information. Access to general as well as specific information about a concept is provided directly from its internal representation. The knowledge that a canary can move (a general propery of animals), can fly (a property shared with other birds), is yellow (a specific fact about the canary), and so on, is all directly accessible from the canary's internal representation. Thus, the model avoids some of the difficulties of the hierarchical propositional model (Collins and Quillian 1969) outlined in chapter 1, including the incorrect prediction that it should generally take longer to verify general than specific properties.

A further important aspect of our PDP approach to semantic inference is that it does not even require explicit categorization during the initial formation of an item representation. In the example above, taken from Rumelhart and Todd 1993, the new information provided about the sparrow did involve explicit categorization (i.e., the network was "told" directly that the sparrow is a bird). However, backprop to representation can assign representations to items based on any kind of information about the item's properties represented in the output. For instance, to form a representation of an unfamiliar item observed to flap its wings and fly away, one could backpropagate error from the output units corresponding to the properties *fly* and *wings* (with the appropriate context units activated). The network would then seek a representation for the item that, given the knowledge stored in its weights, strongly activates these properties, and the representation so discovered would be similar to other familiar items known to have wings and to fly. In general, backprop to representation from any property characteristic of a set of known items will lead to an item representation similar to that of other items in the set. The verbal category labels that pick out the members of such a set are not special to the model in this regard.

The final point is that even the discovery of the underlying hierarchical domain structure reflected in the similarities among the learned representations does not depend on explicit category labels. We will see in the next chapter that this structure arises from the pattern of covariation of properties of objects, and does not depend on the explicit labeling of the objects with taxonomically organized category labels.

Discussion of the Rumelhart Network

Rumelhart's initial simulation demonstrated that distributed representations are capable of carrying out one of the most fundamental operations accomplished by taxonomically organized categorization theories, namely, the attribution of properties of a set of related items to a novel instance. Obviously, the model's behavior in this respect depends on the state of its weight matrix at any given point during learning. The accumulation of small weight changes in the network as it learns leads its internal representations of objects to evolve in interesting ways, with consequences for the network's ability to perform semantic tasks in various contexts. These consequences extend to the network's performance after training, and to its behavior under damage. In the simulations to come, we will show that the gradual weight changes that occur when the network is exposed to a set of propositions about a subdomain of conceptual knowledge, the resulting progressive differentiation of its internal representations, and the consequent change over time in its generalization and induction behavior, together provide a set of processes that allow us to understand a range of empirical phenomena in conceptual development, adult cognition, expertise, and dementia. Prior to embarking on the discussion of these simulations, however, it will be useful to consider some of the simplifications entailed by our use of Rumelhart's model, and how this model and our general approach relate to other connectionist proposals that have been put forward in the literature.

Simplificiations Involved in the Use of the Rumelhart Network

A notable characteristic of the Rumelhart network is its simplicity; given the richness and complexity of human semantic abilities, it must seem to most readers that something far richer and more complex is required to investigate semantic cognition. We certainly acknowledge that the network, and perhaps more importantly, the experiences on which it is trained, vastly underrepresent the content of human semantic knowledge. If, however, the network can in fact provide a basis for addressing important aspects of human semantic cognition, then its simplicity may turn out to be one of its greatest virtues. Connectionist networks can often seem opaque (McCloskey 1991). The comparatively simple feed-forward architecture of the Rumelhart network, and the small corpus of training experiences that appear in its virtual environment, make it possible to gain a fairly complete understanding of its characteristics and properties. Where these characteristics and properties are useful for addressing certain long-standing puzzles and theoretical issues in the study of human semantic abilities, the model can help to further our understanding of the essential nature of human cognition generally.

With that said, it still seems useful to bring out some of the ways the model is simpler than what we take to be the real mechanism underlying human semantic cognition. Here we consider what we feel are the most important of these simplifications.

First, the model uses localist representations in the input and output layers. We believe that representations throughout the system are in fact distributed, just as are the representations in the hidden layers of the Rumelhart network (and all representations in Hinton 1981). The use of localist input and output units simplifies the analysis and interpretation of the model's behavior, and we believe this design choice does not undermine the particular points we want to make. Nevertheless, it may be useful to inquire to what extent we can consider localist input and output units to provide adequate proxies of distributed representations.

If we conceive of the localist units as corresponding to the spoken words people use in uttering propositions—themselves construed as schematic versions of sentences about objects, relations, and attributes—the use of local representations seems quite reasonable. Since the mapping from (monomorphemic) word forms to semantics is largely unsystematic, the surface similarities in the sounds of words do not directly capture the similarities among internal semantic representations of the objects denoted by the words. The use of localist input units in this case is tantamount to the assumption that these surface similarities are discarded by the system, in favor of a representation in which items are treated as completely different, whether or not their sounds are similar.

However, we do not believe that verbal semantic knowledge is isolated from semantic knowledge acquired through other modalities, and we intend our model to bear on tasks such as object naming where the input is visual, not verbal. Furthermore, and perhaps more important, we also intend the model to shed light on the acquisition of semantic information from nonverbal experience. Along with others we assume that information from different modalities converges in a common semantic representational system, and that both verbal and nonverbal experience influence

the formation of semantic representations. We might instead construe the inputs and outputs in the network as directly encoding
perceptual representations of items, situational contexts, and
observed properties (rather than coding spoken words referring to
these items, contexts, and properties). In this case, the use of
localist units can be viewed as providing a coarse discretization of
the "perceptual" similarity relations among individual items, contexts, and attributes. For example, all roses are treated as identical
in the input, and are equally distinct from all other types of objects
in the world. Similarly all cases of "having leaves" are treated as
identical and completely distinct from any other properties. Indeed, the use of localist units (under this construal) seems to presuppose a kind of binary perceptual categorization that greatly
simplifies the similarity relations among experienced objects. This
is an important issue to which we will return in chapter 4, where
we will explicitly be concerned with the differentiation of conceptual representations in preverbal infants. We will see there that
similar results are obtained using distributed representations for
item inputs that capture similarities and differences among them in
a more realistic way.

One technical drawback of the use of localist inputs relates to
the treatment of novel items. When distributed representations
are used, a novel object can be represented by a novel pattern of
activity across the same set of units used to represent previously
familiar items, and similarity of a novel test input to previously
experienced items can be directly represented in the input. In
adopting local input representations we cannot exploit these properties. Instead we must rely on adding a new input unit to represent an unfamiliar object in the environment. All information
about this new item is then provided in the form of target information across the output units, which can be used to assign a representation to the new item using backprop to representation, as in
the case of the sparrow considered above. Again, this approach
seems like a reasonable approximation for new information presented verbally (as in telling someone "a sparrow is a bird"). For

information presented visually, where visual similarity to known objects is known to be important (Sloutsky 2003) the use of localist inputs for novel test items is again more problematic. However, the backprop-to-representation technique provides a way of assigning representations based on an item's observed visual properties (specifically, the visual properties coded by the output units, such as *has fur*, *is yellow*, and so on). We will see in chapter 4 that similarity to known items introduced in this way works similarly to the use of direct overlap in distributed input representations.

A second simplification of the Rumelhart architecture is that "activation" only propagates in one direction, from inputs toward outputs. Thus, the activation process does not allow information specified across the attribute units to influence the states of the *Representation* and *Hidden* units in this model. Again, this choice is a simplification of the state of affairs we imagine actually holds in the human semantic system, where we would assume as in Hinton's (1981) model that all aspects of a proposition or other experience can influence or be influenced by all other aspects. A recurrent implementation incorporating weights that project back from the *Attribute* layer to the *Hidden* units (and from *Hidden* to *Representation* units) would enable us to model this using propagation of activation per se. Such a model has been used by O'Reilly (1996), and in related work of ours (Rogers et al. forthcoming). However, we have found that it is possible to capture this aspect of semantic processing in the feed-forward model, by using the backprop-to-representation method previously described. Although some properties of recurrent networks cannot be captured without fully recurrent connections, we have found that the capabilities of the feed-forward network are sufficient for our purposes, and that the feed-forward instantiation greatly facilitates analysis and interpretation of the network's behavior, making it an especially useful tool for conveying the key points we wish to emphasize in this monograph. Research in the domain of word reading suggests that recurrent and feed-forward networks that use distributed representations share similar tendencies to generalize, allowing the feed-forward models (which require far less computer time to train) to serve as reasonable proxies for fully recurrent networks in many situations (Plaut et al. 1996).

Third, as previously mentioned, we view the Rumelhart network as a model of only one of two complementary learning systems, as proposed by McClelland, McNaughton, and O'Reilly (1995). This approach assumes that human learning and memory are based on two interacting systems with very different properties. One of these, the hippocampal system, allows the rapid formation of a memory for the content of a specific experience, while the cortical system (approximated by the Rumelhart network) learns very gradually so that it extracts the underlying structure present across ensembles of individual experiences. This structure is latent in the entire ensemble of events and experiences, and it is a tenet of this theory that the brain discovers this structure by a gradual, interleaved learning process.

We expect that performance on some semantic tasks reflects contributions from both the hippocampal and the cortical memory systems. Rather than adding a hippocampal component to our models, we approximate its role by making use of proxies available within the Rumelhart network formulation. For example, consider a situation where subjects are taught that a familiar object has an unfamiliar property (e.g., that a robin has a *queem*). We believe that the ability to rapidly associate a new fact with a familiar object is mediated by the hippocampal system—the hippocampus associates the hidden unit representation corresponding to *robin has* with the representation of the novel property *queem*. In the Rumelhart network, we approximate this by creating a new output unit to represent the novel property, and adjusting the weights received by this unit so that it will be activated by the appropriate inputs. Because the representation of the new property is localist, these weights can be rapidly updated without disrupting the knowledge stored in the rest of the network, approximating one of the important functions of hippocampal learning in the McClelland, McNaughton, and O'Reilly (1995) model. A similar situation arises in the case previously discussed, in which the network is exposed to a new proposition *sparrow ISA bird*. As noted above, backprop to representation is used to assign a representation to the sparrow (approximating, in the feed-forward framework, a process that would occur through the settling process in a fully recurrent implementation). In reality, we assume that the rapid association of this representation with the input corresponding to the sparrow would be mediated by the fast-learning hippocampal component. As a proxy for this process, we store the association between novel input and assigned representation directly in connections between a (new) localist input unit for *sparrow* and the representation layer in the network. Again, the fact that the input units are localist means that this learning does not disrupt the rest of the knowledge stored in the network, approximating the characteristics of hippocamal learning. Note that eventually, according to the complementary learning-systems view, new hippocampal-system dependent knowledge will be integrated into the cortical semantic network. This consolidation process would occur through repeatedly training the cortical network with the newly learned association, interleaved with other, previously familiar propositions, as discussed in McClelland, McNaughton, and O'Reilly 1995.

Finally, it will become clear that the network's behavior depends on the frequency and similarity structure of the patterns on which it is trained. As stated above, we conceive of the information contained in the training patterns as originating in the environment (as sampled by the learner, through activity and exposure to various objects and events). The extent to which the network provides a good model of human performance on semantic tasks, then, depends on the degree to which its training patterns constitute a valid model of the environment. Rather than attempting to justify any particular choice of patterns for the training corpus, we have instead adopted the following strategy. We will first explore the behavior of the model using the database employed by Rumelhart (1990; Rumelhart and Todd 1993). Using these patterns, we will see that the Rumelhart network provides a qualitative match to many of the empirical phenomena listed in tables 1.1 through 1.4. We will investigate how certain aspects of the similarity relations among the training patterns used influence these results, and we will explore the effects of using a somewhat more complex corpus, in which we manipulate the frequency and similarity structure of the patterns used to train the network. These simulations will allow us to determine the range of conditions under which the model exhibits the effects of interest, and to suggest how human performance might vary in domains with different frequency and similarity structure. Rather than fitting data, our focus is first to capture the qualitative patterns in the data, and second, to point out the mechanisms that give rise to these patterns. In subsequent chapters, we will apply the principles that arise from this work to the many challenges facing a theory of semantic cognition, identified in chapter 1.

Relationship to Other Work

As a final matter before we turn to our investigations of semantic cognition, it seems important to situate this work within the large body of related efforts that others have brought to bear on the study of human semantic abilities. In this section we discuss other theoretical efforts that we consider most related, including both connectionist and nonconnectionist approaches.

The idea that the semantic representation of an object should be treated as a pattern of activity across simple representational elements has been adopted, in one form or another, by a very wide range of models, targeting various aspects of semantic cognition. The distributed representations used in connectionist networks bear some relation to the feature vectors employed in many psychological models of categorization and memory (e.g., Rips, Shoben, and Smith 1973; Medin and Shaffer 1978; Shiffrin and Steyvers 1997). There are several differences between the patterns used in connectionist models and those used in these other approaches, however.

First, some nonconnectionist models treat the elements of the vectors as corresponding to explicit, nameable features or properties of objects. These features are sometimes not actually named by the modeler, but are nevertheless construed as directly representing particular object properties. In some cases the features are assumed to be statistically independent, or to correspond to psychologically realistic dimensions of the item inputs. In contrast, our approach makes use of activation vectors whose elements are not understood to represent explicit content. Psychologically meaningful "features" or "dimensions" may be represented in a distributed fashion across many units, with salient or important psychological distinctions leading to robust and widely dispersed differences between patterns of activation. As one simple example (and in spite of early suggestions by Hinton 1986, and Rumelhart 1990 that individual units sometimes correspond to such distinctions), the distinction between plant and animal in these networks is not carried by a single unit but is generally widely distributed and redundantly represented across many units, as can be seen by examining the patterns assigned to plants and animals in figure 3.1.

Second, nonconnectionist models that rely on activation vectors often treat these vectors as being stored directly in memory, whereas in connectionist models, the patterns arise as a result of a process that depends on the values of the connection weights.

Third, nonconnectionist models often compare activation patterns directly, whereas the similarity-based effects in connectionist model arise from the fact that similar patterns produce similar results when processed by a network.

Fourth and finally, a very important difference is that the patterns used in the models we will be describing here arise from a learning process, and change gradually as learning proceeds, so that their similarity relations also change with increasing experience. This allows the connectionist approach to address conceptual development as an experience-driven process. Some alternative frameworks provide methods for adjusting the relative weights of the contributions of particular feature dimensions, thereby addressing knowledge acquisition in development (Nosofsky 1986; Kruschke 1992). In many frameworks, however, feature vector representations and their similarity relations are specified directly by the modeler, and the processes governing developmental change are opaque.

There is nevertheless a fundamental similarity across these different approaches, in that they all rely extensively on similarity between patterns as the basis for categorization, inference, and other types of semantic task performance.

One aspect of PDP networks related to other approaches is the notion that similarity is an inherently continuous variable, a matter of degree. We will see throughout the chapters to come that this idea plays an important role in accounting for various findings. The notion that categorization and category-based inference should similarly be viewed as graded, continuous processes was captured in the influential studies of Rosch (1975) on typicality effects. Rosch also was among the first to ask questions about what made some categories better than others, and to pose an answer to this question in terms of their coherence (Rosch et al. 1976a). Though Rosch eschewed quantitative and computational formulations, we nevertheless see part of the grounding of our effort in her work.

Our approach bears some relation to explicitly Bayesian perspectives on categorization, developed from principles of optimal inference in the face of probabilistic relationships between categories and their properties (Anderson 1990; Heit 1998). Bayesian models have been used to address basic aspects of categorization, and to develop models of induction (if a dog has an omentum, does a duck have one too?) (Heit 2000). Also, Sloutsky (2003) is developing a similarity-based theory of categorization, inference, and generalization of conceptual knowledge in development, supported by a considerable body of relevant experimental findings, that is consistent with the theory we develop here in many ways.

The framework we have described also shares some ideas with an approach explored extensively by Landauer and Dumais (1997), which has been termed *latent semantic analysis* (LSA; see Burgess and Lund 1997 for a similar proposal). In this approach, patterns in an abstract representational space are assigned to words based on their tendency to co-occur with other words, and the similarities among these patterns are used to model performance in various tests of verbal knowledge and comprehension, such as analogies or comprehension tests. LSA uses a one-time computation to assign semantic representations based on a table of word co-occurrences. This differs from the gradual learning in our model, which allows as to address specific aspects of the time-course of development. Yet there are important similarities. Common to both frameworks is the idea that semantic task performance depends on similarity relationships among abstract representations extracted from data.

Within the connectionist or PDP framework, Hinton's early work spawned a number of efforts to apply connectionist models to a wide range of issues in language processing, text comprehension, and analogical reasoning. The relationship between this class of models and schema theory was articulated early on by Rumelhart et al. (1986). Miikkulainen introduced the backprop-to-representation technique and used it effectively within connectionist models of sentence processing and language comprehension (Miikkulainen and Dyer 1987; Miikkulainen 1993, 1996). St. John and McClelland (1990) pursued a related approach to sentence comprehension, which was also applied to the interpretation of multisentence descriptions of typical events by St. John (1992). A model by Rohde (2002) extends the approach to sentences with embedded clauses, and MacDonald and collaborators (e.g., MacDonald, Pearlmutter, and Seidenberg 1994) have shown how a PDP approach addresses the resolution of ambiguities that arise in the interpretation of such sentences. Hummel and Holyoak (1997) and others have addressed analogical reasoning in a model that uses dynamic synchrony to bind distributed representations to their appropriate roles. Whether some explicit representation of structure is necessary to capture all the relevant data in these cases remains an important issue of discussion (Marcus 2001).

Connectionist models with distributed semantic representations have frequently been used to address semantic priming effects (e.g., Becker et al. 1997; McRae, De Sa, and Seidenberg 1997; Plaut 1997; Plaut and Booth 2000) and patterns of semantic impairment after brain damage in a variety of tasks, including reading (Plaut and Shallice 1993a), spelling-sound transformations (Plaut et al. 1996), past-tense formation (Joanisse and Seidenberg 1999), and picture naming (Plaut and Shallice 1993b; Rogers et al. forthcoming). Several distributed models of category-specific semantic deficits have also been developed, beginning with Farah and McClelland 1991. Some of these models have demonstrated that representational similarity structure can have a dramatic impact on naming in different semantic domains for patients with impaired semantic knowledge (e.g., Devlin et al. 1998), and others have related such effects to the correlational structure of the environment (McRae and Cree 2002; Moss et al. 1998; Plaut 1999; Rogers and Plaut 2002).

Finally, many researchers have now investigated the potential of network-based learning algorithms to explain aspects of conceptual development. For example, Schyns (1991) developed a model in which a self-organizing learning algorithm is used to construct distributed internal representations in a two-dimensional cortical "semantic map." Taking these representations as input, the model was then trained with a supervised algorithm to produce the correct name for each item. Schyns (1991) has brought this approach to bear on naming data in conceptual development and expertise, and our account of this data will be similar in many respects to his (though without the topographic organization Schyns proposed). There is now a considerable body of work addressing aspects of conceptual representation and development within the PDP framework, including many studies of infant category learning (Mareschal, French, and Quinn 2000; Quinn and Johnson 1997, 2000) and work on the relationship between conceptual development and object naming (Colunga and Smith 2002).

There have also been many applications of parallel distributed processing or related approaches to other aspects of cognitive development, particularly focusing on issues related to object permanence (Mareschal, French, and Quinn 2000; Mareschal, Plunkett, and Harris 1999; Munakata et al. 1997; Munakata 1997) and causal attribution (Cohen, Chaput, and Cashon 2002) in infancy, as well as naive physical reasoning in children and adults (McClelland 1989; Shultz, Mareschal, and Schmidt 1994). Many of these applications are reviewed in Munakata and McClelland 2003. All of this work reflects a growing appreciation of the tools provided by the PDP framework for understanding how structured representations might emerge from experience, and how the mechanisms that govern knowledge acquisition can explain observed patterns of cognitive change during childhood.

In sum, the approach to semantic cognition suggested by Rumelhart's (1990; Rumelhart and Todd 1993) and Hinton's (1981, 1986) early work, sketched out in the current chapter and developed in the remaining chapters of this book, relates closely to a broad range of ongoing efforts to understand human semantic abilities and other fundamental aspects of human cognition. The sheer breadth of these various endeavors precludes us from giving each the full attention it deserves. Instead, our aim has been to acknowledge some of the influences on our own thinking about semantic cognition, reflected in the many points of contact between our approach and those of others, which will be apparent through the book. Also, we hope this brief overview convinces the reader that our own efforts form a small part of a wide-ranging program of research, targeted at explaining cognitive abilities with reference to neurocognitive principles of information processing inherent in the PDP framework. We now turn to the task of using the specific model we have presented here to illustrate how the principles of parallel distributed processing might address fundamental aspects of the development and disintegration of semantic cognition.

3 Latent Hierarchies in Distributed Representations

Among the phenomena we discussed in chapter 1 are those pertaining to the commonly held notion that concepts stored in memory are organized within a taxonomic hierarchy. Specifically, we reviewed evidence that conceptual knowledge undergoes a progressive differentiation in development, resulting in the gradual elaboration of a conceptual hierarchy, and that this process is reversed in dementia, resulting in a progressive loss of first the finest and later the coarser branching structure of the tree. In this chapter we will consider some properties of the Rumelhart model that can help us understand these phenomena. In particular, we consider why development may begin with very broad conceptual distinctions, progressing to finer and finer ones, and why general semantic information appears more robust to damage in neurodegenerative syndromes. We begin with these issues because they will allow us to investigate some fundamental properties of the model that will be crucial for understanding several different aspects of semantic cognition in later chapters.

To this end, we will describe some preliminary simulations we conducted with the Rumelhart model (figure 2.2). We will first consider how the network's internal representations of objects change as the model is exposed to information about the items in its training environment. To understand how knowledge structured by gradual learning in a connectionist system degrades in the face of neurodegeneration, we then explore the effect of simulated lesions in the network on its representations and its performance in model analogs of semantic tasks. The simulations reported in this chapter are based on the very small training environment used originally by Rumelhart and Todd, and as such they do not allow us to address all aspects of developmental and neuropsychological data. The advantage of this simplicity is that it makes it possible to focus attention on very basic but critical aspects of the model's behavior. Later chapters examine particular experimental findings in more detail, using a somewhat larger set of concepts and properties, which we will introduce at the end of this chapter.

All simulations in the book were carried out using the PDP++ software created by O'Reilly, Dawson, and McClelland (1995), which is documented on the web at http://psych.colorado.edu/ oreilly/PDP++/PDP++.html, and which may be downloaded there free of charge. O'Reilly and Munakata (2000) offer an excellent introduction to the simulator and overview of general theoretical issues pertaining to PDP modeling of cognitive processes. Parameterization details for all simulations throughout our work, and methodological details specific to particular simulations, are summarized in appendix A.

Simulation 3.1: Progressive Differentiation of Concept Representations

The progressive differentiation of semantic representations in the Rumelhart and Todd network was previously considered in a simulation reported in McClelland et al. 1995, and similar phenomena have been described by other investigators interested in differentiation of perceptual and conceptual representations in infancy (Quinn and Johnson 1997; Miikkulainen and Dyer 1991; Schyns 1991). Understanding the precise reasons for such phenomena is an important aim of this chapter, since the forces that give rise to progressive differentiation in the model will play an important role in our explanation of several different aspects of semantic cognition throughout the book. In this section, we replicate the progressive differentiation simulation of McClelland et al. 1995 and examine the process in considerable detail to determine how and why it occurs.

We trained the network shown in figure 2.2 with the same corpus of propositions used by Rumelhart and Todd (1993). These are all the true propositions derivable from the Quillian propositional hierarchy in figure 1.2. A table listing the complete set of items and attributes is presented in appendix B, table AB.2. The weights were initialized to small random values selected from a uniform distribution with a mean of zero and range of -0.9–0.9. With each pattern presentation, a single unit was activated in each of the *Item* and *Relation* layers, and activation was propagated through the network. The discrepancy between the pattern produced and the correct pattern was calculated, and weights were adjusted by a small amount (learning rate $= 0.1$) to reduce the sum-squared error across output units, using the backpropagation algorithm. The network processed each input-relation pair once in each training epoch, but the order of patterns within an epoch was randomized. In this simulation, the simplest version of backpropagation was used: the model was trained without noise, weight decay, or momentum. Weights were updated after each processing trial. To ensure that the model's output responses relied entirely on input from other units in the network, we assigned to all units in the model a fixed, untrainable bias of -2. Thus, in the absence of input, each unit's state would rest at approximately 0.19. We trained the network for 3,500 epochs, at which point each output unit was within 0.1 of its target activation (0 or 1) on every pattern.

To see how internal representations develop in the network, we stopped training at different points during learning and stepped through the eight items, recording the states of the representation units for each.

In figure 3.1 we show the activations of the representation units for each of the eight item inputs at three points in learning. Each pattern of activation at each time point is shown using eight bars, with each bar representing the activation of one of the representation units. Initially, and even after 50 epochs of training as shown, the patterns representing the different items are all very similar, with activations hovering around 0.5. At epoch 100, the patterns corresponding to various animal instances are similar to one another, but are distinct from the plants. At epoch 150, items from

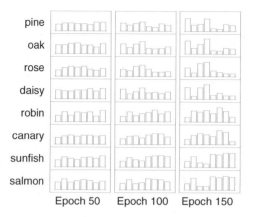

pine
oak
rose
daisy
robin
canary
sunfish
salmon

Epoch 50   Epoch 100   Epoch 150

Figure 3.1   Learned internal representations of eight items at three points during learning, using the network shown in figure 2.2. The height of each vertical bar indicates the degree of activation for one of the eight units in the network's *Representation* layer, in response to the activation of a single *Item* unit in the model's input. Early in learning (50 epochs), the pattern of activation across these units is similar for all eight objects. After 100 epochs of training, the plants are still similar to one another, but are distinct from the animals. By 150 epochs, further differentiation into trees and flowers is evident. Similar results were previously reported in McClelland, McNaughton, and O'Reilly 1995.

the same intermediate cluster, such as *robin* and *canary*, have similar but distinguishable patterns, and are now easily differentiated from their nearest neighbors (e.g., *sunfish* and *salmon*). Thus, each item has a unique representation, but semantic relations are preserved in the similarity structure across representations.

The arrangement and grouping of the representations shown in figure 3.2 reflect the similarity structure among the internal representations, as determined by a hierarchical clustering analysis using Euclidean distance as the measure of similarity between patterns. At 50 epochs the tree is very flat and any similarity structure revealed in the plot is weak and random. By epoch 100 the clustering analysis reveals that the network has differentiated plants from animals: all the plants are grouped under one node, while all the animals are grouped under another. At this point, more fine-grained structure is not yet clear. For example, oak is grouped with

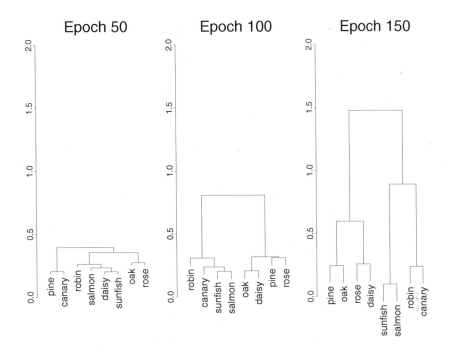

Figure 3.2   Hierarchical cluster plots of the learned internal representations at three points during training. The cluster analysis makes the similarity relations shown in figure 3.1 explicit. The clustering algorithm recursively links a pattern or a previously linked group of patterns to another pattern or previously formed group. The process begins with the pair that is most similar, whose elements are then replaced by the resulting group. These steps are repeated until all items have been joined in a single superordinate group. Similarity is measured by the Euclidean distance metric. The results show that the network is first sensitive to broad semantic distinctions, and only gradually picks up on more specific ones. Similar results have previously been reported by McClelland, McNaughton, and O'Reilly (1995) and Quinn and Johnson (1997).

rose, indicating that these representations are more similar to one another than oak is to pine. By epoch 150, the network has learned the correct similarities, and we can see that the hierarchical relations among concepts made explicit in Quillian's *ISA* hierarchy are fully captured in the similarities among the learned distributed representations.

To better visualize the process of conceptual differentiation that takes place in this model, we performed a multidimensional scaling of the internal representations for all items at 10 equally spaced points during the first 1,500 epochs of training. Specifically, the *Representation*-layer activation vector for each item at each point in time was treated as a vector in an eight-dimensional space. The Euclidean distances between all vectors at all points over development were calculated. Each vector was then assigned a two-dimensional coordinate, such that the pairwise distances in the two-dimensional space were as similar as possible to the distances in the original eight-dimensional space.

The solution is plotted in figure 3.3. The lines trace the trajectory of each item throughout learning in the two-dimensional compression of the representation state space. The labeled end points of the lines denote the internal representations learned after 1,500 epochs of training, at which point the network is able to activate all of the correct output properties for all items above 0.6. The figure shows that the items, which initially are bunched together in the middle of the space, soon divide into two global clusters (plant or animal) based on animacy. Next, the global categories split into smaller intermediate clusters, and finally the individual items are pulled apart.

Discussion of Differentiation Results

Our simulation replicates the previous demonstration (McClelland, McNaughton, and O'Reilly 1995) showing that when a back-propagation network is trained on a set of patterns with a hierarchical similarity structure, it will exhibit a pattern of progres-

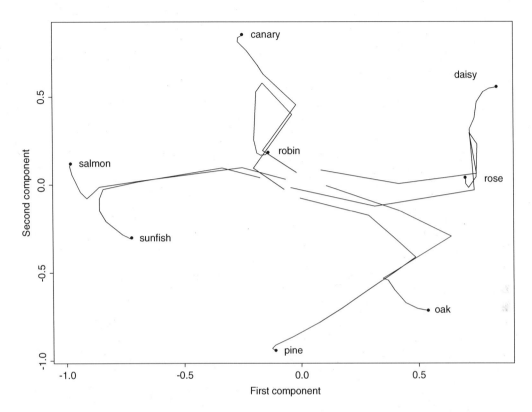

Figure 3.3 Trajectory of learned internal representations during learning. The Euclidean distance matrix for all item representations was calculated at ten different points throughout training. A multidimresional scaling was performed on these data to find corresponding points in a two-dimensional space that preserve, as closely as possible, the pairwise distances among representations across training. Thus, the proximity of two points in the figure approximates the actual Euclidean distance between the network's internal representations of the corresponding objects at a particular point in training. The lines indicate the path traversed by a particular item representation over the course of development.

sive differentiation. Similar demonstrations with other types of training sets have been made by others (e.g., Quinn and Johnson 1997). One interesting aspect of this process is the tendency for the different levels to differentiate in relatively discrete stages, first completing differentiation at the most general level before progressing to successively more fine-grained levels. This tendency to exhibit stagelike learning is a feature of connectionist models that has been considered extensively elsewhere (McClelland 1989; Plunkett and Sinha 1992; McClelland 1994b). Our present task is to try to provide the reader with a mechanistic understanding of the progressive differentiation process, drawing on insights expressed in the publications just cited (see also McClelland and Rumelhart 1988) to explain how stagelike progressive differentiation works in the present case.

With the training set used here, very early in learning, the network comes to represent all the animals as similar to one another, and as quite distinct from the plants. Only later does it come to differentiate the patterns at an intermediate level, and only after that does it learn to differentiate the items from each other at the subordinate level. Why does this occur? To begin to gain an intuitive understanding of this, let us consider how the network learns about the following four objects: the oak, the pine, the daisy, and the salmon. Early in learning, when the weights are small and random, all of these inputs produce a similar meaningless pattern of activity throughout the network. Since oaks and pines share many output properties, this pattern results in a similar error signal for the two items, and the weights leaving the *oak* and *pine* units move in similar directions. Because the salmon shares few properties with the oak and pine, the same initial pattern of output activations produces a different error signal, and the weights leaving the *salmon* input unit move in a different direction. What about the daisy? It shares more properties with the oak and the pine than it does with the salmon or any of the other animals, and so it tends to move in a similar direction as the other plants. Similarly, the rose tends to be pushed in the same direction as all of the other plants, and the other animals tend to be pushed in the same direction as the salmon. As a consequence, on the next pass, the pattern of activity across the representation units will remain similar for all the plants, but will tend to differ between the plants and the animals.

This explanation captures part of what is going on in the early stages of learning in the model, but does not fully explain why there is such a strong tendency to learn the superordinate structure first. Why is it that so little intermediate-level information is acquired until after the superordinate-level information? Put another way, why don't the points in similarity space for different items move in straight lines toward their final locations? Several factors appear to be at work, but one is key:

For items with similar representations, coherent covariation of properties across these items tends to move connections consistently in the same direction, while idiosyncratic variation tends to move weights in opposing directions that cancel each other out.

To see how this happens in the model, let us consider the fact that the animals all share some properties (e.g., they all can move, they all have skin, they are all called animals). Early in training, all the animals have the same representation. When this is so, if the weights going forward from the *Representation* layer "work" to capture these shared properties for one of the animals, they must simultaneously work to capture them for all of the others. Similarly, any weight change that is made to capture the shared properties for one of the items will produce the same benefit in capturing these properties for all of the other items. If the representations of all of the items are the same, then changes applied to the forward-projecting weights for one of the items will affect all of the other items equally, and so the changes made when processing each individual item will tend to accumulate with those made in processing the others. On the other hand, weight changes made to capture a property of an item that is not shared by others with the same representation will tend to be detrimental for the other items, and when these other items are processed the changes will actually be reversed. For example, two of the animals (the canary and robin) can fly but not swim, and the other two (the salmon and sunfish) can swim but not fly. If the four animals all have the same representation, what is right for half of the animals is wrong for the other half, and the weight changes across different patterns will tend to cancel each other out. The consequence is that:

Properties shared by items with similar representations will be learned faster than properties that differentiate such items.

The preceding paragraph considers the effects of coherent covariation in the weights forward from the *Representation* layer in the Rumelhart network. What about the weights from the input units to the *Representation* layer? As previously stated, items with similar outputs will have their representations pushed in the same direction, while items with dissimilar outputs will have their representations pushed in different directions. The question remaining is why the dissimilarity between, say, the fish and the birds does not push the representations apart very much from the very beginning. The answer is somewhat complex, but understanding it is crucial, since it is fundamental to understanding the progressive nature of the differentiation process.

The key to this question lies in understanding that the magnitude of the changes made to the representation weights depends on the extent to which these changes will reduce the error at the output level. The extent to which change in the representation weights will reduce the error at the output in turn depends on whether the forward weights from the *Representation* layer to the output are able to make use of any changes in the activations of the representation units. Their ability to make use of such changes depends on their already being at least partially organized to do so. Put in other words, we can point out a further very important aspect of the way the model learns:

Error backpropagates much more strongly through weights already structured to perform useful forward mappings.

We can illustrate this by observing the error signal propagated back to the representation units for the *canary* item, from three different kinds of output units: those that reliably discriminate plants from animals (such as *can move* and *has roots*), those that reliably discriminate birds from fish (such as *can fly* and *has gills*), and those that differentiate the canary from the robin (such as *is yellow* and *can sing*). In figure 3.4, we show the mean error reaching the *Representation* layer throughout training, across each of these types of output units when the model is given the *canary* as input (middle plot). We graph this alongside measures of the distance between the two bird representations, between the birds and the fish, and between the animals and the plants (bottom plot). We also indicate the activation of the output units for *yellow*, *sing*, *wings*, and *move* throughout training (top plot). We can see that there comes a point at which the network is beginning to differentiate the plants and the animals, and is beginning to activate *move* correctly for all of the animals. At this time the average error information from output properties like *can move* is producing a much stronger signal than the average error information from properties like *has wings* or *can sing*. As a consequence, the information that the canary can move is contributing much more strongly to changing the representation weights than is the information that the canary has wings and can sing. Put differently, the knowledge that the canary can move is more "important" for determining how it should be represented than the information that it has wings and can sing, at this stage of learning. (The error signal for *move* eventually dies out as the correct activation reaches asymptote, since there is no longer any error signal to propagate once the model has learned to produce the correct activation.)

Figure 3.4 also indicates that the rapid learning of coherently covarying properties is not solely a function of the frequency with which the property is experienced in the environment. In this training corpus, the property *is yellow* is true of three objects (the canary, the daisy, and the sunfish), whereas the property *has wings* is true of only two (the robin and the canary). Nevertheless, the

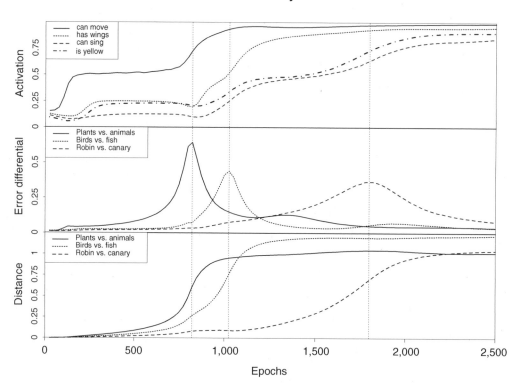

Figure 3.4   *Bottom:* Mean distance between plant and animal, bird and fish, and canary and robin internal representations throughout training. *Middle:* average magnitude of the error signal propagating back from properties that reliably discriminate plants from animals, birds from fish, or the canary from the robin, at different points throughout training when the model is presented with the canary as input. *Top:* Activation of different properties throughout training when the network is probed for information about the canary in different contexts. The properties tested include one shared by animals (*can move*), one shared by birds (*has wings*), one unique to the canary (*can sing*), and one shared by the canary and other nonbirds (*is yellow*).

network learns that the canary has wings more rapidly than it learns that the canary is yellow. The reason is that *has wings* varies coherently with several other properties, and this coherent co-variation drives the model to represent the two birds as similar to one another and as different from the two fish. This structure in turn allows learning about the robin to generalize to the canary (and vice versa), and boosts the rapidity with which properties shared by the two birds are acquired. Comparing *is yellow* with *can sing* (also shown in the figure), we can see that in spite of its greater frequency, the time course of learning *is yellow* mirrors that of *can sing*. Learning about both properties depends on (and contributes to) the differentiation of the canary from the robin. The greater frequency of *is yellow* compared to *can sing* does exert a slight effect, but it only influences the relative degree of activation within a given level of differentiation—not the timing of when the information is mastered.

Properties shared by all items in the model's environment (e.g., *can grow*, *is living*, *ISA living thing*) behave slightly differently than other properties in the training corpus. The network learns to activate these properties most rapidly, but they end up contributing almost nothing to the model's learned internal representations. Both phenomena may be understood with reference to the principles outlined above. Properties common to all objects are learned rapidly because all items have similar internal representations at the outset of training. Learning that one item can grow thus generalizes to all other items, and because there are no items for which this is an incorrect attribution, there are no learning episodes that will "cancel" these weight changes out. The model comes very quickly to activate these properties, even before internal representations have differentiated to any great extent. Despite being rapidly learned, however, common properties exert very little influence on the way representations change with learning. Because the target states for these properties are the same for all items, the error derivatives propagating back from them in early phases of learning will induce the internal representations to change in almost exactly the same direction—they will not serve to differentiate representations at all. The properties can be mastered quickly even without differentiation, and once they have been learned, they generate very little error and will not contribute strongly to any further representational change.

These phenomena suggest that there may be good computational reasons for the semantic system to begin with very similar, undifferentiated internal representations. Specifically, such an initial state would permit very rapid learning about properties common to all things—for example, that they are bounded, they fall if unsupported, they do not vanish and reappear spontaneously, and so on. Certainly infants are known to show signs of such knowledge at very young ages (Spelke et al. 1992; Baillargeon 1995), a finding that has often been taken to indicate that infants are innately imbued with a "naive physics." However, the simulations suggest that even if such knowledge was not innate, it could be acquired very rapidly if infants begin life with very similar and undifferentiated internal representations of all objects.

The Importance of High-Order Covariation

These developmental changes are driven by the model's sensitivity to patterns of high-order covariation among the attributes of items in its environment. The properties to which the model first becomes sensitive, and that organize its nascent conceptual distinctions, are precisely those that consistently vary together across contexts.

To begin to see this, consider figure 3.5, which shows the covariances among all pairs of properties in the training corpus for simulation 3.1 (summarized in appendix B, table AB.2). The properties are ordered according to the magnitude and direction of their mean covariance with other attributes, so that property pairs with strong positive covariances appear in the upper-left and lower-right quadrants, those with strong negative covariances appear in

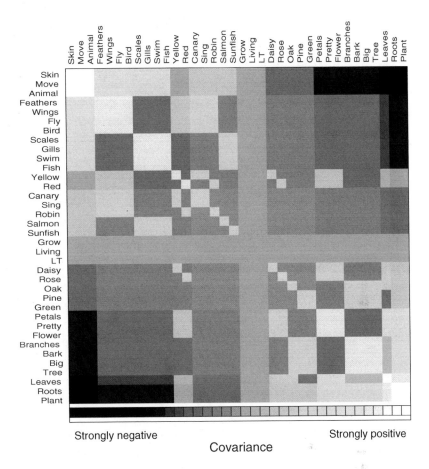

Figure 3.5 Matrix showing the covariances among all pairs of properties in the training corpus. Light colors indicate strong positive covariances; dark colors indicate strong negative covariances. LT refers to living thing.

the lower-left and upper-right quadrants, and those with covariances near zero appear toward the middle of the plot. The strongest covariances observed in the training corpus occur among properties that reliably discriminate broad conceptual domains (e.g., *has skin*, *has roots*). The covariance of properties shared by intermediate groupings of items is moderately strong and positive, whereas the covariance between properties characteristic of different clusters (e.g., between *has wings* and *has gills*) is moderately strong and negative. The weakest covariances are observed among properties common to all items in the training corpus (e.g., *can grow*), and among properties idiodyncratic to one or two items (e.g., *can sing*). From the figure, it is clear that the order in which the network acquires sensitivity to different sets of properties is closely linked to the covariance structure of the items appearing in its training environment. Properties with the strongest covariances are precisely those to which the model first becomes sensitive during training.

While this inspection of the raw covariance matrix is informative, it only provides part of the story. The reason is that the covariance matrix only shows the relationships between individual pairs of properties, but the network's weights are shaped, not solely by *pairs* of properties that reliably covary together, but by *coherent sets* of multiple properties that all covary reliably together. The pairwise covariance of *has skin* and *can move* is certainly one factor that determines their contribution to learning and representation in the network. But more important is the fact that both of these properties also covary strongly and positively with *ISA animal*, moderately strongly and positively with properties that typify birds or fish, and strongly and negatively with characeristic plant properties. The model's stagelike mastery of conceptual structure at different levels, and its tendency to weight object attributes differently at different stages, result from its sensitivity to the complete system of covariation across all sets of properties. Pairs of properties that covary strongly with one another, but that have no systematic relationship with other attributes, will not contribute strongly to the learning and representation that take place in the network.

This is an important point, which we will take up again in considerable detail in later chapters. Here, we would simply like to introduce a second way of looking at the covariance structure of the training corpus in the current simulation, which more transparently reveals higher-order patterns of covariation. Figure 3.6 shows an eigenvector decomposition of the covariance matrix shown above, with the first eight eigenvectors represented.

Mathematically, an *eigenvector* of a matrix is any vector that does not change direction when multiplied by that matrix. For the present purposes it is most useful to understand each eigenvector as a set of weightings for the properties in the model, selected to account as closely as possible for patterns of property covariation shown in figure 3.5. The first eigenvector contains one element for each property in the model, chosen in such a way that the product of any two elements comes as close as possible to the observed covariance of the corresponding two properties in figure 3.5. For example, the element in the first eigenvector that corresponds to *can move* is large and positive, whereas the element that corresponds to *has roots* is large and negative. The product of these numbers is itself large and negative, matching the observed large, negative covariance between the properties *can move* and *has roots* in figure 3.5. In general, properties that, on average, tend to have large covariances with other properties will receive large weightings on this eigenvector. Idiosyncratic properties such as *is yellow* do not covary strongly with any other properties, and contribute little to the covariance matrix itself—hence they receive low weightings in the first eigenvector. Similarly, properties like *can grow* or *is living*, despite being very frequent, do not vary at all and hence do not covary strongly with other properties. Consequently, these properties do not receive strong weightings in the first (or any subsequent) eigenvector. In this sense, the first eigenvector "picks out" properties that account for as much of the property covariation matrix as possible. As figure 3.6 illustrates, these

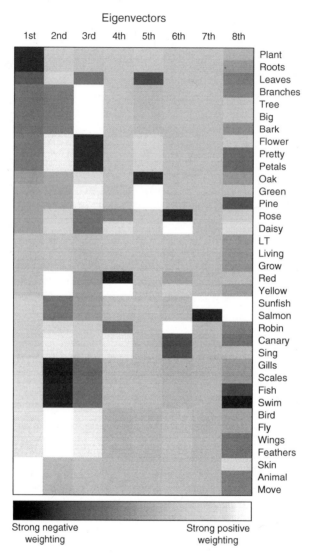

Figure 3.6   Eigenvector decomposition of the covariance matrix for properties in the training corpus. Each vector was normalised to span the same range, and properties were ordered according to their values on the first eigenvector. LT refers to living thing.

tend to be the properties that reliably discriminate plants and animals in the current training corpus.

To derive the second eigenvector, the algorithm calculates the difference between the observed covariances, and those predicted from the first eigenvector alone (a *residual* matrix). The second eigenvector then consists of a set of weightings for each property, such that the product of any two weightings comes as close as possible to the corresponding elements of the residual matrix. Cells in the original covariance matrix that closely match the values predicted from the first eigenvector will yield residual values near zero, and thus will cease contributing to the calculation of further eigenvectors. Cells in the original matrix that were not well predicted from the first eigenvector will yield large positive or negative values in the residual matrix, and so will contribute strongly to the calculation of values for the second eigenvector. Thus, the second eigenvector "explains" covariances that are not well accounted for by the first. When the second vector has been calculated, a new residual matrix is computed, and a third vector is derived from it, and so on.

In figure 3.6, the first eight eigenvectors are shown. Each vector was normalized to span the same range, so that it is easy to compare the relative contributions of different features to each vector. As noted, the first vector weights properties according to the degree to which they discriminate between plant and animal items in the training corpus. The second vector strongly weights properties that discriminate birds from fish, whereas the third picks out properties that differentiate trees from flowers. Notably, attributes characteristic of animals or plants generally do not contribute to these vectors at all. Vector 4 differentiates red from yellow items, which is useful for discriminating between robins and canaries as well as between roses and daisies. Note that these properties, despite being more frequent overall in the training corpus, do not account for as much covariation as less frequent but more coherent properties (such as *has wings*), which are picked out by earlier eigenvectors. Vectors 5–7 weight properties that serve to individuate pairs of items: vector 5 discriminates the pine from the oak;

vector 6 separates both the rose and daisy and the robin and canary; and vector 7 differentiates the salmon from the sunfish. At this point, the residual matrix has effectively been reduced to very small random values, so the eighth vector (and all subsequent vectors) do not contain systematic weightings.

It is clear from figure 3.6 that there is a close correspondence between the eigenvector decomposition of the property covariance matrix, and the model's discovery of representational structure. Features that are strongly weighted by the first eigenvector are those that are first emphasized by the model as it learns. Their values determine on which side of the network's first conceptual boundary each concept will fall. Subsequent vectors, as ordered, match the further discrimination of finer-grained conceptual categories in the network—the properties that receive strong weightings on these vectors determine on which side of further conceptual boundaries a given concept will fall. The reason for this close correspondence is simply that the models' weights are shaped predominantly by patterns of higher-order covariation among sets of attributes in the environment, as discussed above. The eigenvector decomposition provides an explicit representation of these patterns.

The overall situation can be summarized as follows. Initially the network is assigning virtually the same representation to all of the items. At this point, the properties that vary systematically with the network's internal representations are only those that are shared across everything—the *is living*, *can grow*, and *ISA living thing* outputs. All other output properties have their effects on the forward weights almost completely canceled out. However, the plants have several properties that none of the animals have, and vice versa. Weak error signals from these properties begin to accumulate, eventually driving the representations of plants and animals apart. At this point, the shared animal representation can begin to drive the activation of output units that are common to all animals, and the shared plant representation can begin to drive activation of outputs common to all plants. The weights so structured in turn allow these coherently varying properties to exert much stronger influences on the representation units than those exerted by the properties that differ between the birds and the fish. The result is that the individual animal representations stay similar to one another, and are rapidly propelled away from the individual plant representations. Very gradually, however, the weak signals backpropagated from properties that reliably discriminate birds from fish begin to accumulate, and cause the representations of these subgroups to differentiate slightly, thereby providing a basis for exploiting this coherent covariation in the forward weights. This process eventually propagates all the way down to the subordinate level, so that idiosyncratic properties of individual items are eventually mastered by the net. In short, there is a kind of symbiosis of the weights into and out of the representation units, such that both sets are sensitive to successive waves of coherent covariation among output properties. Each wave begins and peaks at a different time, with the peaks occurring at times that depend on the strengths of the corresponding patterns of variation. The timing of different waves of differentiation, and the particular groupings of internal representations that result, are governed by high-order patterns of property covariation in the training environment.

From this analysis, we can see that the network's tendency to differentiate its internal representations in a coarse-to-fine manner does not arise from some general bias toward discovering general or superordinate category structure per se. The network will not be strongly pressured to differentiate superordinate categories that do not have very cohesive structure, even if these are typically considered to form fairly broad superordinate classes (e.g., toys versus tools). Its first conceptual distinctions will always correspond to those that capture the strongest patterns of coherent covariation across all of the items it encounters. The model thus suggests that not all superordinate categories will be discriminated with equal facility early in life—distinctions between items that share coherently covarying sets of properties are mostly likely to be acquired by young infants.

We believe that the dynamics of learning we have reviewed in this section can help us to understand several different aspects of semantic representation in development and in adulthood, and will return to this theme in various places throughout the book. In the next chapter, we will consider in greater detail how the properties of our network might shed light on the differentiation of conceptual representations in infancy. For now we turn our attention to the other basic aspect of the network's performance, namely, its tendency to exhibit a reversal of the progressive differentiation process when subjected to degradation.

Simulation 3.2: Simulating Loss of Differentiation in Dementia

Recall from the introduction that patients with progressive semantic impairments typically show more robust memory for the general names and properties of objects than for their more specific attributes (Warrington 1975). In confrontation naming paradigms, this pattern is reflected in the tendency of patients to give increasingly general naming responses as their semantic impairment worsens. In table 3.1 we show the responses given over several testing sessions by patient J. L. when he was asked to name a variety of bird drawings taken from the Snodgrass and Vanderwart (1980) set. Though J. L., like normal control subjects, initially named many of the birds at a subordinate level, he soon began naming them with the more general label *bird*, and eventually with the still more general label *animal*. The table also shows that J. L. made a number of what are typically called *semantic errors*—that is, errors in which an incorrect name was given rather than the correct name or a valid superordinate response. In earlier sessions, he produced incorrect but closely related names (e.g., *chicken* instead of *rooster*), and in later sessions, he gave more distantly related names (e.g., *horse* instead of *eagle*). However, J. L.'s naming errors almost never crossed superordinate semantic boundaries. Warrington (1975) has suggested that such a pattern reflects the bottom-up

Table 3.1   Naming responses given by J. L. (Hodges, Graham, and Patterson 1995)

ITEM	SEPT 91	MARCH 92	SEPT 92	MARCH 93
bird	+	+	+	animal
chicken	+	+	bird	animal
duck	+	bird	bird	dog
swan	+	bird	bird	animal
eagle	duck	bird	bird	horse
ostrich	swan	bird	cat	animal
peacock	duck	bird	cat	vehicle
penguin	duck	bird	cat	pt of animal
rooster	chicken	chicken	bird	dog

Note: Plus signs indicate correct responses.

deterioration of a taxonomic processing hierarchy. How might the Rumelhart network explain these data?

To simulate the progressive deterioration of semantic knowledge in dementia, we examined how the network's ability to activate the correct output units degrades as these representations progressively deteriorate. We simulated damage in the model as follows. On each damage trial, we added a random value (selected from a Gaussian distribution with a mean of zero and a fixed variance) to each weight projecting from the *Item* to the *Representation* layer, effectively distorting the model's internal representations of individual items. Next we stepped through all the patterns in the network's environment, and recorded the states of its *Representation* and *Attribute* units in response to each input. Then we reloaded the correct, learned set of weights, and started a new damage trial. For each level of damage, we conducted fifty damage trials, and evaluated the network's average performance across these trials.

To administer increasingly severe lesions to the model, we simply raised the variance of the noise added to the weights for a given trial. The main idea was to assess how the model's ability to complete particular propositions degraded as its internal representations were distorted by increasing amounts of noise.

We studied the effects of damage on the model's behavior in an analog of the picture-naming task. In the case of the model, the "picture" was presented to the system by activating the appropriate item input unit. The network's knowledge for naming was probed by activating the *ISA* relation unit in the input. In the trained, unlesioned model, this caused the correct name units to activate in the output. Note that since the input and output units are completely separate, the relation between the input unit for *pine* and the corresponding name output is arbitrary, just as is the relationship between a word and a picture that exemplifies it.

The network's naming response was determined by the strength of activation of the name output units. The healthy, trained network strongly activated three correct names for each item, at increasing levels of inclusiveness. For example, when probed with the input *pine ISA*, the network activated the output units "Pine," "Tree," and "Plant." To assess the network's performance under damage, we examined the activation of the three correct name units for each item under increasing amounts of noise.

Figure 3.7 plots the average (across items and damage trials) activations of the correct name output units at general, intermediate, and specific levels. As the amount of damage increased, activation of the correct name unit fell off most quickly for the most specific names, showing that the network's naming response was most robust for general names, least for specific names, and somewhere in between for intermediate names.

To relate the behavior of the network to picture-naming data, we simply chose as the network's response the most specific name unit active above a threshold of 0.7 (Levelt 1989).[1] If there was no unit active above threshold, the network was considered to have made no response. In the trained, undamaged network, the correct

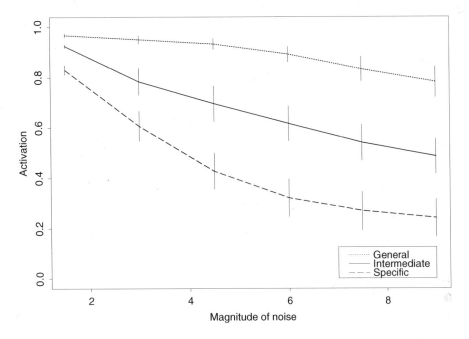

Figure 3.7 Activation of the correct name units under increasing amounts of simulated damage, averaged across all items and trials of damage. Units along the abscissa correspond to the magnitude of the noise added to the net inputs of units in the representation layer.

name units at every level of specificity are strongly activated, and no incorrect units have appreciable activation. The response selection heuristic chooses the most specific of these, so that, in the absence of noise, the network always names each item at the most specific level.

For this analysis, we counted the number of correct responses and the various kinds of errors made by the network across all fifty damage trials. The responses from the model under increasing amounts of damage were examined, and classified in the following way:

1. *Correct response* when the damaged model produced the correct specific name corresponding to the presented item.

2. *Superordinate error* when the damaged model provided a correct but more general response (either at the intermediate or general level).
3. *Semantic error* when the damaged model provided an incorrect response from within the correct superordinate category.
4. *Cross-category error* when the damaged network provided a response from the incorrect superordinate category.
5. *No response* when no name unit was active above threshold.

The network's naming responses under damage are shown in figure 3.8. The graph shows that the likelihood of producing the correct specific name is 100 percent in the undamaged network. As noise is added to the network's internal representations, its performance is compromised: correct responses drop off, and the network begins to make superordinate and semantic errors. Greater amounts of noise have an increasingly deleterious effect, so that by the time the magnitude reaches 6.0, the network produces very few correct responses—most responses are either superordinate, semantic, or no-response errors. The number of seemingly random cross-category errors also increases with damage, though the network makes fewer such responses.

An examination of the superordinate errors made by the network shows that the specific naming responses produced by the intact network gradually give way to more general responses, first at the intermediate level, and later at the general level, as shown in table 3.2.

A more detailed consideration of the network's naming responses reveals a progressive de-differentiation of items as representations degrade. In table 3.3 we show the difference between the activation of the correct name output unit and its closest neighbor at the same level, for the input *rose ISA*. The difference in activation for the *rose* and *daisy* name units begins to shrink at low levels of damage, showing that the network's ability to maintain distinctions between specific concepts erodes quickly. The difference between the *plant* and *animal* name units diminishes at a much slower rate, while the difference between *tree* and *flower* shows an intermediate progression.

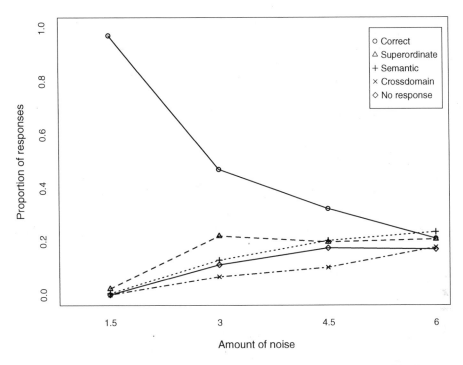

Figure 3.8 Model's naming performance as its internal representations deteriorate. We chose as the network's naming response the name unit with the greatest activity above a threshold of 0.7. When no unit was active above threshold, it was considered to have given no response. The model shows a pattern of deterioration in its naming behavior that is qualitatively similar to that witnessed in semantic dementia (Hodges, Graham, and Patterson 1995). See text for a discussion of how responses were classified.

This fine-to-coarse deterioration of concept knowledge in the network is not limited to naming responses—names are just one among many kinds of attributes that may be attributed to objects. In table 3.4 we show the activation of a general (*can move*), intermediate (*has wings*), and specific (*can sing*) output property for the input *canary* paired with appropriate relations. It is clear that the network's performance degrades gracefully for other types of semantic knowledge as well, replicating the pattern reported for semantic dementia patients by Warrington (1975). The properties common to many items, such as *can move*, are most robust.

Table 3.2 Proportion of the model's total naming responses that were intermediate- or general-level superordinate errors

	LEVEL	
NOISE	*Intermediate*	*General*
1.5	0.07	0.00
3.0	0.16	0.14
4.5	0.15	0.14
6.0	0.09	0.18
7.5	0.09	0.16
9.0	0.07	0.14

Table 3.3 Difference in activation between the correct name response and its closest neighbor

	SPECIFICITY		
NOISE	*Specific*	*Intermediate*	*General*
1.5	0.61	0.81	0.81
3.0	0.19	0.43	0.55
4.5	0.14	0.25	0.40
6.0	0.00	0.15	0.38
7.5	0.02	0.11	0.25
9.0	0.01	0.06	0.06

Table 3.4 Activation of output units for specific and general properties of *canary*

NOISE	can sing	has wings	can move
0.5	0.77	0.92	0.92
1.5	0.61	0.82	0.90
3.0	0.43	0.47	0.63
4.5	0.34	0.37	0.58

Idiosyncratic properties serving to differentiate subordinate items, such as *can sing*, are the first to be lost. Properties common to members of an intermediate-level category (e.g., *has wings*) degrade at an intermediate rate.

Discussion of Progressive Disintegration

To understand why general information is most robust in this simulation, consider the distribution of item representations in the trained, intact model, as shown in the MDS plot in figure 3.9. The shading in this diagram provides an approximate characterization of the way different predicates (such as names) are distributed across regions of the representaion space. For example, the predicate *ISA animal* applies to a large region of space depicted here as the entire upper-left portion of the representational space. The predicate *ISA fish* applies to a smaller region, depicted here as a medium-sized blob on the left-hand side, and the predicate *ISA salmon* applies only to the learned representation of *salmon* itself and a closely neighboring region indicated by the small circle surrounding the location of the *salmon* representation. From this depiction, we can see that the items predicated by *ISA animal* span a larger subspace than those predicated by *ISA fish*.

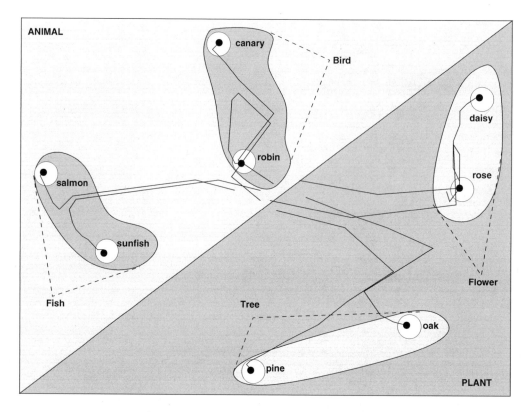

Figure 3.9   Learned distribution of predicates in representation space. The shading is illustrative, and suggests characteristics of the regions of the representation space to which particular predicates may apply. More general names apply to items in a broader region of the space.

The effect of noise in the representation units is to move the items around in this space. This effect must be very large to move an animal item out of the subspace spanned by the predicate *ISA animal*. Consequently, under low levels of damage, the network will continue to produce the response *animal* for such items when probed in the appropriate relation context. However, for the predicate *ISA salmon*, a small amount of noise is likely to move it out of the subspace for which *salmon* is a correct response, and thus the network's ability to correctly activate this specific name deteriorates most rapidly.

In general, we may consider the weights from the *Item* to the *Representation* layer to be sending a signal indicating where in the representation space an item is located. As these weights deteriorate, the signal is degraded. Small amounts of degradation are sufficient to compromise the network's ability to perform correctly when it must discriminate nearby points semantic space, as when naming at a specific level. However, when naming at more general levels, the effect of noise must be considerably stronger in order to drown the signal. Thus, as a consequence of the way that the model has learned to map from its internal representations to particular output properties:

Properties that span a large, contiguous volume of the representation space are more robust to impairment than properties that span narrower and noncontiguous regions of the space.

This account also allows us to understand why the model makes semantic errors. When its internal representations are subjected to noise, it grows increasingly likely that items with neighboring representations will be confused with one another. For example, because *pine* and *oak* are represented similarly in the network, the effect of damage may lead *pine* to fall into the region of representation space to which the name "oak" applies. When this happens, the network makes a semantic error. By contrast, because *pine* and *salmon* receive representations that are very far apart, it is unlikely under small amounts of damage that *pine* will fall into the representation subspace across which the names "salmon," "fish," and "animal" apply. Consequently the model makes comparatively few cross-domain naming errors.

Summary of Basic Simulations

In the simulations described in this chapter, we have seen how progressive general-to-specific differentiation arises from coherent covariation of properties among ensembles of items, how the dynamics of learning influence which properties contribute to learning and representation at different points during development, and how progressive specific-to-general deterioration arises from greater and greater degrees of degradation to acquired semantic representations. We view these phenomena as central to our investigation, and the extreme simplicity of the training corpus adopted from Collins and Quillian (1969) has had the virtue of allowing us to focus on understanding these effects in considerable detail. However, the effects of training on this corpus and of damage to the resulting network only capture the most basic aspects of the developmental and neuropsychological data. There are many additional phenomena that coexist with these aspects of development and dementia, and many further issues that we have not so far addressed, to which we will turn in subsequent chapters.

Extended Training Corpus for Use in Subsequent Simulations

For this effort, the Rumelhart training corpus is a bit too simple to address all of the phenomena of interest. With only two items per intermediate-level category, for example, it is not really possible to investigate typicality effects, since any two items are always equidistant from their average. A more complex corpus is certainly required to investigate effects of typicality, and in general we felt it would be desirable to have a somewhat larger set of items, and a few additional differentiating properties, in the training set. Accordingly, the bulk of the remaining simulations are built around an extended version of the Rumelhart training corpus, and around a correspondingly extended version of the network, illustrated in figure 3.10. In the extended corpus, we added land animals to the birds, fish, flowers, and trees of the original Rumelhart network. There are five different land animals, and four members of each of the four other intermediate-level groups. To allow differentiation of the individual items, and to capture the properties of the land animals, several additional property units were required. These are all indicated in the figure. The full set of attributes associated with each item is provided in appendix B, table AB.3.

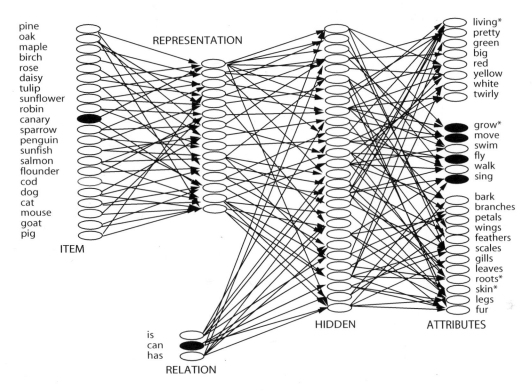

pine
oak
maple
birch
rose
daisy
tulip
sunflower
robin
canary
sparrow
penguin
sunfish
salmon
flounder
cod
dog
cat
mouse
goat
pig

ITEM

REPRESENTATION

HIDDEN

RELATION

is
can
has

ATTRIBUTES

living*
pretty
green
big
red
yellow
white
twirly

grow*
move
swim
fly
walk
sing

bark
branches
petals
wings
feathers
scales
gills
leaves
roots*
skin*
legs
fur

Figure 3.10   Base architecture used for many of the simulations in later chapters. Not shown are output units for names at different levels of generality (e.g., oak, tree, plant) as well as the corresponding context units to probe the network for names at different levels. Such units were included in some but not all of the subsequent simulations. Asterisks by the output units indicate properties not likely available to infants through direct perception, except through verbal statements. However, the particular property labels chosen, as in Collins and Quillian's original work, are only intended to be suggestive of the kinds of facts people know about objects. What is essential to the model's behavior is not the labels chosen, but the pattern of property overlap across items in different contexts. Thus the starred properties in the figure could be replaced with alternative labels to indicate attributes available to infants directly through perception, with no change to the network's behavior. See text for further discussion.

While we have extended the training corpus, the reader will note that we have not gone all the way to producing a fully realistic training environment. First of all, there are many more kinds of things in the world that are not included in this training corpus, and indeed many more examples of each of the kinds that we are actually using. Second, though the properties are in some sense correctly assigned to the items, it is also true that the set of properties is far from complete, and it is not at all clear that the properties included are necessarily the most salient, informative, or likely to be available from the environment. As one example, from Collins and Quillian's original data set we retain the property *has skin*—a feature probably not as salient or readily available from the environment as, say, the missing property *has eyes*. Moreover, other properties in the set are clearly not available to infants until they have begun to master language—for example, the property *is living* is included, even though this is a highly abstract property unlikely to be directly discernible from perceptual input. Many readers may wonder what insights can come from a model based on such inherently incomplete and even somewhat inaccurate training data. Our response to this question is as follows.

As emphasized in the first half of the chapter, the fundamental force that drives learning in our network is not the particular set of properties we have chosen, but the patterns of covariation that occur among the properties used in the model's training environment. To see this, imagine that we relabeled all of the input and output units with completely arbitrary symbols, such as I1–I21 (for the twenty-one different items), R1–R4 (for the four different relation types), and A1–A34 for the thirty-four different attributes. None of this would have the slightest consequence for the process of learning in the network, which depends only on the degree of overlap in the properties shared across the range of items. Thus, we may agree that *has skin* is not really a salient feature of animals, but we might also agree that animals do nevertheless share some other salient attribute (e.g., *has eyes*). The crucial point is that it is not the labels attached to the output units, but the patterns of covariation across output units, that is essential to the model's behavior.

Through conversations with other researchers we have come to understand that the particular property labels the Rumelhart model inherited from Collins and Quillian sometimes pose a barrier to acceptance of the more general framework. The particular attributes that might pose a problem in this respect are those flagged with an asterisk in figure 3.10. In each case, the labels we have employed could be replaced with alternatives that covary with other properties in the same way, but that are more likely to be available through direct experience. For instance, *is living* and *can grow*, common to all items in the training set, could be replaced with the properties *is solid* and *can be touched*—properties that are true of all concrete objects. As already mentioned, *has skin* could be replaced with *has eyes*, and *has roots* could be replaced with the perceptible (but often not stated) property of branching upward and outward from a main stem emerging from the ground.

Neither the original set nor these alternatives are intended as a complete or comprehensive description of the information to which human beings might be exposed. We provide them to help the reader understand that it does not matter whether the output units are construed as corresponding to directly observable properties of objects, propositional statements about objects, or both. What is important to the model's behavior is the propensity for various sets of properties to covary across different items and contexts, regardless of whether the properties are conveyed through spoken statements or through other perceptual information. It is not the identity of the properties themselves, but their patterns of covariation that is essential to the model's behavior.

Because the pattern of covariation is essential to the model, we have chosen to display here a representation of the degree to which different items in the extended training set (from appendix B, table AB.3) tend to share similar sets of properties, across all contexts (figure 3.11). The figure shows that the individual trees all have very similar sets of attributes, as do the flowers, the birds, the fish,

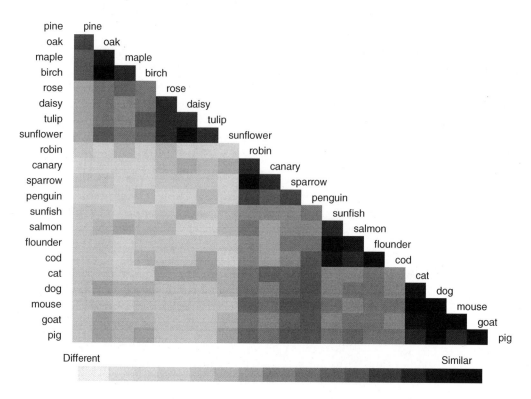

Figure 3.11   Matrix indicating the similarities among the different items in their attribute structures. The shading indicates the degree to which two items have similar attributes, with dark colors signifying items with higher degrees of similarity. The measure of similarity is obtained by concatenating the output patterns for the *is*, *can*, and *has* contexts into a single vector for each item, with 1s for attributes that are present and 0s for attributes that are absent, then computing the normalized dot product among the item representations.

and the land animals; that there is considerable similarity between the trees and the flowers and among the three types of animals; and that there is very little similarity between the various plants on the one hand and the various animals on the other. Furthermore, one can see that two of the items (the pine and the penguin) are fairly atypical, in that the similarity of the pine to the other trees and of the penguin to the other birds is low. It is the structure present in this similarity matrix, rather than the particular sets of item, relation, and attribute labels used, that governs the model's learning and performance. We will have plenty of occasion to refer back to this structure as we proceed, and to consider its interaction with manipulations of frequency of exposure to particular items, sets of items, or types of properties of items.

In the preceding chapter we considered how the Rumelhart model exhibited a progressive differentiation of conceptual knowledge, paralleling the progressive differentiation of conceptual knowledge seen in the predicability trees of Keil 1979, using a training corpus of propositional information modeled on the database employed by Quillian in his taxonomically organized processing model. In the present chapter we will consider how the basic Rumelhart framework might be extended to encompass the early acquisition of semantic knowledge and representations in preverbal infants, and how the principles investigated in chapter 3 might help to explain infants' earliest conceptual abilities. We focus in particular on knowledge acquired over the first year of life, before infants typically learn to speak. Accordingly, the models we will discuss in this chapter are not trained to produce names, or any other explicitly verbal output. The phenomena we will review, and the account of these phenomena suggested by our modeling efforts, are viewed as flowing from nonverbal learning about the properties of objects as they are experienced during the first 12–14 months of life.

The crucial issue we will address is how infants between 7 and 10 months of age sometimes seem to respond to objects on the basis of their nonobvious and abstract conceptual properties, rather than relying solely on their immediately observed perceptual properties. In a series of studies employing several related methods, Mandler and her collaborators (e.g., Mandler and Bauer 1988; Mandler, Bauer, and McDonough 1991; Mandler and McDonough 1993, 1996; Mandler 1997, 2000a) and other investigators (e.g., Pauen 2002b, 2002a) have argued that preverbal children's choices of replicas of objects to touch, to play with, and to use in imitations of actions performed by others, suggest that at the earliest testable ages (about 7 months) infants treat objects that share certain informative but abstract properties (such as self-initiated movement) as similar to one another, even if the objects happen to differ in many other perceptible respects. Moreover, infants at this age seem sensitive predominantly to very general conceptual distinctions among perceptually varying items, and only later come to honor finer distinctions when perceptual and conceptual relations do not happen to coincide (e.g., Mandler and Bauer 1988; Mandler 2002). There is considerable dispute regarding the interpretation of these data—specifically, whether they can be explained solely with reference to perceptual learning mechanisms; whether confounding factors have been adequately controlled; and whether the infant behavior really reveals the first emergence of conceptual knowledge structures. But whichever position one takes on these issues, the data raise two important questions about conceptual development in infancy. First, how do infants come to construe semantically related items as similar to one another when they have few (or perhaps no) directly perceived properties in common? Second, why are coarse-grained conceptual distinctions available before finer-grained distinctions?

Other investigators have offered answers to one or both of these questions. These answers come with somewhat different slants on the empirical evidence, and both the evidence itself and the theories are the subject of considerable current discussion (see for example the commentaries on Mandler 2000a, and the collection of articles in Rakison and Oakes 2003). Here, we would like to raise the possibility that a process not considered by any of these investigators needs to be added to the mix of possible bases for the characteristics of children's early conceptual abilities. Specifically, we will suggest that the learning mechanisms that give rise to infants' earliest concepts are sensitive to coherent covariation among stimulus properties, as investigated in chapter 3. We will also suggest that this sensitivity influences the first conceptual distinctions that emerge in infancy, as well as constraining the particular properties of objects to which infants lend weight in their behavior. Our goal will be first to show that children's initial conceptual distinctions may reflect the effects of this sensitivity, and second, that the importance they assign to particular cues may reflect the fact that these cues vary coherently with others, and *acquire* salience as a result of this coherent covariation. These points will not and cannot refute the possibility that factors raised by other investigators are also at work. However, if we are able to establish that coherent covariation can play a role in shaping children's conceptual distinctions and in determining what cues they are sensitive to, our account suggests that some of the proposals offered by others, heretofore understood to be mutually incompatible, may in fact be reconciled with one another.

A Brief Overview of the Literature

Conceptual development in infancy is a wide and varying field of study that encompasses many different points of view. It is difficult to do justice to the richness of the literature in this regard; however, it will be useful for us to briefly survey some of the stances others have taken on this issue. Accordingly, we will outline four positions regarding the nature of the knowledge that permits older infants to treat items from the same conceptual domain as similar, regardless of whether they share directly perceived properties.

Perceptual Enrichment

One possibility offered by several researchers (e.g., Quinn and Eimas 1997; Quinn and Johnson 1997; Mareschal 2000) is that older infants come to discern conceptual relationships on the basis of learned associations among directly perceived properties of items across different episodes and situations. For example, older infants, on the basis of their encounters with particular dogs, cats, birds, and other animals, have learned to associate the various

perceptual properties that co-occur together in these encounters—
including some properties that may be directly observable in static
photographs and toy replicas (such as eyes, legs, and fur) as well as
some that are not (such as patterns of movement and behavior).
Capitalizing on this stored knowledge, older infants in experiments
like Mandler's make inferences about properties of the stimulus
objects that cannot be directly observed in the experiment, but that
have been directly observed on past occasions. In this view, semantically related items come to be associated with similar sets of
properties, and as children gain experience they can come to exploit conceptual similarity relations on this basis.

Investigators who adopt this perspective emphasize studies of
perceptual categorization in infancy, which have convincingly
demonstrated that by 3–4 months of age infants are sensitive to
visual similarities among discriminably different stimulus items,
and can employ these similarities to direct their expectations in
preferential-looking and dishabituation procedures (e.g., Younger
and Fearing 2000; Behl-Chada 1996; Eimas and Quinn 1994). For
example, when young infants are habituated with a series of cat
photographs, habituation generalizes to novel cat photos, but not to
photographs of dogs (Quinn, Eimas, and Rosenkrantz 1991). A series of related studies has demonstrated that infant behavior in this
respect depends on the visual similarity and variability of the specific items viewed during habituation, and it has been noted that it
is not necessary to assume they reflect any prior knowledge about
the classes to which the stimuli belong (Mareschal, French, and
Quinn 2000). Nevertheless, these studies are viewed as being important for understanding conceptual development, because they
demonstrate that in many cases, the visual similarities apparent
from photographs of real objects can be sufficient to allow the discrimination of semantic categories. The suggestion is that the same
perceptual-learning mechanisms observed in such experiments,
operating over a much longer interval, may be sufficient to explain
the ultimate acquisition of conceptual representations (Quinn and

Eimas 1997, 2000; Quinn 2002) through day-to-day perceptual experience.

Advocates of the perceptual-enrichment view have tended to focus on understanding the perceptual-learning skills of very young infants, and on putting forth the argument that within-experiment perceptual learning could be the basis of successful discrimination of both fairly broad semantic categories (such as mammals versus furniture; see Behl-Chada 1996; Younger and Fearing 2000; Quinn and Johnson 1997) and somewhat narrower categories (such as cats versus dogs, as cited above), based on the perceptual structure of the items encountered during the experiment (Quinn and Eimas 2000). There has been less detailed emphasis on understanding how infant behavior changes with increasing age, and less acceptance of claims by others that performance on various tasks is conceptually rather than perceptually based.

Initial Salience of Particular Perceptual Properties

A related possibility put forward by Rakison and colleagues is that, when infants first appear to demonstrate knowledge of conceptual relationships, they are in fact relying on certain directly observed perceptual properties that are inherently salient (Rakison 2003). For example, 12-month-olds may tend to treat toy replicas of animals as similar to one another, and as different from artifacts, because the animals all share legs where most artifacts do not, and legs are especially salient to infants at this age. Specifically, Rakison proposes that at the end of the first year of life, infants assess similarity based mainly or even exclusively on whether objects share the same large external parts, and whether they are seen to exhibit the same patterns of movement. Subsequent conceptual development arises from a process of association-based enrichment, as children learn the correlations among these salient properties.

The idea that observed patterns of motion might provide the initial impetus for discriminating animate from inanimate objects was proposed in earlier work by Mandler (1988, 1992). The hypothesis also received some support from Bertenthal's (1993) finding that, even at 3 months of age, infants discriminate mechanical from biological patterns of motion. Rakison has extended the notion that movement patterns form the first basis for conceptual distinctions by raising the possibility that children might notice that items with one kind of large external part (legs) tend to move in one way, whereas items with another kind of large external part (wheels) tend to move in a different way. Such correlations among highly salient properties, which Rakison suggests are shared among category members at a fairly superordinate level (animals have legs and move in one way, vehicles have wheels and move in another), would lead to an early emergence of relatively broad category distinctions. Once these sets of salient properties became associated with other properties that are less salient initially, the infant would be able to treat diverse members of a superordinate category the same way, even if none of the highly salient features were actually present in the test stimulus (see Rakison 2003).

Evidence for Rakison's view stems from experiments that follow up on some of Mandler's own work, in which semantic domain (e.g., animal or artifact) is pitted against the external parts possessed by the objects (e.g., whether or not they have legs or wheels). Across a set of such studies, Rakison and colleagues find that 12-month-old infants discriminate wheeled objects from objects with legs, but do not otherwise discriminate animals from artifacts (Rakison and Butterworth 1998b, 1998a; Rakison and Poulin-Dubois 2001; Rakison and Cohen 1999). For example, when confronted with hybrid objects, such as truck bodies with animal legs or cows with wheels, the infants appear to treat artifacts with legs as no different from normal animals, and animals with wheels as no different from wheeled artifacts. The main factor determining their selection of objects to touch or to use for imitation appears to be whether the object has wheels or legs. Thus, Rakison suggests that wheels and legs are among the set of properties that infants find especially salient at 12 months of age. When tested with normal animals and vehicles, infants may appear to be discriminating items on the basis of their semantic relationships, but in fact they are attending only to particular salient properties, according to Rakison (2003).

Rakison also suggests that the inherent salience of external parts and patterns of motion may provide an explanation of why broad semantic distinctions are the first to appear in development. Specifically, the initial salience of certain object properties makes these easier to attend to and learn about than other, less salient properties that happen to differentiate more fine-grained categories. As in the perceptual-enrichment view, infants first discern broad semantic distinctions because they first acquire the associations among properties shared by items in the same semantic domain. However, in Rakison's view, the reason these associations are the first to be learned is that such properties are initially and inherently more salient to infants (Rakison 2003).

The interpretation of Rakison's findings is challenged to some degree by data from other studies suggesting that infants can discriminate animate from inanimate objects, even when they share similar large external parts and are not observed to be moving. For example, Pauen (2002a) found that 11-month-olds reliably discriminate toy animals from toy furniture in an object-examination paradigm, even when the replicas are stylized in such a way that items in both categories have similar-looking "legs," similar textures, and similar salient parts (e.g., the "eyes" on the animals are physically the same as the "knobs" on the furniture, and so on). In fact, infants in this experiment were just as likely to discriminate animals from furniture as was a second group of 11-month-olds who were tested with realistic toy replicas that were perceptually quite different from one another. The results suggest that the conceptual judgments of 11-month-olds are not always influenced by perceptual similarities and differences, and reflect instead an appreciation of what kind of thing the object is.

A key factor contributing to the difference between Rakison's and Pauen's results may be that Pauen did not pit two highly salient and informative cues (such as legs and wheels) against other factors that may be weaker. When faced with some items that have wheels and others that have legs, infants may tend to group items on the basis of these features to the exclusion of other informative similarities and differences. However, Pauen's data demonstrate that 11-month-old infants are nonetheless capable of discriminating animals from artifacts when there are no obvious single features that differentiate the domains—a finding difficult to attribute to the inherent salience of large external moving parts. Thus her findings appear consistent with the two approaches considered below, in which children rely on their emerging conceptual knowledge, at least on some tasks.

Conceptual vs. Perceptual Knowledge

According to the approach taken by Mandler (e.g., Mandler 1990, 1992, 1997, 2000a, 2000b), the competencies exhibited by older preverbal infants reflect a form of knowledge representation qualitatively different from that apparent earlier in life. Specifically, Mandler distinguishes between two forms of knowledge possessed by infants: perceptual and conceptual knowledge. Perceptual knowledge encompasses knowledge about what things look like, and on the basis of the dishabituation studies described above, is available to infants by at least 3 months of age. Conceptual knowledge encompasses knowledge about object kinds: it allows infants (as well as older children and adults) to understand that different objects are of the same kind, regardless of whether they are perceptually similar. In this view, the ability of 7- to 9-month-old infants to treat perceptually disparate items as similar to one another (and perceptually similar items from different domains as distinct) provides the earliest evidence for an influence of conceptual knowledge on behavior. As discussed in the introduction, Mandler's claims have sometimes been controversial because of uncertainties about whether perceptual factors could account for some aspects of her results. The findings of Pauen's recent studies go some way toward addressing these uncertainties, and support the claim that children in the second half of the first year of life show sensitivity to conceptual distinctions in object-manipulation tasks.

According to Mandler, early conceptual representations are built on representational primitives that she calls *image schemas* (Lakoff 1987). Image schemas are structures that capture knowledge about relatively abstract spatiotemporal characteristics of objects and events, such as containment, self-initiated movement, and contingency. Mandler differentiates image schemas from perceptual representations precisely because they capture similarities among inputs that may be superficially quite different. For example, a dog and a bird may move in ways that are perceptually quite distinct, but in both cases the movement is self-initiated. An image schema for self-initiated movement thus permits infants to represent an element of similarity across these perceptually distinct events. Accordingly, initial concepts are built from such primitives, when infants notice and represent relationships among them. For example, the initial concept *animal* might be built from image schemas such as *moves-by-itself*, *moves-irregularly*, *moves-contingently*, *interacts-at-a-distance*, and so on. Infants arrive at the concept *animal* through observing that self-moving objects also happen to be those that behave contingently, show irregular patterns of motion, interact with objects at a distance, and so forth. That is, the initial animal concept results from noticing and representing the relationships amongst these image-schematic primitives. The further ability to discriminate replicas of animals from artifacts, even when these are completely static, similarly arises when infants become sensitive to the fact that things that move by themselves also tend to have limbs on the bottom, faces, and other directly observable properties. On the basis of such knowledge, infants understand that different self-moving, contingently interacting objects are of the same kind, and that such items tend to have certain observable external parts. Subsequently, they no longer need to observe an object in motion, or behaving contingently, to "categorize" it as such.

It is not fully clear to us whether Mandler believes that the set of image schemas children first apply are predetermined by innate characteristics of their perceptual or conceptual systems, or whether she believes that they are discovered through the application of some sort of very general purpose mechanism of acquisition. Relatedly it is not clear how early in life the first image schemas are available to differentiate concepts. Mandler believes that the data from infants under about 7 months cannot shed light on these matters, because the looking tasks with which very young infants are tested only tap perceptual representations, and not conceptual or image-schematic knowledge. Thus it is difficult to know whether young infants possess conceptual knowledge but do not express it in laboratory tasks, or whether this knowledge first emerges at about 7 months.

In any case, Mandler's view is that by 7–9 months children conceptualize all instances of self-initiated movement as effectively the same, and from this knowledge the early distinction between animate and inanimate things falls out. Thus in this view, the competencies displayed by infants at 7–9 months of age reveal the presence of knowledge structures that, though they may or may not be abstracted from perceptual experience, are qualitatively different from perceptual representations in that they allow the infant to ignore irrelevant perceptual variability and to zero in on the more abstract commonalities and differences that reliably discriminate kinds. Items that have different overall shapes, parts, colors, and textures may be treated as similar to one another if they exhibit the same motion characteristics, or if they share other observable properties that have been incorporated into the infant's image schemas. Conversely, items with similar outward appearances may be treated differently if they engage different image schemas. The first image schemas available to infants describe patterns of motion, and hence the first concepts represented discriminate animate from inanimate objects. Further conceptual development, and the progressive differentiation of concept representations, arise from a continuing process that yields new image schemas as well as new knowledge about the relationships among image schemas, although the precise mechanism by which this process occurs is not spelled out.

Emergence of an Initial Domain Theory

A fourth possibility derives from the theory-theory approach to cognition (Carey 1985; Gopnik and Meltzoff 1997; Keil 1989; Gelman and Williams 1998). In this view, different entities are construed as being the same kind of thing when they are understood to share certain "core" properties—that is, nonobservable characteristics that are causal in the sense that they give rise to the item's observable attributes and behaviors. For example, the concept *animal* might include such core properties as agency, rationality, and goal-directedness (e.g., Gergely et al. 1995).

Core properties in the theory-theory tradition serve a function similar to that of Mandler's image schemas—that is, they permit infants (and older children and adults) to conceive as similar items that may differ in many peripheral respects. If the core properties of animacy include agency and goal-directedness, for example, then any items assigned these characteristics will be understood to be the same kind of thing, regardless of how perceptually dissimilar they may be. However, where Mandler stresses that new image schemas and conceptual representations may be discovered by the infant through development, theory-theorists often emphasize that some important core properties cannot be acquired through experience, and must be specified innately (e.g., Carey and Spelke 1994, 1996).

In principle this addresses the question of why certain very broad distinctions are apparent early in life—they are based, in this view, on initially available core properties, rather than on less essential properties that must be learned. However, this stance still raises questions about how young children happen to know that a given object with particular directly observable properties also possesses certain crucial but nonobservable core properties. One answer (Gelman 1990; Carey and Spelke 1994) is that there are initial tendencies to associate certain perceivable properties (e.g., legs) with certain core properties (e.g., agency). Under this position, one can see how the results reported by Rakison might be explained. Specifically, the 12-month-old's judgments would rely on certain directly perceived object properties (legs again), which by virtue of an innate mechanism, have been associated with the relevant core properties (e.g., agency). Learning could then allow the infant to associate the noncore properties of objects (such as their surface features, for example) with their core properties, allowing subsequent judgments to be based on nonobservable properties.

The Essence of Our Argument

The positions we have reviewed offer different answers to what is effectively the same question: On what basis do infants treat different objects as being of the same kind? For Quinn, Johnson, Mareschal, and colleagues, the answer is that conceptually related items come to be associated with similar constellations of attributes on the basis of perceptual learning. For Rakison, conceptually related items share certain inherently salient perceptual properties, including large external parts and patterns of movement. According to Mandler, an understanding of conceptual relations arises from descriptions of objects provided by image schemas, some of which may be innate and some of which are acquired with experience. According to Carey, conceptual relations are determined by nonobservable core causal properties, at least some of which cannot be acquired from perceptual learning and must be innate.

To these ideas we would like to add one further suggestion: perhaps infants treat objects as being of the same kind because they are sensitive to patterns of experienced coherent covariation of properties across objects. This proposal appears to be distinct from the proposals that have been offered by the investigators whose work we have reviewed above. Although many of them discuss the idea that correlational learning plays a role in category formation, none of these accounts really consider anything beyond the role of pairwise correlations.

Many of the arguments offered by proponents of other approaches are explicitly or implicitly sensitive to the concern expressed by some proponents of theory-theory (e.g., Keil 1989; Murphy and Medin 1985; Gelman and Williams 1998; Ahn 1998), that correlation-based learning mechanisms are too underconstrained to provide a basis for concept acquisition. The reason is that there are simply far too many spurious or uninformative pairwise correlations in the world for such correlations to provide a good basis for concept learning (e.g., Ahn et al. 1995). For example, Keil et al. (1998) point out that although virtually all washing machines are white in color, being white is not critical to the concept *washing machine*. By contrast, all polar bears are white, and in this case, "whiteness" seems to be more important to the concept *polar bear*. How do people know that the former pairwise correlation (between whiteness and washing machines) is not particularly important, whereas the latter correlation (between whiteness and polar bears) is?

On the basis of such arguments, investigators who may otherwise have little common ground often agree that infants must begin life with what R. Gelman (Gelman 1990; Gelman and Williams 1998) calls *enabling constraints*—that is, an initial state that constrains which correlations infants will notice and become sensitive to. Thus, for example, Rakison addresses Keil's critique by suggesting that children initially learn about correlations among highly salient properties—effectively giving some correlations a privileged status relative to others. Similarly, Mandler promotes image schemas as providing descriptors that shine through the welter of detail captured directly by perception, and Carey explicitly contends that innate knowledge provides the necessary guidance to bootstrap concept acquisition in the face of an overwhelming amount of irrelevant perceptual information.

What we would like to add to these ideas is the following principle:

Infants' sensitivity to a property, as indexed by attention, ease of learning, and other measures, is affected by the extent of its coherent covariation with other properties.

The simulations reported below are intended to show that this principle holds in our PDP model, and to indicate that many aspects of the developmental findings reviewed above may reflect its role in infants' conceptual development. According to this principle, properties that vary coherently with other properties will be relatively more salient to infants and relatively easier to learn to associate with other properties, compared to properties that vary independently of each other. This does not preclude a role for other contributing factors to concept development, including additional assumptions similar to those that other investigators have offered. We believe that more than one of the alternative positions can be partially correct; indeed, we believe it is likely that all of them have at least some partial validity. This validity stems in part from the fact that the child's perceptual experience reflects, not just the structure present in the world, but the ways this structure is filtered by the child's perceptual system.

Consider, first, the suggestion of Rakison that some kinds of perceptual information may be more salient than others. This idea is a very old one and is almost certain to have some validity. For example, it is clear that the brain has specialized mechanisms for motion detection (e.g., Zeki 1978), and that motion strongly engages attention. The training materials used in our modeling efforts could not be justified without accepting that they presuppose a selection of certain properties for inclusion, and that the basis for inclusion reflects assumptions about the availability and salience of information in the input. That is, the model's behavior depends on the particular training patterns to which it is exposed, and these training patterns incorporate implicit or explicit assumptions about which properties of objects are available or salient in the input, and which are not. It should perhaps be noted that salience can be manipulated explicitly in connectionist networks —for example, by introducing a scalar "salience" parameter that determines the strength with which each property can drive learning in the network. We have refrained from doing this, for the sake of simplicity. One can, however, view the inclusion of some properties and not others in the training set as tantamount to an extreme manipulation of salience, in which all included properties are assigned a uniformly high salience and all those excluded are assigned a null salience value.

Consider, second, the suggestion of Mandler that conceptual knowledge emerges from a process that generates conceptual descriptors, which represent certain stimulus events as similar despite differences in perceptual details. For example, as we have seen, different instances of self-initiated movement, in Mandler's view, come to be treated as conceptually the same, even though they may be quite distinct perceptually: a flounder and a gazelle seem to move in very different ways, but somehow the fact that they are both self-propelled becomes apparent to infants, and provides the basis for forming the concept *animal*. For Mandler, the problem of understanding how infants arrive at this realization is solved by supposing that a process exists (which she calls *perceptual analysis*) that yields up descriptions of the flounder's movement and the gazelle's movement that have something in common. Our analysis, like Mandler's, also depends on the assumption that different kinds of animal movement share some common representational element. We include a unit in the model that corresponds to the attribute *can move*—an attribute shared by all animals and none of the plants. To use such a unit in our simulations is essentially to specify that all forms of animal movement overlap in some perceptually detectable way, thereby providing a basis for seeing them as having something in common. Similar points can be made about all of the attributes in our training set.

It is important to realize, however, that in imbuing the network with these perceptual skills, we have not predisposed it to assign special weight or salience to some attributes rather than others. The network must still discover the category structure inherent in its inputs, and must still determine which of the attributes are "important" for organizing its internal representations. To see this, consider what happens when the network described in the previous chapter is exposed to three different events—a red robin, flying; a white goat, walking; and a red rose, growing. The target representations used in this network "build in" similarities and differences between experiences with these different events. The *move* attribute unit in the model encodes a degree of similarity between the goat's walking and the robin's flying, while the *walk* and *fly* units code a degree of difference between these as well. The *red* unit codes an aspect of similarity between the robin and the rose, which differentiate both from the goat. All of these elements of similarity and difference are coded in target patterns provided for the model's attribute units. However, feedback from the environment does not indicate which of them the model should use to "group together" the different items in its internal conceptual representations. In fact, on the basis of their movement patterns and colors, there is no perceptual basis provided by the environment for determining which two items are of the same "kind" in this example. What this will depend on, instead, is the fact that moving covaries coherently with other properties, whereas being red does not—thus the learning process will assign a greater salience to movement.

At issue is the young infant's (and the model's) capacity to "choose" which of the many different kinds of detectable similarities and differences among stimulus objects should be used to determine which items are of the same kind. While the model "builds in" an initial ability to detect various elements of similarity and difference between experiences (and could be further augmented to reflect differential salience, as previously noted), there is nothing in the initial state as we have specified it for these simulations that inherently lends more weight or importance to (for example) the *move* attribute relative to others. Hence the model has no greater "built-in" basis to represent as similar two items that share the capacity to move than two items that share the attribute *is red*. The competencies exhibited by infants at 9 months of age in the studies described above—their ability to zero in on such properties as self-initiated movement, or movement-enabling parts, and to employ these as the basis for representing objects as similar to one another—thus are not given to the network in its initial state. As we will see, however, such competencies emerge in the network as a consequence of its sensitivity to coherent covariation, as explored in the previous chapter.

Prior to moving on to the simulations, there remains, in our view, a fundamental unresolved question: To what extent do our assumptions about the structure that drives early conceptual differentiation amount to building in domain-specific knowledge? This is where we anticipate that the opinions of other investigators will differ, with Carey, Spelke, and some of the other theory-theorists lining up behind the view that it does, and with Quinn, Rakison, and others whose perspectives we have considered perhaps leaning toward the view that it does not. We would like to adopt an intermediate position on this point. We accept that children's perceptual processing systems can act as "filters" that influence the degree to which distinct events will be perceived as similar or different. At the same time, we see less reason to believe that different perceptual filtering systems are brought to bear on different "kinds" of things. To be sure, different "kinds" of things draw on different types of information (e.g., some objects move, while others have more distinctive shapes), and different types of information may be filtered in different ways from birth. We do not deny that such filtering can influence the knowledge infants acquire about different kinds of things. But it may not be necessary to assume that perceptual filtering systems are wired up in advance to apply different filters to the very same type of information, depending only on knowledge of what "kind" of object or event is being processed by the filter.

We would add as a further and separate point that we do not view perceptual filtering systems as necessarily immutable; rather we tend to view them as being shaped by experience. We will see in this and later chapters that the representations formed inside the model do in fact "filter" the inputs they receive in an experience-dependent way, and that such experience-dependent filtering can vary for different kinds of things. Such kind-specific filtering could also arise in perceptual processes, if these processes were mutable by experience. We have used a fixed encoding of the inputs and learning targets of our network, in effect treating them as immutable products of fixed perceptual filtering systems. This choice does not reflect our views about the nature of perceptual processing, but it is useful for simplicity.

Simulating Preverbal Conceptual Development in the Rumelhart Model

With the above background in place, we are ready to turn to the specific details of our use of the Rumelhart model as a vehicle for illustrating the key points of our argument. To launch our discussion of these issues, consider the following abstract formulation of the Rumelhart-model architecture. Here we envision that the two parts of the input represent a perceived object (perhaps foregrounded for some reason, to be the focus of attention) and a context provided by other information available together with the perceived object. Perhaps the situation is analogous to one in which a young child is looking at a robin on a branch of a tree, and, as a cat approaches, sees it suddenly fly away. The object and the situation together provide a context in which it would be possible for an experienced observer to anticipate that the robin will fly away, and the observation that it does would provide input allowing a less experienced observer to develop such an anticipation. Conceptually speaking, this is how we see learning occurring in preverbal conceptual development. An object and a situation or context afford the basis for implicit predictions (which may initially be null or weak), and observed events then provide the basis for adjusting the connection weights underlying these predictions, allowing the experience to drive change in both underlying representations and predictions of observable outcomes.

With this scenario in front of us, we can consider the wide range of different contexts in which the child might encounter an object. Some such contexts will be ones in which the child is watching the object and observing what others might do with it (pick it up, eat it, use it to sweep the floor, and so on); another context (as in the example above) might be one in which the child is simply observing the object itself, watching the things it does in various situations. Several contexts will be ones in which someone engages the child in language-related interactions concerning the object. Some such encounters may involve naming, as when an adult points to an object and says to a child "Look, Sally, it's a bunny rabbit." Others may include indicating for the child the various parts of the object ("OK, Sally, let's pat the bunny's tail. Can you see the tail? Here it is!"). Each encounter with a particular object in a given context will give rise to certain observed consequences, and we suggest that the child learns to assign a conceptual representation to each object based on the consequences observed in different situations. The contexts or situations include linguistic ones as well as non-linguistic situations in which the child observes the object either alone or in interaction with other objects. We suggest that conceptual development arises from the learning that occurs across many such situations.[1]

We can now consider how our modeling framework allows us to capture aspects of this learning process, and in particular how useful conceptual representations can be acquired on the basis of such learning. The presentation of the "object" corresponds to the activation of the appropriate pattern of activity over the input units in the Rumelhart model; the context can be represented via the activation of an appropriate pattern over the context units; the child's expectations about the outcome of the event may be equated with the model's outputs; and the presentation of the actual observed outcome is analogous to the presentation of the target for the output units in the network.

In this view, the environment provides the input that characterizes a situation as well as the information about the outcome that then drives the process of learning. In the example above, the item input corresponds to the visual appearance of the object, and the context input provides the additional source of information that constrains the child's predictions about what will happen next, which take the form of a pattern of activation across the output units. The weights and representations that mediate between the inputs and the outputs constitute the state of knowledge that allows the system to anticipate the outcome of the event, by activating the units that correspond to the predicted conclusion, but the environment contributes again by providing the actual observed event outcome, yielding information the system can use to determine whether its predictions were accurate or not. This outcome information will consist sometimes of verbal, sometimes of nonverbal information, and in general is construed as information filtered through perceptual systems, no different in any essential way from the information that drives the *Item* and *Context* units in the network. What this means is that this information is provided by nonconceptual (perceptual, motor feedback, and so on) systems and serves as input that drives the learning that results in the formation of conceptual representations. It will of course be obvious that this is a drastic simplification of perceptual, motoric, attentional, and other processes, but we believe the resulting model is useful in that it brings out some aspects of the processes that may underlie conceptual development.

We can also see that there is a natural analog in the model for the distinction drawn between the perceptual information available from an item in a given situation, and the conceptual representations derived from this information. Specifically, the model's input, context, and targets code the "perceptual" information available from the environment in a given episode, and the intermediating units in the *Representation* and *Hidden* layers correspond to the "conceptual" representations that allow the semantic system to accurately perform semantic tasks.

The Choice of Input and Target Representations

As should be evident from the preceding discussion, several issues arise as we contemplate this application of the model, especially with regard to determining an acceptable choice of input and target representations. Let us begin with the item input, becuase it is perhaps the most apparent case. Consider the use of localist input representations in the simulations discussed previously, in which one unit is used to represent each type of object that might be encountered. A network trained on our expanded corpus might include a separate input unit for *pine*, another for *oak*, another for *daisy*, another for *canary*, another for *robin*, and so on. This choice treats all cases of (say) pine trees as identical, while treating all cases of any other kind of tree, or flower, or anything else at all as completely different. It seems to presuppose a prior categorization of inputs at a certain specific granularity. No distinctions at all can be made at a finer grain, no similarities are represented among distinct objects that yet might have much in common perceptually, and no differences in degrees of similarity are made directly available in the coding of inputs to the perceptual system.

What difference does this choice of input representation make? Obviously, it prevents differentiation beyond a certain level; the network can never learn to respond differently to things that are represented identically in the input. It may be useful, however, to see that it is primarily the targets, rather than the inputs themselves, that govern the differentiation of the conceptual representations used in the model. One simulation exploring this issue is presented in appendix C. The simulation made use of the database introduced at the end of chapter 3. It contrasts the performance of a standard version of the model with localist input units for each for the types of objects listed in figure 3.10 with a comparison version in which the unit for one of the different types of inputs (*cat*) was replaced by a bank of five units, intended to represent each of five specific cats. The training was the same in both models, and each specific cat in the comparison model had the same set of properties as the single cat in the standard model. The only difference was that training patterns for each specific cat in the comparison model occurred one-fifth as often as training patterns for the generic cat in the standard model, so that in both simulations, the total number of training patterns involving cats and their properties was the same. The results from the comparison model were indistinguishable from those from the standard: the network assigned the same representation to each of the specific cats in the comparison model, and produced the same similarity structure overall in both cases. In the same simulation we also found that the network was able to learn a fine-grain differentiation when it was present, and this was illustrated in the comparison model by including a set of five individual *dog* units to replace the single generic dog from the standard simulation. In this case the dogs differed slightly in their target properties. As we might expect based on the results in chapter 3, all of the dogs were treated identically for quite some time in the simulation, but late in training some differentiation did occur, consistent with the findings on progressive differentiation presented in chapter 3.

These simulation results underscore an important basic point about the model, which is that the conceptual representations of different inputs are treated the same at first, even though with localist input representations, the "perceptual" inputs are completely nonoverlapping. *All conceptual representations start out the same in the model, even though perceptual inputs are distinct, and differentiation only occurs insofar as items are differentiated by having distinct output properties.* This follows from the fact that when the model is initialized, we use small random values for the connection weights. Since the weights could be initialized differently—for example, we could use weights that assigned distinct idiosyncratic representations to each item initially—this can be viewed as one of the assumptions we have built into the model about the starting place of conceptual development: all things are represented as the same until we encounter reasons to treat them as different.

We will explore the effects of choices of the item input representations a bit further in the main simulations of this chapter, which are directed toward modeling conceptual differentiation like that obtained in Mandler's experiments. For now, let us turn our attention to the policies we have adopted in assigning the same output units to represent related attributes of particular objects.

For the sake of concreteness, consider some of the units representing what various objects can do—move, swim, fly, and walk—and some of the parts that various objects have—roots, leaves, legs, and fur. When the inputs to the network are treated as words (constitutents of propositions), then it is natural to think that the unit for *move* should be the same unit whether the proposition involves birds, fish, or mammals; it is the same word, after all ("move") that is occurring in each of these propositions. Another way of saying this is simply to point out that the propositions "a salmon can move," "a canary can move," and "a cat can move" are ipso facto propositions that predicate the very same property (ability to move) to all three kinds of animals. Thus if we think of cases in which the information driving learning is propositional in nature, it seems natural to treat different cases of movement as the same.

But if the attribute units in the network are to be treated as perceptual inputs arising from observation of behaviors of objects, then the critical issues raised above become apparent. Treating different kinds of movement as the same in the model (with respect to a particular attribute unit) effectively solves the problem of seeing an underlying similarity of the different specific movements observed in different cases. Similarly, if the teaching inputs to the network are to be treated as representations of parts of objects, then treating different kinds of appendages as the same (e.g., legs) is to solve the problem of perceiving different examples of legs (the legs of a robin and the legs of a dog, for instance) as similar to one another. While it seems relatively unproblematic to treat the predicates "can move" and "has legs" as the same wherever they occur in sentences, it is far less clear that all the things we call "legs" are initially perceivable as similar by young children, and therefore provide the basis for extracting common structure between, say, birds and dogs. This issue is an important one for the model in that its differentiation behavior does depend on the degree to which the teaching input treats the attributes of different objects as the same or different. As previously noted, some protagonists of nativist points of view might assert that it is precisely the ability to detect such similarities that confers on a learning system an innate preparation to acquire just the kinds of things we want to see it acquire. We have no quarrel with this argument, but we remind the reader that nothing in the network's initial state predisposes it to lend special weight to some properties over others in forming its internal representations. Though the model is imbued in its architecture with the ability to detect various aspects of similarity and difference among the items in its environment, all properties are initially given equal weight or salience in the following simulations. Any tendency to emphasize some properties over others after training emerges from knowledge acquired through learning, predicated on these "built-in" perceptual abilities.

Simulation 4.1: Capturing Conceptual Differentiation in Infancy

To investigate how the earliest conceptual abilities might emerge and develop in infancy, we conducted simulations with two versions of the Rumelhart model. These simulations were designed to illustrate how the model comes to represent semantically related items as similar on the basis of coherently covarying target properties, even if these are few in number, and even if the items differ in many other respects. Specifically, we will see that:

1. The model "groups together" items that share the same coherently covarying target properties, even when they differ in many other

properties, and when there are no shared "coherent" properties in the input.

2. The model is first sensitive to broad semantic distinctions, and only later to more subtle distinctions.

3. The model learns to assign greater weight in its representations to coherent properties; it comes to treat items that differ on a coherent property as more distinct than items that differ on other, noncoherent properties.

4. The same effects are observed whether inputs are presented as nonoverlapping localist representations, or as distributed representations that capture "perceptual" but not "conceptual" similarity structure.

5. The same effects are observed both for familiar items from the training corpus and for novel test items that do not appear in the training corpus.

After establishing these phenomena in the model, we will consider how they can help to explain data from particular infant experiments.

The first version of the model employs localist input representations and the expanded training corpus, as shown in figure 3.10 and appendix B, table AB.3. The second uses the same items and attributes, but employs distributed input representations intended to capture differences between items that are available from static perceptual inputs. We construe both input and target properties not as verbal, propositional information but as observable properties of objects in the environment. Additionally, because these simulations are meant to address preverbal conceptual learning, the models were not trained to name objects in either simulation —they were exposed to only the *is*, *can*, and *has* information. Though we believe that experience with spoken language may play some role in concept acquisition prior to the infant's ability to produce speech, it will be useful to see that the progressive differentiation of representations in the model does not depend on its being trained to name the objects or to explicitly categorize them according to their position in the taxonomic hierarchy.

We emphasize that the particular attributes that are included in the training corpus were not chosen with the goal of addressing infancy findings per se. Rather, this expanded version is used throughout the rest of the book as a basis on which to explore a wide range of different issues. Accepting that the particular perceptual properties to which infants are sensitive may not be precisely those that are expressed by the labeled attributes in the model, recall that it is the pattern of property covariation across items in the training corpus that determines the model's behavior. The units in the network could be relabeled to better express the particular kinds of perceptual information to which real infants are actually exposed (as mentioned in chapter 3), but of course this would not influence the behavior of the model. Addition or deletion of properties, alterations of the assignments of particular properties to particular objects, and manipulations of salience could alter the results, but only to the extent that these alterations influence the particular pattern of coherent covariation of properties that gives rise to the item similarity structure seen in figure 3.11. Furthermore, it may be worth noting that properties that are the same for all concepts (e.g., *can grow*) are very easy to learn and do not contribute to the conceptual differentiation process as dicussed in chapter 3.

Model Versions Using Localist vs. Distributed Input Representations

Localist Version   The localist version of the model employs the model architecture and training corpus described at the end of the last chapter, with all of the naming patterns omitted. The complete list of items, contexts, and attributes can be found in appendix B. The similarity structure, as shown in figure 3.11, has the property that there is a two-level hierarchical structure embedded in it. That is, all of the plants (four flowers and four trees) are very different from all of the animals (four fish, four birds, and five land animals). All the plants are more similar to each other than they are to any of the animals, and all the animals are more similar to each other than they are to any of the plants. However, within the plants, the various trees are more similar to each other than they are to any of the flowers, and vice versa. Correspondingly within the animals, the fish, birds, and land animals are all more similar to each other than they are to either of the other kinds of animals. This structure is apparent across the complete set of attributes observed in all three contexts (*is*, *can*, and *has*), but it is not exactly replicated in each context independently. For example, trees are not differentiated from flowers in the *can* context, since all trees and flowers have only one *can* property (*grow*). Similarly, *is* properties are more arbitrarily assigned to all the various items, and do not capture the conceptual relationships among the different items to any great extent. The similarities illustrated in figure 3.11 are only apparent taking into consideration all attributes across all of the contexts.

Distributed Version The distributed version of the model uses the same corpus of training items and a similar model architecture. However, in place of the twenty-one *Item* units employed in the localist version (with one unit standing for each item), we instead construe the input units as representing the subset of each object's attributes that are apparent from its visual appearance—for example, features such as *red*, *big*, and *legs*. A particular item is presented to the model by instantiating a pattern of activation across this set of "perceptual" input units. The model might be shown a picture of a robin, for instance, by activating input units corresponding to *red*, *legs*, and *wings*. Each item in the training corpus is represented with a different pattern of activity across input features, rather than by the activation of a single input unit. The extent of feature overlap in these input representations provides a model analog of "visual" similarity in the input. These input patterns still give rise to patterns of activity across the *Representation* and *Hidden* units via learned connection weights, so that these still correspond to internal "conceptual" representations as in the localist version.

In generating "visual" input patterns for the twenty-one items in the distributed-inputs version, one is immediately faced with the question of which attributes to include in the input. We have argued that, in principle, all of the properties included in the training corpus are potentially observable, at least in certain circumstances—for example, the property *can move* can be considered "perceptual" information available from the input whenever one is directly observing a moving object. In other situations, this information is not available directly from perception, but must be inferred—for example, when one observes a stationary cat. Should the property be coded, then, in the input, the output, or both? In fact, we do not think there is a categorical distinction between properties that are available as the basis for making predictions, and those that should be predicted. In recurrent networks, where a given unit can be at once both an input and an output unit, all attributes can serve both as inputs and as targets, and as stated in chapter 2, we believe that the "real" system is just such a recurrent network (Rogers et al. forthcoming). For simplicity we have stayed with the feed-forward architecture, however, so we must adopt a specific policy on the allocation of attributes to input and output.

The policy chosen reflects our primary aim in the current simulation, which is to investigate how the model comes to represent semantically related items as similar, even when they have few or no directly perceived properties in common in the test situation. To this end, we employed as "perceptual" input attributes seven of the eight *is* properties from the training corpus—excluding *living*, but including *big*, *pretty*, *green*, *red*, *yellow*, *white*, and *twirly*—as well as a subset of the *has* properties: specifically, *wings*, *legs*, *gills*, *petals*, and *branches*. Note that these properties are also included as output attributes, along with *is living*, the remaining *has* properties, and the *can* properties for all twenty-one instances.

This choice accomplished three ends. First, the set of attributes chosen were intended to correspond at least approximately to those that might be directly observable in almost any encounter with the item or a picture of it, and thus could provide a simple analog to the visible properties of real-world objects that are likely to be seen regardless of the task or situation. We do not intend to suggest by this that the specific attributes we have chosen correspond to the actual visual attributes of real objects. We simply note that, of the complete set of perceptual properties that one could potentially observe in an object, a relatively small subset are likely to be frequently visible (for example, outside parts and colors), whereas others are likely to be perceived only in certain limited circumstances (for instance, inside parts or particular behaviors). In the present context, the complete range of potentially observable attributes is coded in the model's output attributes, and the subset of attributes that are treated as observable in all contexts and situations are coded in the distributed input.

Second, to the extent that the set of attributes used are the ones available in a picture or a scale replica of the object, they provide patterns that can be used as inputs in simulation analogs of experimental tests performed on children, which commonly use pictures or scale replicas as stimuli.

Third, and of central importance for the key points we wish to make, the "perceptual" similarities expressed by this subset of attributes do not specify any superordinate similarity structure above the intermediate category level. As shown in figure 4.1, items from the same intermediate categories (birds, fish, mammals, flowers, and trees) are "perceptually" similar to one another, but no superordinate similarity between the trees and flowers, or between the birds, fish, and mammals, is available in this subset of properties. Thus the "perceptual" similarities captured by our choice of input patterns provide no impetus for the distributed-inputs simulation to develop a superordinate distinction between plants on the one hand and animals on the other. Yet as we will see, the model does still learn to differentiate the inputs on this basis, since the superordinate structure is still present in the set of target attributes.

Simulation Details Both networks were trained much as described in chapter 3, with each pattern appearing once in every training

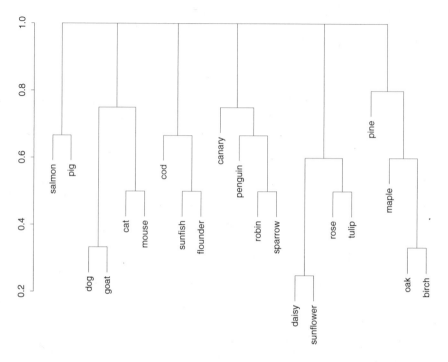

Figure 4.1   Hierarchical cluster plot of the similarities expressed by the overlap of input features used in the distributed-inputs implementation.

epoch, without momentum or weight decay, and with output units assigned a fixed, untrainable bias weight of −2. However, in this and subsequent simulations throughout the book, we adopted the following slight changes to the training procedure, as detailed in appendix A. First, a small amount of noise selected from a Gaussian distribution with a mean of zero and a variance of 0.05 was injected into the inputs of all the hidden units throughout training. As has been argued elsewhere, we take noisy activation to be an intrinsic property of neural processing that promotes robustness, generalization, and graceful degradation (McClelland 1993). Second, the model was trained with a learning rate of 0.01 instead of 0.1; with the larger training corpus and the noisy hidden units, a larger learning rate occasionally prevented the model from completely mastering the training corpus. Third, weights were updated after every ten pattern presentations (rather than at the end of each epoch). This approximates patternwise updating, which we take to be what happens in the brain, while being computationally more efficient. The order in which patterns were presented to the network was determined randomly in each epoch, as previously. Finally, because the model's internal representations in the early epochs of training can be influenced by the particular configuration of random weights with which it is initialized, the results we describe here are averaged across five network runs trained with different random starting weights.

Differentiation of Representations for Familiar Items

To see how the two models' internal "conceptual" representations for the familiar items in the training corpus change over development, we stopped training after every 125 epochs in both versions, and stepped through all 21 items, recording the patterns of activation across *Representation* units. Figure 4.2 shows hierarchical cluster plots of the distances among representations at three different points during learning, averaged across the five training runs. The top row shows results for the localist version, and the bottom row shows the distributed version. In both cases, items differentiated in a coarse-to-fine manner, despite our withholding the name patterns during training. For many items, when names are excluded, no single feature is sufficient to determine specific category membership; nevertheless, the network was able to learn the correct similarities. Thus the simulations establish that explicit training with names is not essential to the discovery of the hierarchical domain structure in either version. The reason is that the hierarchical domain structure is present in the pattern of covariation of target attributes, across contexts. This accords with our belief that concept names are largely reflections, rather than the main determinants, of the organization of conceptual representations.

Localist inputs

Epoch 625

Epoch 2,125

Epoch 4,250

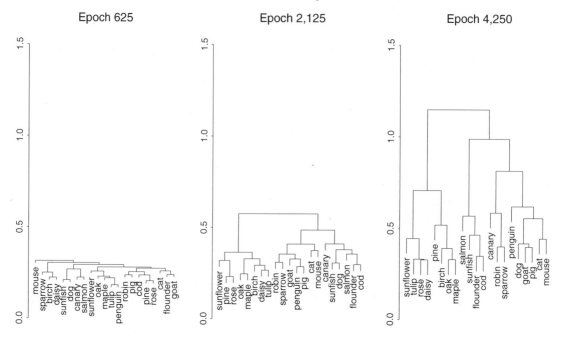

Distributed inputs

Epoch 125

Epoch 1,000

Epoch 2,500

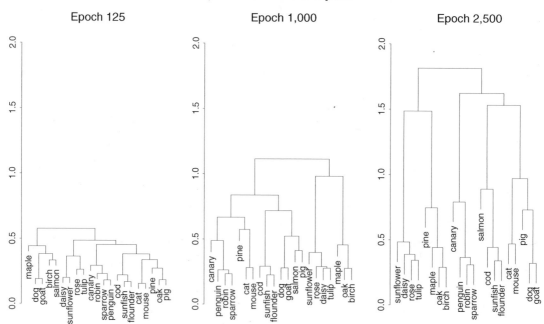

Note that at epoch 2,125 in the localist-inputs version and epoch 1000 in the distributed-inputs version, the two models behave in a manner analogous to Mandler's 9-month-old infants. That is, they "group together" items that share the few properties that reliably discriminate broad semantic domains—properties such as *can move*, *has skin*, *has roots*, and *has leaves*. In the localist-inputs version, this structure has been imposed on completely nonoverlapping inputs. In the case of the distributed-inputs version, the model may appear as though it is "using" these attributes as its basis for grouping items, even though none of these properties is coded in the input. In fact, there are no properties shared by all plants or all animals represented in the input, but nevertheless the model first differentiates its internal representations with respect to this broad semantic distinction. Thus in the distributed-inputs version, the weights that project from the *Input* to the *Representation* layer effectively serve the function that Mandler (2000a) attributes to image schemas and that Carey (2000) attributes to core causal properties: they allow the model to "group together" a set of items that have disparate visual appearances, on the basis of a few abstract shared properties that are not directly represented in the input.

Both models show progressive differentiation for the same reasons outlined in the previous chapter. Initially all items are represented as similar to one another by virtue of the intital small random weights, and the model reduces error by learning to activate output units shared by all items in the environment (e.g., *can grow*). However, plants and animals, because they have few properties in common in the output, generate quite different error

Figure 4.2 Hierarchical cluster plot of the internal representations for both versions of the network at three different points in learning. In both cases the networks were trained with the extended corpus and without name properties. The distance matrices were generated by calculating the mean pairwise Euclidean distances among representations across five different network runs in each version. As in the previous chapter, the model first learned to differentiate superordinate categories, and learned more fine-grained distinctions later in development.

signals, and these gradually lead the model to distinguish them slightly. As the plants and animals slowly come to receive different internal representations, a kind of bootstrapping effect arises in the learning mechanism: the weights projecting forward from the *Representation* layer are able to use the dimension of variability that separates plants and animals to reduce error on the sets of output properties shared across items in each domain. Consequently the error derivatives that come back from these properties to the *Representation* units grow increasingly large, propelling the plant and animal representations further apart. This in turn gives the forward weights even more information to work with, and they adjust to captialize still further on the growing distinction represented between plants and animals.

In both models, the constellation of output properties that reliably discriminate plants from animals become more "salient" to the model early in training, in the sense that only these properties generate a coherent error signal across the training corpus in the early epochs of learning. That is, the property *can move* is not initially predisposed to be any more salient or informative than any other attribute. But as the model begins to learn, the coherent covariation between *can move* and other attributes that reliably discriminate animate from inanimate objects in the training environment leads these properties to dominate learning in the model in the early epochs of training, as shown in chapter 3. As a consequence, these properties more strongly constrain the model's internal representations—leading both versions to discover an early weight configuration that "filters" input similarities in such a way that differences between items in the same domain are minimized, and differences between items in different domains are emphasized.

As the network masters properties that vary coherently across domains, and as the smaller weight changes that accumulate across other output units very gradually allow the model to differentiate more fine-grained categories such as *bird* and *fish*, the dynamics shift in favor of learning about the properties that vary coherently with these intermediate categories. That is, as the *bird* and *fish* representations pull apart from one another, properties such as *can fly* and *can swim* begin to produce error signals that produce large derivatives and therefore large weight changes, at which point this learning comes to strongly influence representational change in the model. The consequence of these dynamics is that different sets of properties dominate the learning that drives representational change in the model at different points during training.

Simulating the Object-Manipulation Experiment

With these ideas in hand, we can begin to see how the model provides a basis for understanding the phenomena reviewed at the beginning of this chapter: the ability to conceive of perceptually disparate stimuli as similar to one another on the basis of properties not present in the input available at the time of test. The explanation offered by the model is similar in some respects to that suggested by other investigators: perceptual properties that reliably discriminate broad semantic domains are more important in determining the model's behavior early in development than are other kinds of perceptual properties, and items that share these properties are represented as conceptually similar, even if they differ in many other respects. What sets our account apart from that offered by others is the basis for the importance of these properties. In the case of our model, the salience of properties like movement emerges as a consequence of the sensitivity of the learning mechanism to coherent covariation.

To provide a concrete illustration of how these phenomena in the model might explain data from infant experiments, we conducted a simulation of the object-examination task conducted by Mandler and McDonough (1993). In this experiment, infants were allowed to play with a series of toy objects belonging to the same semantic category. After habituation, they were presented with two new test objects in succession: first, a novel item from the same semantic category, and second, a novel item from a different category. The authors then measured the amount of time the infant spent examining each. They used the difference in looking time between the last habituation trial and the novel same-category item to measure sensitivity to within-category item differences. Similarly, they used the difference in looking time between the novel different-category item and the novel same-category item as a measure of the infants' sensitivity to the category-level distinction.

Three different experimental conditions are of particular interest in this experiment. First, the authors habituated 9- and 11-month-olds to items from the same broad semantic domain (e.g., a series of animals, or a series of vehicles), which had broadly different overall shapes. In this case, infants of both ages did not look longer at the novel same-category item compared to the last habituation trial, but did look longer at the different-category item, indicating that (a) they treated as similar items from the same general category, even though they were perceptually fairly dissimilar, and (b) they treated such items as different from an out-of-category item. In the second condition, the authors habituated 9- and 11-month-olds to a set of items from the same intermediate category (e.g., a series of dogs), and then tested them with an item from a different category, but within the same broad domain (e.g., a fish). In this case, the different-category test item had a fairly different shape and some different parts from the habituation items; but nevertheless, 9-month-olds did not dishabituate to this test item—indicating to the authors that they did not construe the dogs and fish as different, despite their perceptual differences. In contrast, 11-month-olds dishabituated to the out-of-category item, indicating successful discrimination of the different kinds of animal. Finally in the third condition, the authors habituated 9- and 11-month-olds to a series of toy birds modeled with their wings outspread, and then tested them with a novel bird (also with wings outspread) or with a toy plane. Infants at both ages dishabituated to the different-category item. Thus in sum, the authors concluded that infants at 9 months always discriminated items from broadly different semantic categories, both when the habituation and test items had variable shapes and parts, and when they had a grossly similar overall shape; but they failed to discriminate dogs from fish, despite the perceptual differences among these items. In contrast, 11-month-olds discriminated both the broader and more specific categories in all conditions. Similar results with further controls for perceptual similarities have recently been reported by Pauen (2002b).

We find the Mandler and McDonough findings and the similar findings of Pauen to be of particular interest because they indicate an early ability to discriminate broad conceptual domains for both perceptually similar and perceptually disparate items, and a developmental change between the ages of 9 and 11 months in the ability to differentiate subcategories within the same conceptual domain (i.e., dogs vs. fish). Infants at both ages were tested with the same stimulus items—hence the different patterns of behavior cannot be explained solely with reference to the perceptual structure of the stimulus materials themselves. While it remains possible to attribute some aspects of the findings to perceptual rather than semantic similarities, the developmental change indicates differences in the representations and/or processing held by infants at different ages—changes that are consistent with the developmental processes that operate in our model as well.

In the model analog of the experiment, we "habituate" the model with novel stimulus items that are perceptually similar to one another, and that belong to one of the four categories with which the model is familiar (birds, fish, trees, and flowers). We then test the model with novel test items that include an item from the same semantic category but with few perceived attributes in common with the habituation items (*same-category item*), and an item from a different category that shares many perceived attributes with the habituation items (*different-category item*). In both versions, we allow the model to derive internal representations of habituation and test items, and examine the similarities among these representations to determine which of the test items the model construes as "novel" with respect to the habituation items, at different stages of learning.

Representing Test Items in the Distributed Version In the case of the distributed-inputs version, presentation of a novel stimulus image to the model is straightforward: we simply create a new pattern of activity across the perceptual input units for each item. On applying this pattern to the model's inputs, we can inspect the resulting pattern of activity across *Representation* units to determine what conceptual representation the model assigns to the item. To simulate the experiment, we needed to create "perceptual" input patterns that express similarity relations analogous to those among the stimuli used in the experiment—specifically, a set of *habituation* items that have many perceptual attributes in common and that belong to the same category; a *same-category* test item perceptually different from the habituation items (like the dogs and fish in the experiment); and a *different-category* test item that shares many perceptual properties with the habituation stimuli, despite being from a different semantic category (like the birds and planes in the experiment).

The input patterns employed in the simulation are shown in figure 4.3. There are four "categories" of items represented. In each category, items 1–4 share many perceptible attributes. The fifth item in each case has few directly perceived attributes in common with its category neighbors, but in all cases it shares one especially useful and informative property with them. For example, *bird 5* shares the property *wings* with the other birds, but otherwise has no perceptible attribute in common with them.

For each of the four categories, there is one "perceptually similar" item from the contrasting domain, and one from the contrasting category in the same domain. For instance, *trees 1–4* have many properties that overlap with *bird 5*, and many that overlap with *flower 5*. In this sense, both *bird 5* and *flower 5* are "perceptually" more similar to *trees 1–4* than is *tree 5*. This construction allows us to pit perceptual-feature overlap in the input against semantic relatedness in our analog of the preference task: we "habituate" the network with four similar items from the same category (e.g., *trees 1–4*), and then "test" it with a perceptually dissimilar

	pretty	big	green	red	yellow	white	twirly	branches	petals	wings	gills	fur
tree 1	0	1	1	1	1	0	0	1	0	0	0	0
tree 2	0	1	1	0	1	1	0	1	0	0	0	0
tree 3	0	1	1	0	1	0	0	1	0	0	0	0
tree 4	0	1	1	0	0	0	0	1	0	0	0	0
tree 5	0	0	0	1	0	1	1	1	0	0	0	0
flower 1	1	0	0	1	0	1	1	0	1	0	0	0
flower 2	1	0	0	0	1	1	1	0	1	0	0	0
flower 3	1	0	0	0	0	1	1	0	1	0	0	0
flower 4	1	0	0	0	0	1	0	0	1	0	0	0
flower 5	0	1	1	0	1	0	0	0	1	0	0	0
bird 1	1	0	1	1	0	0	1	0	0	1	0	0
bird 2	1	0	0	1	1	1	0	0	0	1	0	0
bird 3	1	0	0	1	0	1	0	0	0	1	0	0
bird 4	1	0	0	0	0	1	1	0	0	1	0	0
bird 5	0	1	1	0	1	0	0	0	0	1	0	0
fish 1	0	1	1	0	0	1	0	0	0	0	1	0
fish 2	0	1	1	1	1	0	0	0	0	0	1	0
fish 3	0	1	1	0	1	0	1	0	0	0	1	0
fish 4	0	1	1	0	1	0	0	0	0	0	1	0
fish 5	1	0	0	1	0	1	1	0	0	0	1	0

Figure 4.3   Attributes of twenty novel items used to simulate Mandler and McDonough's infant-preference experiment. Associated with each category are four perceptually similar exemplars that constitute habituation items, one perceptually dissimilar exemplar employed as a test item, and two perceptually similar out-of-category distractors: one from the contrasting category in the same domain, and one in the opposite domain.

item from the same category (e.g., *tree 5*) and a perceptually similar item from the contrasting category (*flower 5*) or domain (*bird 5*).

Figure 4.4 shows the similarities among some of the habituation and test items that are determined by the overlap in attributes shown in figure 4.3. In each case the "habituation" items are those labeled 1–4 in the tree. As is apparent from the figure, the fifth category member is less similar to the four habituation items than is the test item from the contrasting category or domain. Using this set of patterns, we can investigate changes in the model's ability to discriminate both broad and more specific conceptual categories as it learns.

Basic Contrast   Global Contrast

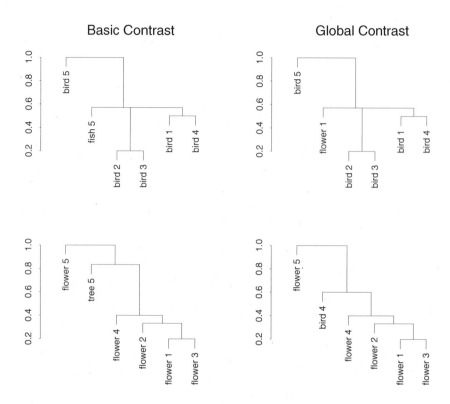

Figure 4.4 Hierarchical cluster plot of the "perceptual" similarities for some of the novel habituation and test items used in the simulation. In each case, the fifth category item is less
similar to its category coordinates than is an out-of-category distractor.

Representing Test Items in the Localist Version The distributed-inputs
version of the model offers a natural means of presenting new
items, but it is less obvious how to accomplish this in the localist-
inputs version—we need a means of allowing the model to use the
knowledge stored in its weights to derive an internal representation of a novel item when given information from the environment
about its observed attributes. To do this, we used the technique of
backpropagation to representation described in chapter 2. In this
case, we use the backpropagated error signal from the observed
attributes of the test item, not to adjust weights in the network, but

to adjust the activations of the *Representation* units in order to find an internal representation that comes as close as possible to generating a pattern of activation across the output units that correspond to the object's observed properties. That is, backpropagation to representation allows us to ask the network: Given that the item has these observed attributes, how should it be represented?

Using this technique, we can backpropagate error from any subset of the output properties in the model. With respect to simulating the infant-preference experiment, we conceive of the output units from which error is propagated as corresponding to the directly perceived attributes of the stimulus item. Specifically, we can employ the same subset of attributes used as input properties in the distributed-inputs version of the model—all of the *is* units except for *is living*, and a subset of the *has* units—and we can use the same patterns shown in figure 4.3 as target patterns for the backprop-to-representation technique, to represent the visual appearance of habituation and test stimuli in modeling the experiment.

Habituation and Test Procedure   In both versions of the model, we simulate the habituation trials by presenting four habituation items (e.g., *birds 1–4*) and recording the representations the network generates for each. We also present a same-category test item (e.g., *bird 5*), and a different-category test item (e.g., *fish 5* or *tree 5*). The models derive internal representations for each item as described above. We then calculate the distance between the centroid of the representations for the four habituation items, and each of the two test items. To map from these distances to an analog of the infant behavior, we adopt the following assumption: we assume that the model construes as more novel, and therefore prefers to manipulate, whichever test item gives rise to a representation that has the largest distance from the centroid of the habituation items, and that the likelihood of preferring one object over another increases with the discrepancy in their respective distances from the habituation centroid. Consistent with this assumption, we use the following formula to determine the likelihood of preferring one test item over another given the relevant mean distances:

$$p_b = \sigma(s(d_b - d_w))$$

In this formula, p_b is the probability of choosing the between-category test item, σ is the logistic function, d_b is the distance from the between-category test item to the centroid of the four habituation items, d_w is the distance from the within-category test item to the habituation centroid, and s is a scaling parameter that determines the degree to which the model is sensitive to the difference $d_b - d_w$. The probability of preferring (i.e., examining for a longer time) the within-category test item, p_w, is just $1 - p_b$. Intuitively, the equation indicates that when the between- and within-category items are equally distant from the habituation items, the model is equally likely to favor either over the other, but as one test item gets further from these relative to the other, the likelihood of preferring it for examination increases.

Simulation Details   Both models were again trained as described earlier in this chapter (see pp. 149–150). Training was halted every 125 epochs, the weights were stored, and the simulation of the habituation experiment was begun. For each of the twenty test items in figure 4.3, the model generated an internal representation, either using the backprop-to-representation method (localist-inputs version) or by simply presenting the appropriate pattern across the input units (distributed-inputs version).

To test the network's tendency to choose a between-category test item, at both the global and intermediate (i.e., basic) levels, the distances among its internal representations of habituation and test items were calculated. Specifically, the centroid was determined for each set of four habituation items (*birds 1–4, fish 1–4, flowers 1–4*, or *trees 1–4*), and the distance between this centroid and each of the corresponding test items was calculated. These distances were then entered into the formula shown above to determine the probability that the model "preferred" the different-category item. Each category (e.g., the bird category) had one perceptually dissimilar same-category test item (e.g., *bird 5*); one perceptually similar global different-category test item (e.g., *flower 1*); and one perceptually similar, intermediate-level different-category test item, from the contrasting category in the same domain (e.g., *fish 5*). This yielded four comparisons testing intermediate category differentiation, and four testing global category differentiation. The simulation was run five times with different starting weights, yielding twenty data points in total for each level of contrast. The data we report are averaged across these trials.

Note that the model was never trained with the items used in the habituation procedure, and no weight changes were made during the habituation process. The representations the model generates for these items simply reflect knowledge the model has accumulated on the basis of learning in the normal training environment.

Results Figure 4.5 shows the similarities among the representations the model generates in the localist-inputs version for one set of habituation items (the birds) and the corresponding test items at three different points throughout learning. Figure 4.6 shows analogous data for the distributed-inputs version. During the very early epochs of training in both cases all items are represented as quite similar to one another, although the organization of items does reflect to some extent the degree of overlap in the perceptual properties from which the internal representations are derived. For instance, *bird 5* is represented as less similar to the other birds than either *flower 1* or *fish 5*. The reason is that at this point, there is no information accumulated in the network's weights that allows it to map reliably between parts of the representation space and the attributes specified by the test input that give rise to the network's internal representations (either by forward or backpropagation). Items with similar attributes specified by the test input thus generate similar internal representations, regardless of the semantic relations among them, which depend on other attributes not available at the time of the test.

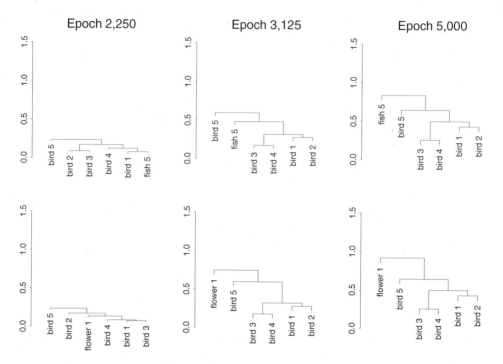

Figure 4.5 Hierarchical cluster plot of the representations derived by the network using the backprop-to-representation method in the localist-inputs version of the network, using the four novel "bird" habituation items (birds 1–4) and the corresponding same- and different-category test items (bird 5, fish 5, flower 1).

As the model learns more about the coherent covariation among properties in the training corpus, this picture begins to change: in both cases, the model first differentiates the global different-category test item (the flower) from the five birds, and later comes to differentiate the intermediate-level different-category item (the fish) from the birds—even though both of these test items share more "perceptual" properties with *birds 1–4* than does *bird 5*. This phenomenon can be observed in the similarities among habituation and test items for the *bird* category shown in figures 4.5 and 4.6. A similar pattern was observed for all four categories in both simulations.

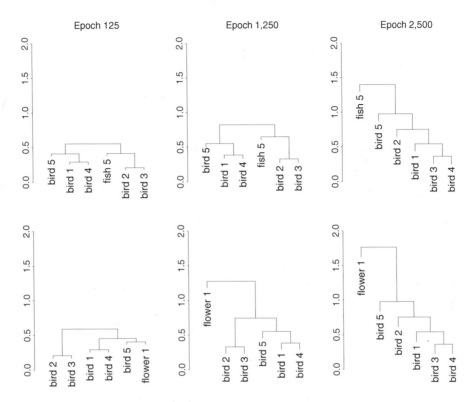

Figure 4.6   Hierarchical cluster plot of the representations derived by the network in the distributed-inputs version, showing the four novel "bird" habituation items (birds 1–4) and the corresponding same- and different-category test items (bird 5, fish 5, flower 1).

Figure 4.7 shows the likelihood of choosing the different-category test item over the same-category test item throughout early training in both simulations, for between-domain test items (e.g., tree or flower versus bird, a global discrimination) or for intermediate-level between-category test items (e.g., tree versus flower or bird versus fish). Early in learning, all items are represented as similar to one another, so same- and different-category test items (at both the global and intermediate levels) are equally distant from the habituation centroid. Consequently, the likelihood of choosing

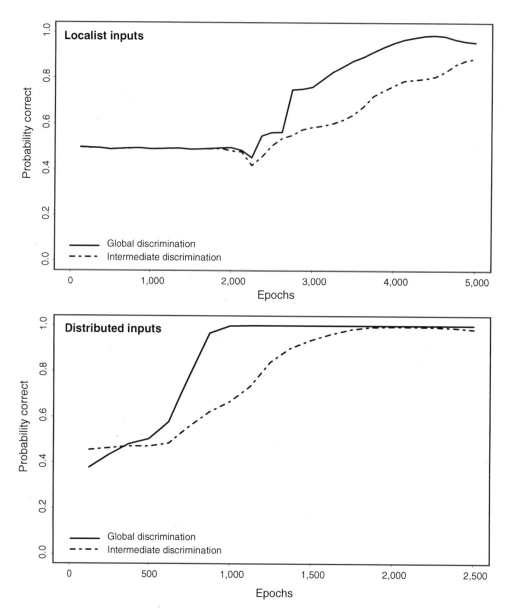

Figure 4.7   Average likelihood of "choosing" the correct item throughout early epochs of learning, in model analogs of the object-manipulation task for localist and distributed versions.

the between-category item is near chance. As training proceeds, this likelihood begins to change—the model first begins to reliably choose the different-category test item from the contrasting global domain from the same domain, and later begins to choose the between-category test item. Like infants, the model's ability to differentiate items on conceptual grounds emerges first for broad semantic distinctions, and only later for more specific ones.

Finally, it is worth noting that, in generating its internal representations of the novel items after learning, the model seems to lend special weight or importance to the properties that covary coherently together in its training environment. This is reflected in the fact that for all categories, both versions of the model continue to group the same-category item with the habituation items through learning—even though it shares very few of its properties with them. For instance, of the four features that describe *bird 5* (shown in figure 4.3), only one is consistently shared by the four other birds seen during habituation. By contrast, the test item *fish 5* shares five of its six properties with at least half of the birds seen during habituation. Considering just the overlap in features, then, *fish 5* is more similar to the habituation items than is *bird 5* (as is clear from figure 4.4). However, the one property that *bird 5* does have in common with the four habituation birds—*wings*—happens to covary coherently with many other properties in the model training corpus. By contrast, the five properties that *fish 5* shares with the habituation birds are all somewhat idiosyncratic in the training corpus, and do not covary coherently together with anything else. As a consequence of the dynamics of learning described in the previous chapter, the coherently covarying property comes to contribute more strongly to representational change than do the various idiosyncratic properties—so that the network treats as similar those items that share the coherent property, even if they do not have many other attributes in common, and treats as different items that differ for the coherent property, even if they share many idiosyncratic attributes. In this sense, the model's sensitivity to coherent covariation leads it to treat some properties as more "important" for semantic representation than others—that is, these properties come to have an acquired salience for the model.

Discussion

We would like to make several points on the basis of the preceding simulations. To begin, one of our aims has been to support the idea that the Rumelhart model, as simple as it is, might nevertheless provide some insight into the acquisition of semantic knowledge from different kinds of perceptual experience across a range of events and situations. Specifically, we have suggested that general principles governing the discovery of representational structure in the Rumelhart network, as explored in the previous two chapters, may have relevance to understanding aspects of the early conceptual development of preverbal infants. One aspect of the results relevant to this point is the fact that the pattern of progressive differentiation observed in chapter 3 did not depend on training the model to name at different levels of specificity. Instead, this phenomenon arises in the model from patterns of covariation among the properties of objects in the model's environment. Whether these properties are construed as corresponding to names and other verbal statements about objects, or to observable perceptual properties, is immaterial to the model's behavior.

On the present construal of the model, both the input and output attributes can be viewed as coding various aspects of similarity and difference among objects encountered in the environment, as detected by perceptual processes across different events and situations. In any given situation, such perceptual similarities may not yield much information about which objects should be treated as the same kind of thing. However, repeated encounters with a range of objects across a variety of contexts leads to a state of knowledge in which some attributes exert particularly strong constraints on the semantic system's internal representations, allowing it to treat items that share these properties as similar even when they differ in many other respects.

The key factor contributing to this state of knowledge is the influence of coherent covariation on the learning processes that govern weight changes in the system. The ease with which the system can learn that a particular item has a certain property depends on the degree to which the property is shared by other items with similar internal representations. However, the similarities represented by the model at any point in time themselves depend on the mappings it has learned between internal representations and particular attributes experienced during training. At a particular time the model treats as salient those properties that covary coherently within the clusters of objects it has learned to differentiate at that time. As we have seen previously, such properties are easiest for the system to acquire, and thus dominate the representational change that occurs as the system learns. Once these properties have been mastered, representational change slows dramatically until, on the basis of minute weight changes accumulating from noncoherent properties, the system finds a new organization of its internal representations that renders a new set of properties salient. Such properties become easier to learn and propel new, rapid representational change until they are mastered. Thus, coherent covariation among stimulus attributes at different levels of hierarchical organization spurs successive waves of differentiation, with different stimulus properties acquiring salience at different points during development. It is this changing sensitivity to patterns of coherent covariation that we propose to add to the repertoire of possible mechanisms that may contribute to the process of conceptual development.

As stated in the introduction to this chapter, the principles illustrated by the Rumelhart model do not and cannot refute other claims about the factors that may potentially contribute to conceptual development. However, accepting that the mechanism we have identified may be a contributing factor, our simulations have implications for each of the other viewpoints we reviewed above.

In agreement with advocates of perceptual enrichment, the PDP framework suggests that conceptual knowledge acquisition is spurred by domain-general learning based on perceptual experience. Our further point here is that the sensitivity of correlation-based learning mechanisms to coherent covariation among stimulus properties, and the resultant influence on acquired feature salience, provide a previously unrecognized mechanism by which such domain-general perceptual learning can give rise to internal representations that capture similarity structure different from that which is available directly from the perceptual input provided by test stimuli.

Rakison's claim that certain directly observed properties are especially salient to 12-month-old infants is not inconsistent with our theory, and indeed, nothing in our approach refutes the possibility that some attributes are initially and inherently more salient to infants than others. However, our simulations also demonstrate that coherent covariation can lead certain properties to have an *acquired* salience. Thus, the empirical demonstration that infants in semantic tasks are most sensitive to large, external parts, or to patterns of motion, need not reflect a learning-independent perceptual salience of these properties—this salience might emerge as a consequence of domain-general learning over the first year of life. If so, this might explain why 12-month-olds are inclined to emphasize external parts such as legs or wheels as a basis for grouping objects (Rakison and Poulin-Dubois 2001). Note that, under this account, there is nothing special about external parts; any properties that varied coherently across domains could potentially provide the basis for differentiating concepts, including overall shape and structural characteristics likely to covary coherently with other properties.

We also suggest that the PDP framework has similarities with some aspects of Mandler's ideas about the emergence of conceptual representations from perceptual experience. The state of knowledge captured by the network at a fairly early point is similar in many respects to that attributed by Mandler to 7- to 9-month-old infants. That is, the model treats as similar perceptually varying items that happen to share characteristics such as self-initiated movement that are not directly available in stimuli used in experiments. In the distributed version of the simulation above, for example, the model first represents animals as similar to one another and as distinct from plants, despite the fact that there are no input properties held in common between the birds and the fish, and many input and target properties that distinguish between these items. One might argue that the model's "conceptual" and "perceptual" representations capture different information about the similarities among objects, as Mandler suggests—immediately available perceptual similarities are captured in the input, and conceptual similarities are captured in the internal representations. Moreover, the learning process captured by our model provides a new mechanistic basis for the extraction of conceptual representations from perceptual experience, different from but not inconsistent with what Mandler refers to as "perceptual analysis."

Finally, Carey (2000) suggests that the conceptual distinctions made by infants early in life cannot be acquired and must reflect initial domain-specific knowledge about nonobvious "core" conceptual attributes. We will address some of Carey's ideas in substantial detail in chapter 7, but for the time being we should point out that there is one sense in which, in our view, infants are biologically prepared to acquire concepts. The influence of coherent covariation on concept development depends on the infant's initial ability to detect elements of similarity and difference among particular events. Without such a facility, there can be no basis for patterns of covariation to influence knowledge acquisition. The theory thus assumes that, among the many elements of similarity to which infants are initially sensitive, some exist that vary coherently across semantic domains. Our simulations suggest that it may not be necessary to attribute to infants initial domain-specific predispositions to lend special salience, weight, or attention to specific core properties, since this salience may emerge as a consequence of coherent covariation.

We would like to close this chapter with a final thought on what will perhaps be viewed as the most difficult contention of our theory: the assumption that "perceptual" input contains elements that remain invariant from one event to another, despite discriminable differences in the particular instantiations of such common elements across different events. To return to an example previously discussed, the use of a single unit to represent the attribute *has legs* amounts to treating all legs as perceptually identical, despite their obvious differences. Making them identical is unlikely to be necessary, but some overlap in the input is likely to influence the success of the simulation. Our network assigns internal representations to objects on the basis of coherent covariation tabulated across such presumed elements of similarity, and the results described here exploit the fact that these elements of overlap are straightforwardly encoded in the input, facilitating the discovery of the category structure of the domain.

Although our simulations do not illustrate it, other work has shown that PDP networks can sometimes discover latent patterns of coherent covariation among items that have no direct feature overlap of any kind. Such a situation is illustrated in the simulations Hinton (1986, 1989) conducted with the family-trees network previously discussed in chapter 2. In these simulations, Hinton trained his network on two isomorphic family trees: one consisting of three generations of an Italian family, and the other consisting of three generations of an English family. When given an individual's name and a relationship as input (e.g., *Joe* and *father*), the model was trained to activate the name of the appropriate individual in the output (e.g., Joe's father, Bill). Each person was represented with a localist unit in the model, both at the input and the output level, so there was no direct overlap of any kind for the various individuals in the two families. Even so, the network discovered internal representations that captured the position of each individual within the respective family tree—for example, assigning corresponding points in the representational space to the English and Italian "grandchildren," to the English and Italian "uncles," and so on. Although there was no direct overlap in the input and target representations for, say, the English and Italian grandfathers, the network's internal representations reflected the commonalities across the two different families—that is, it assigned corresponding representations to corresponding members of the two family trees. In the Hinton simulations there was overlap across families in the specific ensembles of relations particular individuals entered into, and this overlap is directly available in the inputs to the relation units. However, there are other simulations (e.g., Altmann and Dienes 1999) in which abstract structural correspondences have been discovered by networks even in the absence of any overlap of the input and target patterns of activation.

While direct feature overlap for different items may not be necessary for coherent covariation to exert an influence on the acquisition of internal representations, we believe such overlap is in fact made available by our perceptual systems, at least for some covarying attributes of objects if not for all of them. In either case, the fundamental point remains the same: the ability of networks to exploit such covariation plays a crucial role in the early emergence of semantic categorization abilities, and in the gradual differentiation of such categories as a result of experience, beginning in infancy and continuing throughout life.

5 Naming Things: Privileged Categories, Familiarity, Typicality, and Expertise

To this point we have considered phenomena in development and in dementia that have been interpreted as supporting the theory that semantic representations are organized hierarchically in memory. Specifically, we have investigated the coarse-to-fine differentiation of object concepts in preverbal infants, and the apparent reversion of this process witnessed in semantic dementia. In the early days of this research, Warrington suggested that these complementary patterns revealed the gradual construction and deterioration of a Quillian-like taxonomic hierarchy in memory. We have in some sense made a similar proposal, in which the "hierarchy" is not reified in the processing architecture that directs semantic task performance, but is instead latent in the similarities across distributed internal representations of objects in a PDP network.

In this chapter we will turn our attention to a set of phenomena that in some ways seem to conflict with the doctrine of progressive differentiation of concepts in development, and the reversal of this process in dementia: so-called *basic-level effects*. As discussed in chapter 1, basic-level effects have often been interpreted as demonstrating that the first conceptual distinctions to be acquired in development, and the most important distinctions in adulthood, are those that discriminate between objects at an intermediate level of specificity (such as *dog* versus *horse*). Such claims have been bolstered by a variety of often-replicated empirical findings that indicate that the properties shared by items in the same "basic" category are more rapidly produced or verified by participants in semantic tasks. For example:

1. Children first learn to label objects with their basic-level name, instead of with more general or more specific names.
2. In free-naming tasks, adults prefer to name at the basic level even when they know more general or specific names.
3. Adults are faster in verifying category membership at the basic level.
4. Adults are quicker to verify properties of objects that are shared by exemplars of a "basic" category.

A predominant view in development and in research in adult semantic cognition has been that "basic-level" concepts are special in two senses: they are the first to be acquired in development (e.g., Mervis 1987b), and they are the first to be activated or accessed in semantic tasks in adulthood (e.g., Jolicoeur, Gluck, and Kosslyn 1984). However, as we discussed in detail in chapter 1, basic-level phenomena raise a number of important questions when considered alongside a broader range of data from semantic task performance.

First, it is difficult to reconcile claims of basic-level primacy in acquisition with the studies of preverbal concept differentiation discussed in the last chapter. As Mandler has pointed out, much of the earliest research demonstrating basic-level primacy effects in development has relied on verbal testing methods that require participants to produce or comprehend the names of objects and their properties (Mandler, Bauer, and McDonough 1991). Though the data from such experiments are of considerable interest, it is difficult to draw conclusions about earlier concept development from them, because these methods cannot be used with infants younger than about 2.5 years. Nevertheless, studies of early language acquisition do clearly show that infants learn to name objects with their basic-level label prior to acquiring more general or specific names. Thus the data suggest that preverbal infants first represent fairly broad semantic distinctions, but with further development, they first learn to name objects with somewhat more specific labels. Relatedly, studies with normal adults show an advantage for naming at the basic level, but in semantic dementia, the superordinate-level naming tends to be best preserved. Thus, there are two paradoxes: in development, it appears that early emergence of naming at the basic level coexists with a general-to-specific progression of underlying semantic representations, while in dementia, it appears that a primacy for the basic level before the disease sets in gives way to an advantage for the superordinate level as the disease progresses. Understanding how these paradoxes can occur will be a main focus of the first part of this chapter.

Second, there are well-known empirical phenomena that complicate the simple view that basic-level names (or other properties) are always the first to be acquired in development and the first to be activated in semantic tasks in adulthood. Basic-level advantages are known to be strongly influenced by typicality, and in some cases these effects can lead to advantages in learning or producing information about atypical objects at a more specific level than the basic level. For example, children often restrict basic-level names solely to typical items in a domain early in lexical acquisition (applying the name "ball" to baseballs but not to footballs), and may learn specific names such as "penguin" prior to basic-level names for such items. Similarly, adults prefer to name atypical items with a specific label, and verify category membership of such items more rapidly at a level subordinate to basic. How does typicality influence the ease with which semantic information is learned in childhood, and the rapidity with which such information is produced in adulthood?

Third, performance on tasks used to measure basic-level effects is known to be influenced by the nature and extent of one's experience with objects in a given domain. A simple example of such an influence is the effect of familiarity on object naming. In early language learning, the names of highly familiar items are often misapplied to less familiar but semantically related objects, as when a child applies the name "dog" to all medium-sized animals. Similarly in semantic dementia, the names of highly familiar objects are typically more robust than less familiar names, and are often inappropriately extended to encompass semantically related objects. Such data are not especially surprising, but should be encompassed by a general theory of basic-level effects. Moreover, findings from the study of expertise suggest that increased familiarity with a domain can have more subtle and interesting effects on semantic task performance. Such studies have shown that basic-level advantages in naming and property verification may be attenuated with expertise, with experts showing increased facility at producing and verifying information at a more specific level (Tanaka and Taylor 1991). Experts also appear to differentiate items from the same basic category to a greater degree than do novices (Boster and Johnson 1989), and different varieties of expertise within a given domain may give rise to differing ideas about the similarity structure of the domain (Medin, Lynch, and Coley 1997). Together these findings suggest that experience plays a crucial role in shaping the representations and processes that give rise to semantic task performance generally, and to basic-level advantages in particular. What is the mechanism by which experience exerts its influence?

Though many of these findings were first reported years ago and have found their place in the canon of robust effects reported in the study of cognition, we are not aware of any mechanistic theory that has successfully reconciled them with the broader literature, and in particular with the studies of progressive differentiation and deterioration considered in the preceding two chapters. In this chapter we will offer the beginnings of such a reconciliation, by investigating how basic-level avantages in naming and other semantic tasks might emerge in the PDP framework, and how such effects might coexist with the progressive differentiation of internal representations and the robust preservation of general knowledge under semantic impairment investigated previously. To foreshadow, we will consider how the changing structure of the Rumelhart model's internal representations influences its ability to activate output units that correspond to names at different levels of specificity. We will see that the strength with which the model activates these units when queried appropriately depends on two factors: the frequency with which it has experienced the item in the relevant relation context, and the degree to which other items with similar internal representations share the property in question. Together, these factors can explain both the apparent advantage in retrieving basic-level information for typical objects, and the absence of such an advantage for atypical objects.

Because basic-level effects span a broad range of empirical and theoretical issues, it will be useful to briefly preview the set of simulations presented in the chapter. Table 5.1 provides a summary of the simulations and the theoretical and empirical issues they are intended to address. We will begin with a simulation that establishes how the primary basic-level phenomena in naming might emerge in the model, and that illustrates how such phenomena can coexist with the progressive differentiation of internal representations in development and the robust preservation of general knowledge in dementia. In two follow-up simulations we investigate the complementary roles of word frequency and the attribute structure of the training corpus in contributing to these effects—an endeavor that allows us to consider how typicality and frequency interact to produce basic-level advantages in the model.

After establishing the primary points, we will go on to consider how the representations and processes that give rise to basic-level effects in the model are influenced by different kinds of training experience. Specifically, in simulation 5.4 we will investigate how increased familiarity with a particular class of objects can lead to the overextension of familiar names to semantically related items during early language learning and in semantic dementia. In simulations 5.5 and 5.6 we will address other effects of extensive experience revealed by the study of expertise. Specifically, simulation 5.5 addresses the attenuation of basic-level advantages with increasing experience, and the increased differentiation of specific

Table 5.1 Summary of the simulations presented in the chapter, with the theoretical and empirical issues they are designed to address

SIMULATION CONDITIONS	THEORETICAL ISSUE	EMPIRICAL PHENOMENA
5.1: Basic-level advantages Model is trained with the corpus from appendix B, table AB.3, but with basic-level names appearing more frequently than more general or specific names.	Establishes how basic-level effects emerge in the model, even as internal representations progressively differentiate, and even though general information continues to be more robust when representations degrade.	Addresses basic-level advantages for typical items in lexical acquisition, free naming, and category and property verification, coincident with progressive differentiation of concepts through learning and the robust preservation of general semantic information in semantic dementia.
5.2: Effects of word frequency and typicality Model is trained with the corpus in table AB.3, but with all names appearing equally frequently in the environment.	Illustrates how word frequency and concept typicality interact to determine the speed and strength which which the model learns to activate names at different levels of specificity.	Addresses the interaction of basic-level effects with typicality in lexical acquisition and adult semantic tasks.
5.3: Effects of attribute structure Model is trained with all names presented equally frequently in the environment, but varying the degree of similarity structure apparent across output properties.	Establishes that the basic-level effects produced by the model are strongly influenced by the tendency for different groups of objects to share properties, and that strong basic-level advantages are observed when basic categories are maximally informative and distinctive.	Addresses the tendency for basic-level advantages to be observed for groupings of objects that are maximally informative and distinctive with respect to their properties.
5.4: Effects of concept familiarity Model is trained with the usual corpus, but with *dog* patterns appearing more frequently than other mammals in the training environment.	Demonstrates how increased familiarity with an item influences the model's naming behavior during early learning and when its representations degrade.	Addresses the misapplication of familiar names to semantically related items in childhood and in semantic dementia.

Table 5.1 (continued)

SIMULATION CONDITIONS	THEORETICAL ISSUE	EMPIRICAL PHENOMENA
5.5: Effects of expertise in different domains Model is trained with the usual corpus and with either *bird* or *fish* patterns presented more frequently than other animals, in order to simulate expertise with a particular domain.	Illustrates how increased experience with a set of related items results in an increased differentiation of internal representations, and a subsequent attenuation of basic-level advantages, for items in the set.	Addresses the increased differentiation of sub-classes in expert domains observed in sorting experiments, and the reduction or elimination of basic-level advantages in naming, as well as category and property verification witnessed in expertise.
5.6: Effects of different kinds of expertise Model is trained with the usual corpus, but with all items appearing more frequently in either the *is* or the *can* relation context, in order to simulate the effects of different kinds of expertise.	Demonstrates how extensive exposure to different aspects of information about a set of objects may give rise to somewhat different internal representations of the same items.	Addresses sorting studies that suggest that different varieties of experience can lead different kinds of experts to derive different similarity relations for the same set of highly familiar objects.

concepts in expert domains; and simulation 5.6 illustrates how different varieties of expertise may give rise to differently structured internal representations for the same set of items.

As we hope will become abundantly clear, frequency of exposure to individual items and to particular kinds of properties (including names at different levels of generality), as well as the similarity structure of object attributes encountered across different experiences, all have a profound influence on the patterns of performance we see in our model. Indeed, the sensitivity of the model to these factors is crucial to our account of the phenomena we plan to address. This sensitivity, however, raises an important methodological issue for the modeling effort: If the pattern of performance we obtain depends so strongly on the structure of the experience built into the model's environment, then shouldn't we take careful account of the details of real experience in constructing the particular set of patterns used in training? Of course, the answer to this question is yes in principle, but in practice it is not at all a simple matter to characterize or quantify the actual experience children have. Rather than attempt this, our approach has been to explore the effects of variation both in the frequency structure and in the similarity structure of the training items. Our investigations begin with the network introduced at the end of chapter 3, using localist input units and the corpus of training experiences from appendix B, table AB.3. Our claim is not that we have faithfully captured the frequency and similarity structure of objects in the world, but that we have produced a model that has the appropriate kinds of sensitivity to frequency and similarity structure, and that this sensitivity is the key to understanding the types of phenomena we are considering.

A PDP Account of Basic-Level Effects

Labeling Conventions

The terms *basic level*, *superordinate*, and *subordinate* are potentially confusing since, as we noted in chapter 1, the basic level does not occupy a fixed level of the conceptual hierarchy in all cases. Accordingly, we adopt the following conventions when referring to the level of inclusiveness at which a particular name applies, both in the model and in the real world. We will use the term *basic name* to indicate labels that identify an object at an intermediate level of specificity, approximating the name commonly given to typical category exemplars by ordinary members of a language community in free-naming tasks. In the model, the basic names are *tree*, *flower*, *bird*, *fish*, *cat*, *dog*, *mouse*, *goat*, and *pig*. Labels that identify an item at a more inclusive level than the basic name will be referred to as *general* names, while those that identify objects at a more specific level will be termed *specific* names. The general names in the model are *animal* and *plant*, and the specific names are *pine*, *oak*, *maple*, *birch*, *rose*, *daisy*, *tulip*, *sunflower*, *robin*, *canary*, *sparrow*, *penguin*, *sunfish*, *salmon*, *flounder*, and *cod*. In the model's environment, there are no specific names for the cat, dog, mouse, goat, or pig.

In Rumelhart's original simulations (and in those presented in chapter 3), the three naming levels mapped transparently onto the clustering structure of the environment—specific names described individual items, basic names applied to sets of items with many properties in common, and general names referred to larger groupings of objects with some shared attributes. However, in reality, labels do not always map so nicely onto the similarity structure of the world. The same name may be given to a small group of dissimilar objects—for example, the word "pet" could refer to a parrot, a dog, or a goldfish, but is not likely to indicate a stork, a deer, or a sturgeon. Conversely, groupings of similar objects may exist for which no common label exists in the language environment. For instance, although *four-legged land animals* seem to form a psychologically natural group of highly similar and distinctive objects in the world, there is no single English word used to refer to this category.

For the sake of clarity, then, it is useful to distinguish between the level of specificity at which an item is named and the level of inclusiveness at which the similarity structure in the domain is described. When discussing the similarity among the training patterns in our simulations at different levels of inclusiveness, we will use the term *global cluster* to refer to groups of similar instances at the most inclusive level; *intermediate cluster* to describe such groupings at an intermediate level of specificity; and *specific cluster* to refer to the very specific set of items represented by individual input units in the *Item* layer.

In the simulations described in this chapter, there are two global clusters—plants and animals—and five intermediate clusters: trees, flowers, birds, fish, and a group of four-legged mammals (henceforth just called mammals). The birds, fish, trees, and flowers were assigned names just as in the previous simulations: each item received a specific, basic, and general name, and these mapped transparently onto the similarity structure of the property vectors. The mammals, though, represent a special case. By virtue of sharing many properties with one another, and relatively few with the birds and fish, these five items constitute an intermediate cluster. However, in our model there is no name used to refer to the group of mammals. Instead, each was assigned a unique basic name as described above. These animals were not given specific names, because the different types were not further differentiated in the input. That is, the model has no basis for distinguishing among different kinds of cats, dogs, mice, goats, or pigs (but see appendix C for a simulation involving a set of five different dogs and five identical cats). Thus, each mammal could be labeled with its basic name, or with the general name *animal*, but not with a more specific name.

Word-Frequency Corpus Analysis

Because our explanation of basic-level naming effects depends partly on the frequency with which items are named at different levels of specificity, it is important that the training regime adopted in the simulation is informed by knowledge of the frequency of these words in the real world. In the simulations in chapter 3, this was clearly not the case: when required to name an item, the network was always trained to simultaneously activate all the correct name units in the output. For example, in response to the input *pine ISA*, the network learned to activate the *pine*, *tree*, and *plant* units. Because general names such as *plant* apply to more items than do specific names like *pine*, they were more often active as targets as the network learned. In effect, the network got more frequent exposure to more inclusive names during learning.

Empirically, it is difficult to make accurate generalizations about the relative frequency of words at different levels of specificity. Some studies of word frequency in children's vocabularies (Brown

1958) and child-directed speech (Mervis and Mervis 1982) show basic names to be most frequent overall in a child's linguistic environment. In contrast, Rosch et al. (1976) argued that basic-level primacy in lexical acquisition could not arise from word frequencies alone, because the superordinate labels used in her experiments were more frequent than the basic-level labels for some categories. However, one may question the validity of this assertion, because Rosch relied on word-frequency data from Kucera and Francis's norms (Kucera and Francis 1967), which derive from a corpus of written documents that are unlikely to be representative of the child's linguistic environment. To help inform our choice of word frequencies used in training the model, we examined a more representative corpus: Brown's corpus of mother-child linguistic interactions in natural settings for Adam, Eve, and Sarah (Brown 1973). This is a corpus of actual conversational exchanges between mother and child, recorded in a variety of natural settings during a three-year span when the children ranged in age from 1 year and 6 months (Eve) to 5 years and 1 month (Sarah). We examined the entire corpus for both Adam and Sarah, and counted the number of times a mother used each of a set of general, basic, or specific nouns.

The nouns we examined appear in table 5.2. They are based on the categories employed by Rosch et al. (1976) in their explorations of basic-level effects, with a few additions. Whereas Rosch initially considered the categories *tree*, *bird*, and *fish* to be superordinates, her experiments demonstrated that these are treated as basic by most North American subjects. Thus, we counted these as basic nouns, and added the words "animal" and "plant" to our list as the corresponding general names. We also added the word "flower" to provide consistency with the model, and a variety of land-animal names selected from the category *four-legged animals* in Battig and Montague's 1969 study of category-listing norms. We did not include more specific nouns for the inanimate categories (such as "wing-back chair"), because a spot check revealed that these were rarely if ever used in child-directed speech. However, we did

Table 5.2   Nouns used in our analysis of word frequency by noun type in child-directed speech

GENERAL	BASIC	SPECIFIC
Musical instrument	Guitar, Piano, Drum, Trumpet, Violin, Clarinet, Flute, Saxophone, Trombone, Oboe	—
Fruit	Apple, Orange, Pear, Banana, Peach, Grapes, Cherry, Plum, Grapefruit, Lemon	—
Tools	Hammer, Saw, Nails, Screwdriver, Level, Plane, Chisel, Ruler, Wrench, Pliers	—
Clothes	Shirt, Socks, Pants, Shoes, Blouse, Skirt, Coat, Dress, Hat, Sweater	—
Furniture	Chair, Table, Bed, Sofa, Desk, Lamp, Couch, Dresser, Television, Stool	—
Vehicle	Car, Bus, Airplane, Train, Truck, Bicycle, Motorcycle, Boat, Scooter, Wagon	—
Plant	Tree	oak, maple, pine, elm, apple, birch, cherry, dogwood, spruce, redwood
	Flower	rose, tulip, carnation, daisy, violet, orchid, chrysanthemum, lily, pansy, petunia
Animal	Fish	trout, bass, shark, herring, catfish, perch, salmon, tuna, goldfish, swordfish
	Bird	robin, sparrow, cardinal, bluejay, eagle, crow, bluebird, canary, parakeet, hawk
	Dog, Cat, Horse, Cow, Lion, Tiger, Elephant, Pig, Bear, Mouse, Goat	

include specific nouns for the four categories of living objects used in the simulations: *birds*, *fish*, *trees*, and *flowers*. For three of these categories (birds, fish, and trees) we chose the same subordinate names used by Rosch et al. (1976). In the case of *flowers*, we selected the ten most frequently listed flowers from Battig and Montague's (1969) category-listing norms.

We then counted the number of times each word was used in child-directed speech according to the Brown corpus, for Adam and Sarah's protocols, using the CHILDES online corpus (MacWhinney 1994). For ambiguous words such as "drum," which may be considered a noun or verb, or "plane," which might refer to a tool or vehicle, we examined the word in context to disambiguate it. We also grouped together variations on a stem, such as "clothes" and "clothing," or "dog" and "doggie." Only nouns were counted, and we included both singular and plural tokens.

Figure 5.1 shows the frequencies of the various words on our list, plotted against a log scale, in Adam's mother's speech. Basic nouns are plotted on the right-hand side of each line, whereas general and specific labels appear on the left. General labels are shown in capital letters, and specific labels are shown in italics.

There are several aspects of this data to note. First, there is considerable variability in the frequency of basic labels—they span the range from least to most frequent in every category. Second, the most frequent basic labels for all categories are more frequent than the general label. In fact, with the exception of "animal," general labels appear infrequently or not at all. Note that this cannot be because exemplars of the category were never discussed. For all categories, some reference was made to some exemplar (as indicated by the presence of the basic names); however, mothers rarely chose to use the general label in doing so. Third, of the forty specific nouns we examined, only three appeared at all in the mothers' speech, and even these occurred only rarely. In this case, it is difficult to tell whether the low frequency of occurrence arises because, for example, there are simply no appropriate items (such as blue jays) to talk about in the experimental setting, or whether

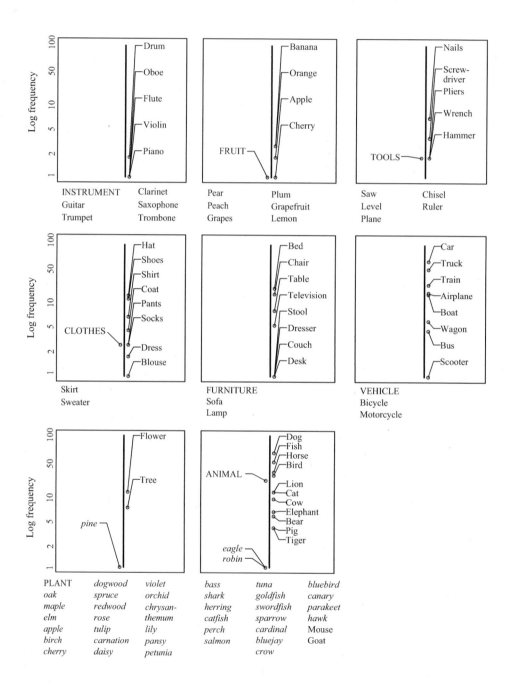

such items abound but the mother prefers to use the label "bird" to describe them.

Given these results, it seems safe (to a first approximation) to conclude that the most frequent basic labels appear more often than do more general or specific labels in the child's linguistic environment. In simulation 5.1, we train the model with frequencies that reflect this observation. To understand how this particular choice influences the model's behavior, we will then train it in an artificial situation, in which names at all levels occur equally frequently in the corpus (simulations 5.2 and 5.3). We will see that word frequency and representational structure interact in the model to explain basic-level effects.

Simulation 5.1: Learning with Basic Names Most Frequent

To manipulate word frequencies in the network's training environment, we added three new units to the *Relation* layer, which we designated *ISA-general*, *ISA-basic*, and *ISA-specific*. These units represent different contexts in which naming can occur. For example, the input unit *ISA-general* indicates a context in which the appropriate response is a general word describing the object in the *Item* layer—for the input *pine ISA-general*, the correct response is *plant*. The input unit *ISA-specific* indicates a context in which a specific name is appropriate (e.g., *pine*), and the input unit *ISA-basic* indicates a context in which the basic name is required (e.g., *tree*). Each item and *ISA*-relation pair uniquely determines a name

Figure 5.1   The figure shows the frequency of the words in table 5.3, as they appeared in speech directed to Adam by his mother, plotted against a log scale. Basic-level nouns appear on the right side of each line, and more general or specific names appear on the left. More general labels are shown in uppercase letters, whereas more specific names are shown in italics. Words that did not appear at all are listed below each plot. Most superordinates and subordinates were not found in the corpus. Where superordinate nouns do appear, they are generally less frequent than the most frequent basic labels. The corresponding frequencies for Sarah, which exhibited the same patterns, are not shown.

response in the output. Thus we were able to manipulate the frequency with which names at different levels of inclusiveness appear in the training environment. (When asked to provide a specific name for one of the mammal items, the model was simply trained to turn all the name units off.)

In simulation 5.1, we trained the model by selecting a set of training patterns from the model's environment at random in each epoch. Associated with each pattern was a probability, which determined the likelihood and frequency with which the pattern was chosen for presentation in a given epoch. We "sampled" each pattern by choosing a random number from a uniform distribution between zero and one, and comparing it to the probability associated with the pattern. If the number was less than this probability, we added the pattern to the set that comprised the epoch. In a single epoch, each pattern was sampled 1,000 times. Hence, a pattern with an associated probability of 0.03 was likely to occur thirty times in a given epoch. The training patterns were resampled independently for each training epoch. Once selected, the order of the patterns within the epoch was randomized.

The pattern probabilities were assigned to satisfy three constraints:

1. Each basic name appeared as a target three times more often than the corresponding general or specific names in the network's training environment.
2. Plant and animal items appeared equally frequently as inputs in the training environment.
3. Only 20 percent of the training trials required the model to produce a name as output. The other three relation contexts appeared equally frequently to one another.

Table 5.3 shows the expected number of presentations for each training pattern across 10,000 training trials (rounded to the nearest integer) for the probabilities we used.[1] Individual items are listed in the columns, and different contexts are shown in the rows. The table indicates the mean number of times in 10,000 trials that a given item was paired with a particular context. For example, the

Table 5.3 Mean number of times each pattern appears in 10,000 pattern presentations (basic names are shown in boldface)

Items	PLANT		ANIMAL		
	tree	flower	bird	fish	
	pine	rose	robin	salmon	**cat**
	oak	daisy	canary	sunfish	**dog**
	maple	tulip	sparrow	flounder	**mouse**
	birch	sunflower	penguin	cod	**goat**
					pig
ISA-specific	40	40	40	40	40
ISA-basic	30	30	30	30	120
ISA-general	5	5	3	3	3
is	167	167	111	111	90
can	167	167	111	111	90
has	167	167	111	111	90

item *pine* was paired with the context *ISA-specific* 40 times, with the context *ISA-basic* 30 times, and with the context *ISA-general* 5 times. This means that overall, the name *pine* occurred as a target 40 times; the name *tree* occurred as a target 120 times (30 times for each of 4 different trees); and the name *plant* occurred 40 times (5 times for each of 8 different plants). A close inspection of table 5.3 will reveal that the same is true for all names—each specific and general name occurred as a target 40 times in 10,000 training trials, whereas each basic name (including the 5 basic mammal names) occurred 120 times. Thus, basic names were three times more frequent in the training corpus than were more general or specific names, providing a rough correspondence to our analysis of word frequencies described above. Note also that the 8 individual plants occurred 167 times each with each of the *is*, *can*, and *has* contexts, so that in each context a plant item appeared as input 1,336 times in 10,000 training trials. The 4 birds and 4 fish all appeared 111 times with each of these contexts, whereas the 5 animals appeared 90 times—thus an animal item appeared as input 1,338 times in 10,000 trials with these contexts $((4*111) + (4*111) + (5*90))$.

As in the simulations described in the previous chapter, we added random noise from a Gaussian distribution centered around zero, with a variance of 0.05, to the net inputs of all the hidden units in the network. We also trained the model with softer targets in this and subsequent simulations. That is, instead of requiring the model to produce either a zero or a one on its output units, we trained it to produce either a 0.05 (for output units that were meant to be off) or a 0.95 (for units that were meant to be on). This prevented the most frequent patterns from dominating learning after they had been more or less mastered by the network. We employed a learning rate of 0.005 to ensure that all properties in the corpus were mastered. Weights were updated after every epoch. The larger training corpus and word-frequency manipulation required that the network be trained for 12,000 epochs before it could activate all the properties to within 0.1 of their targets. See appendix A for a summary of the training details.

Naming at Different Levels of Specificity

To investigate the model's ability to name at different points during development, we turned off learning in the model and probed it with each item/*ISA*-relation pair. In figure 5.2 we show the activation of the correct name units at each level of specificity, averaged across all items. Because the five mammals were not assigned specific names, these instances were not included in the analysis (inclusion of these items in the results for the basic and general levels does not alter the pattern of results). In general the basic name is the most strongly activated throughout training.

To simulate the picture-naming task, in which there is no context constraining which level of response is appropriate, we again adopted the heuristic suggested by Levelt (1989), and selected the

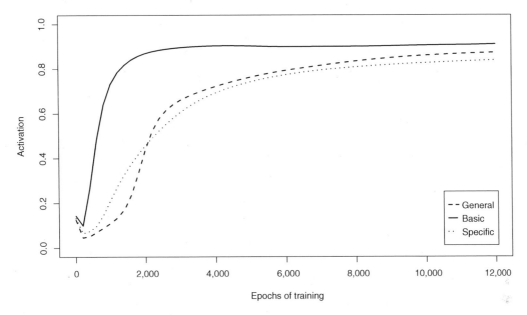

Figure 5.2   Average activation of the correct name units across training, for all items excluding mammals at each level of specificity. Each point corresponds to the activation of the correct general, basic, or specific name unit, averaged across the sixteen nonmammal items, after a given amount of training.

most specific response active above threshold when the network was queried with each *ISA* relation in turn. Table 5.4 shows that, like children, the network learned to name each item with its basic name first.

As discussed previously, Rosch et al. (1976) found that, for many objects, subjects are quicker to verify membership in basic categories, relative to more general or specific categories. Though our model is a simple feed-forward network whose unit states do not build up over time, we can take the strength of activation for each output unit to indicate how quickly a cascaded implementation would be able to activate the corresponding properties (Plaut et al. 1996). In a cascaded network, the stronger the net input, the more quickly the unit will activate. Hence, the strength of activation of an output unit in our model can be interpreted as a proxy for the

Table 5.4   Model's naming response when the name-selection heuristic is applied with a threshold of 0.7

OBJECT	200 EPOCHS	2,000 EPOCHS	4,000 EPOCHS	6,000 EPOCHS	8,000 EPOCHS
pine	No response	tree	tree	pine	pine
oak	No response	tree	tree	tree	oak
maple	No response	tree	maple	maple	maple
birch	No response	tree	birch	birch	birch
rose	No response	flower	flower	rose	rose
daisy	No response	flower	flower	daisy	daisy
tulip	No response	flower	tulip	tulip	tulip
sunflower	No response	flower	sunflower	sunflower	sunflower
robin	No response	bird	robin	robin	robin
canary	No response	bird	bird	canary	canary
sparrow	No response	bird	sparrow	sparrow	sparrow
penguin	No response	bird	penguin	penguin	penguin
sunfish	No response	fish	sunfish	sunfish	sunfish
salmon	No response	fish	fish	salmon	salmon
flounder	No response	fish	fish	flounder	flounder
cod	No response	fish	fish	cod	cod

time taken to retrieve the corresponding name or property, with stronger activations indicating a faster reaction time.

By inspecting figure 5.2, we can see the average activation of the correct name units, at different points during learning. The basic name is most active on average at each stage, even after 12,000 epochs of learning. Taking the strength of activation to indicate the speed with which the model can verify category membership, the model is "fastest" to verify information at the basic level. The effect does become smaller over time, as the network gradually continues to improve its overall performance toward ceiling levels.

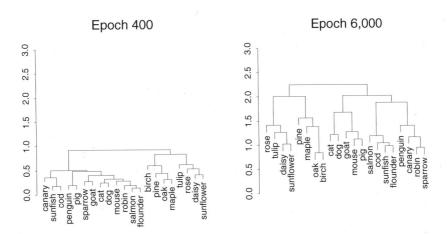

Figure 5.3   Hierarchical cluster analysis of the model's internal representations after 400 and 6,000 epochs of training. Despite the advantage shown by the network in learning to name at the basic level, its internal representations undergo the same coarse-to-fine differentiation described in simulations 3.1 and 4.1.

Despite this advantage for learning and activating names at the basic level, the network's internal representations undergo the same coarse-to-fine differentiation seen in simulations 3.1 and 4.1. Figure 5.3 shows that, after 400 epochs of training, the model correctly differentiates items in global categories, but confuses more specific distinctions. By 6,000 epochs, the network correctly represents the semantic relationships among objects at all levels of granularity.

Naming in Dementia

Figure 5.4 shows the network's average naming performance over the course of deterioration. Initially, basic names are most active, followed by more general and then more specific names. As damage increases, however, activation drops off more quickly for the basic names than for the general names. With large amounts of damage, the network's ability to produce the correct general name is more robust than its ability to produce the correct basic name.

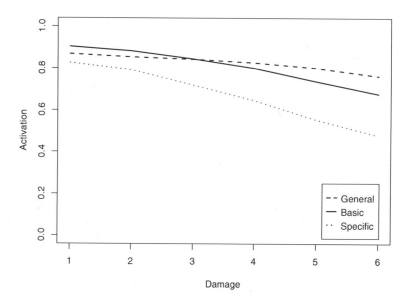

Figure 5.4 Average activation of correct name units for all items excluding mammals, at different levels of specificity under increasing amounts of damage in simulation 5.1. Though the undamaged network most strongly activates the basic name for each item, its ability to name under damage is most robust for more general labels.

Thus, although basic names were the first to be learned, and were the most strongly active in the undamaged network, they were more vulnerable to damage than were general names.

The results show that the robustness of general naming in response to degradation of internal representations found previously was not caused by the unrealistically high general "word frequencies" employed during training in the earlier simulation. The network's ability to name at the most inclusive level degrades least rapidly, even when general labels are one-third as frequent as basic labels in the training corpus. Whereas the network's general-naming responses were the best preserved under damage, basic-naming responses were the first to be acquired, and the most robustly activated at the end of training. Thus the robust preservation of general knowledge in patients with semantic dementia need not conflict with data supporting basic-level primacy in lexical acquisition and category verification. Similarly, the idea that concepts differentiate in a coarse-to-fine manner coexists with basic-level primacy phenomena in naming in the context of the model.

Simulation 5.2: Learning with All Names Equally Frequent

In simulation 5.1, the model first learned to activate each item's basic name (and to activate it most strongly) when these labels were more frequent in the linguistic environment. However, Rosch et al. (1976) argued that word frequency alone could not explain basic-level advantages in naming, because at least for some objects, more general names are more frequent in the linguistic environment than are basic labels. To what extent do the basic-level effects we observed simply reflect the frequency with which the network was trained to produce basic labels?

To address this question, we trained the network in an artificial situation, in which all names at every level of specificity appeared as targets equally often in the training environment. Thus the name units *animal*, *bird*, and *robin* occurred as targets in the corpus an equal number of times in every epoch. Note that, to achieve this, each individual item was named most frequently with its specific name, least frequently with its general name, and at an intermediate frequency with its basic name. For example, because there are thirteen items to which the name *animal* applies, and only a single item to which the name *robin* applies, the input pattern *robin ISA-specific* was shown to the network thirteen times more often than the pattern *robin ISA-general*. As a consequence, across the entire training corpus, the name *animal* and the name *robin* appeared as targets an equal number of times. Table 5.5 shows the expected number of times each pattern appeared in 10,000 trials, rounded to the nearest integer. The training proceeded exactly as described in the last section.

Table 5.5 Mean number of times each pattern appears in 10,000 pattern presentations in simulation 5.2 (basic names are shown in boldface)

	PLANT		ANIMAL		
	tree	*flower*	*bird*	*fish*	
Items	pine	rose	robin	salmon	**cat**
	oak	daisy	canary	sunfish	**dog**
	maple	tulip	sparrow	flounder	**mouse**
	birch	sunflower	penguin	cod	**goat**
					pig
ISA-specific	63	63	63	63	63
ISA-basic	16	16	16	16	63
ISA-general	8	8	5	5	5
is	167	167	111	111	90
can	167	167	111	111	90
has	167	167	111	111	90

Naming Behavior

The left-hand graph in figure 5.5 displays, at different epochs of training, the activation of the correct name unit at each level of specificity, averaged across the sixteen nonmammal items. With frequencies equalized, we see that the network still produces a slight basic-level advantage, but the effect is considerably smaller than before, and after about 2,000 epochs differences between the levels become negligible. When damaged, general-naming responses continued to be the most robust, as expected (see the right-hand side of figure 5.5).

The small overall advantage for basic- over subordinate-level names varies considerably across items in the training set, reflecting typicality effects. Figure 5.6 considers the activation of the correct basic and specific name units throughout learning for two of the birds: the *penguin* and the *sparrow*. Given the features used in our corpus, *sparrow* is a very typical bird and *penguin* is much less

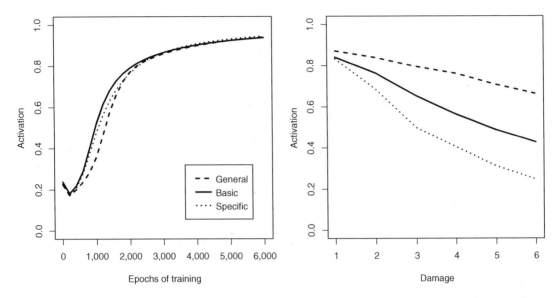

Figure 5.5 Average activation of correct name units during training and under damage when the word frequencies are made equal in the corpus. Unlike simulation 5.1, the network shows little tendency to activate the basic name most strongly on average. General naming responses are still most robust in the face of damage.

typical. By *typicality*, we refer to the degree to which an item shares properties with other items predicated by the same basic name. *Penguin* is an atypical bird, because it lacks a property shared by the other birds (*can fly*), and has other properties that differentiate it from the other birds (*can swim, is big*). *Sparrow* is fairly typical, because it has all of the properties generally common to birds, and few differentiating properties. For the atypical item *penguin*, its specific name *penguin* was learned more quickly than the basic name *bird*, but the basic name *bird* was learned more quickly for the typical item *sparrow*.

   To more systematically investigate these typicality effects, we calculated a basic-level typicality score for each item, designed to measure the extent to which each item shares properties with other objects described by the same basic name. Our measure of basic-level typicality was calculated as follows. For all the items

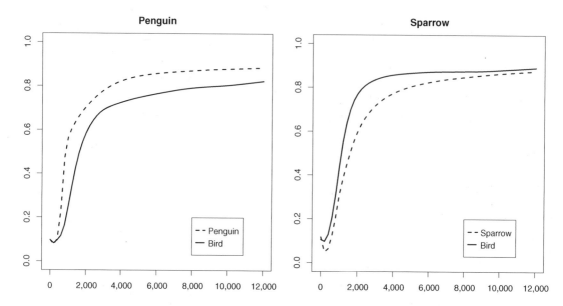

Figure 5.6   Activation of the correct name units at basic and specific levels for the atypical item *penguin* and the typical item *sparrow* when the network is trained with all words equally frequent in the corpus.

described by a basic name—for example, all the trees—we averaged the attribute vectors, to find the group centroid. To assess typicality for each object in the group, we took the normalized dot product of its attribute vector with the group centroid. Intuitively, this measure describes the extent to which a given item deviates from the group's central tendency in its attributes. The score ranges from 0 to 1, with 1 indicating a highly typical item—that is, an item with many properties in common with the other items in the group.

Of interest is how the network's ability to learn and strongly activate an object's specific or basic name varies with the item's typicality. Thus, we also assigned to each item a *lexical specificity index* based on the relative activations of its specific and basic name units over the course of learning. Every 200 epochs during learning, we assessed the network's ability to name each item at basic and specific levels, by querying it with the appropriate item-relation pair. At each point, we subtracted the activation of the correct basic name from the activation of the correct specific name. Thus, for the item *pine*, if the name *pine* was more active than the name *tree* for the *pine* item at a given point during training, the difference at that point was positive. For each item, we calculated this difference averaged across the entire course of learning:

$$\text{LSI} = \frac{\Sigma_e(s_e - b_e)}{n_e}$$

where e indexes the points during training where performance was assessed (once every 200 epochs for 12,000 epochs), n_e indicates the total number of times performance was assessed, s_e is the activation of the correct specific name unit at epoch e when the network is queried with the input *ISA-specific*, and b_e is the activation of the correct basic name unit at epoch e when the network is queried with the input *ISA-basic*.

We ran this simulation ten times, with different random initial starting weights, and calculated the average LSI across all ten runs to ensure that the results we report are not due to a chance configuration of starting weights.

Figure 5.7 shows the relationship between typicality and LSI for the sixteen nonmammal items in the model, averaged across ten simulation runs. Mammals were excluded from the analysis, because they did not have specific names. Points above the zero line represent concepts for which the specific name was most strongly activated, while points below indicate concepts for which the basic name was most strongly activated. The plot shows a strong relationship between typicality and LSI: atypical items activated specific names more strongly on average, while typical items tended to activate names at the basic level most strongly. Every name appeared as a target equally often during training, so these differences do not result from differences in word frequencies.

This interaction between an item's typicality and the rate at which the model learns names at different levels of specificity may also

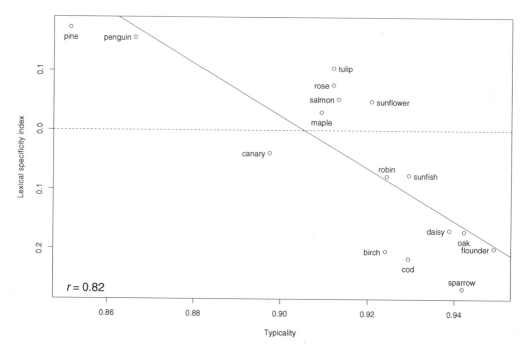

Figure 5.7 Relationship between typicality and the lexical specificity index. Points above the zero line indicate items for which the network activated the specific name most strongly (averaged across all points during training). Points below the line indicate items for which the network tended to activate the basic name most strongly across learning. The figure shows a strong relationship between typicality and the lexical specificity index, with highly typical objects most strongly activating basic names, and atypical items most strongly activating specific names.

help to explain another aspect of children's early naming behavior: their tendency to restrict basic names to typical category members only. Recall from the introduction that, during early word learning, children can inappropriately restrict their use of names to typical members of a category only—denying, for example, that the name "ball" could apply to a football (Chapman and Mervis 1989). Could an item's typicality also affect whether the model can name it correctly at the basic level during early learning? To answer this question, we calculated how many epochs of training the network required on average to activate the correct basic name for each item

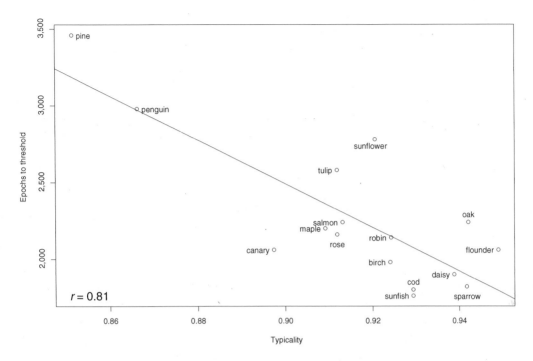

Figure 5.8 Relationship between typicality and the number of epochs the network took to activate the correct basic name above a threshold of 0.7. Note that between epochs 2,400 and 3,000, the network passed through a period in which the name *bird* exceeded threshold for all birds except the penguin, and the name *tree* exceeded threshold for all trees except the pine. Like children, the network restricted these names to typical items during this period.

above a threshold of 0.7 in simulation 5.2. We then plotted this data against the item's typicality score.

The results, shown in figure 5.8, indicate a strong relationship between typicality and the number of epochs needed to activate the correct basic name above threshold. The network generally takes longer to learn the basic name for atypical items. By epoch 2,400, the model learned to correctly apply the name *bird* to all of the birds except the penguin, and the name *tree* to all of the trees except the pine. During the period of learning between 2,400 and 3,000 epochs, then, the network inappropriately restricted the names *tree* and *bird* to typical items only, similar to the pattern often seen in children (e.g., Chapman and Mervis 1989).

Simulation 5.3: Effects of the Attribute Structure of the Training Corpus

These results suggest that the basic-level advantages described in simulation 5.1 were due in part to the greater frequency of basic names relative to other names across the training corpus in that experiment. However, the finding that typicality strongly influences the rate at which the network learns basic relative to specific names suggests that the attribute structure of the environment also plays a role in the model's naming behavior. In simulation 5.3, our goal was to systematically investigate these effects, to understand how the model's behavior changes as the attribute structure of its environment varies. We again trained the network in an artificial situation, in which all names appeared equally often in the corpus. However, in this simulation, we also systematically varied the assignment of properties to items. We ran four simulations, each with a different training corpus.

The similarity matrices for each training set are shown in figure 5.9. Each matrix shows how similar the various items were to one another, considering their *is*, *can*, and *has* properties but not their names. In the *original structure* condition, we used the same output training patterns as in simulation 5.2. In the *intermediate structure only* condition, items from the same intermediate category (trees, flowers, birds, fish, or mammals) were made highly similar to one another, but global similarities were eliminated. To accomplish this, we simply turned off all of the attributes that reliably discriminated between global categories. For example, properties such as *can move* (which is shared by all the animals but by none of the trees) and *has roots* (shared by the plants) were set to zero. Also, properties that tended to be shared by members of an intermediate category were made perfectly regular in this respect —that is, they were made to be shared by all members of the cate-

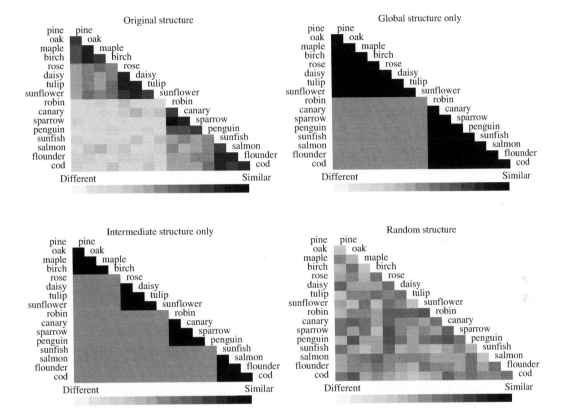

Figure 5.9 Dot-product measure of similarity across output property vectors in the four conditions of simulation 5.3. Dark squares indicate pairs of items with similar sets of output properties.

gory and by no members of contrasting categories. For instance, in our original corpus, the property *can fly* was true of three of the four birds, but not true of the penguin, whereas *can swim* was true of the penguin in addition to all four fish. In the *intermediate structure only* condition, *can fly* was assigned to all of the birds including the penguin, and *can swim* was assigned to all four fish but not to the penguin. Finally, all individuating features (save the specific names) were turned off for each item. For example, the property *is yellow*, which distinguishes the canary from its neighbors, was turned off. The consequence of these manipulations was to make items from the same intermediate category very similar to one another, but dissimilar to items from the same domain—for instance, flowers were no more similar to trees than to fish. The network continued to receive some pressure to differentiate items, because it was required to name them all with a unique specific name.

In the *global structure only* condition, global similarities were preserved, and intermediate structure eliminated. In this case, properties such as *can move* (which reliably differentiate plants from animals) were made perfectly regular, while properties such as *can fly* and *has petals* (which discriminate among intermediate categories) were set to zero. Individuating features were again turned off. Hence, items from the same global category were very similar to one another, but intermediate category structure was eliminated: while *pine* was more similar to *rose* than to *salmon*, it was no more similar to *oak* than to *rose*.

In the *random structure* condition, features were assigned to items randomly: we assigned to each item 20 percent of the attributes, selected at random. Category membership did not influence output similarity in any way. In each of the four conditions, the network was trained as described in simulation 5.2, with each name occurring as a target an equal number of times in every epoch.

Figure 5.10 shows the average activation of the correct name units for the nonmammal items during learning for each training condition. As shown previously, the network learned to activate basic names a bit more rapidly than specific names and somewhat more rapidly than general names in the *original structure* condition. However, a very different pattern of acquisition was obtained in the other conditions. In the *global structure only* condition, the network activated the correct general name most strongly on average throughout learning. In the *intermediate structure only* condition, basic names were more highly activated at all points in

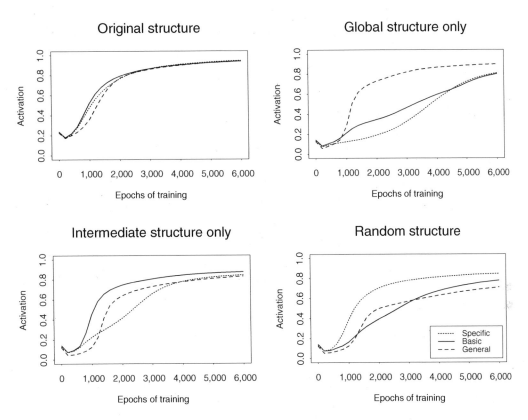

Figure 5.10   Average activation of the correct name units for nonmammal items in four simulations with different degrees of structure across output properties. When global but not basic structure is retained, the network first learns to activate the correct general name. When intermediate but not superordinate structure is retained, the model shows an advantage for learning the basic name. When the structure is completely random, the model learns the specific name most quickly and easily. In each simulation, all names were presented with equal frequency across the training corpus; hence, the observed differences did not result from differences in word frequency.

training. The network learned to activate specific names most quickly and strongly when there was no structure in the output properties.

Despite the fact that all names appeared equally often in the four conditions of this simulation, the network showed four different patterns of name acquisition. These results can be understood with reference to the similarity-based generalization that results from distributed representations. As we have seen, the structure of the output properties across items in the network's environment determines the similarity of the model's internal representations. In turn, these representations constrain how new learning generalizes from one item to another. When the network is trained to produce the output *tree* in response to the input *oak ISA-basic*, this response generalizes to the other typical trees in the set by virtue of their having similar internal representations. For most properties, such similarity-based generalization is appropriate, and the network benefits. However, when the network must learn how related items differ—for example, when it must learn to name at the specific level—similarity-based generalization can hinder its performance. The weights in the forward part of the network must grow comparatively large in order to work against the learned similarities between semantically related items. Thus, when groups of similar items share the same name, lexical acquisition is facilitated; when similar items have different names, similarity based generalization makes it difficult for the network to learn them. In the model, these effects interact with the frequency of the different naming responses produced for a particular input, to determine the strength with which a given name is activated. In simulation 5.2, to ensure that general names such as *animal* occurred with the same frequency as specific names like *sparrow* across the corpus, we required the network to name each individual item most often with its specific name. When the animal items had similar attributes, as they did in the *global structure only* condition in simulation 5.3, similarity-based generalization effects caused the general names to be learned first despite this choice of word frequencies. However, in the *random structure* condition, when few properties were shared across animals, there were no consistent facilitation or interference effects, and specific names were learned first. In the *intermediate structure only* condition, generalization and word frequency effects combined to give the basic names the upper hand.

Conclusions from Simulations 5.1–5.3

Simulation 5.3 demonstrates that basic-level advantages in acquisition can arise in the model when within-category similarities in the training set are high at the basic level, and low at the superordinate level—in other words, when basic categories are maximally informative and distinctive. The network showed this effect even when all names occurred equally frequently in the training corpus. The fact that we found a relatively small effect in simulation 5.2, then, resulted from our relatively arbitrary assignment of properties to items—in effect, the basic categories were not distinct and informative enough to produce a strong basic-level advantage when overall word frequencies were controlled.

More generally, these simulations suggest an explanation of basic-level advantages in semantic tasks, which builds on our analysis of conceptual differentiation in infancy. In this view, the attribute structure of the environment constrains the similarities among items represented in the semantic system as it learns. These similarities in turn interact with the frequency with which individual items are labeled with a given name, to determine how readily the name "comes to mind" in a given context. Though we have focused primarily on naming in the simulations, the same account applies equally well to other kinds of attributes. From this perspective, names are not special in any way—the same forces affect the ease with which the system can generate the correct response in reaction to any query. "Basic" categories are the groups of items for which similarity-based generalization results in the greatest benefit and the least interference in learning most properties. The fact that such categories are informative—their exemplars have many properties in common—means that similarity-based facilitation will enable the semantic system to quickly learn these common properties. That basic categories are distinctive means that they encounter little interference as the system learns about objects in neighboring categories. Thus, under this account, basic-level advantages in lexical acquisition and category verification arise from precisely those characteristics of basic categories first identified by Rosch—maximal informativeness and distinctiveness—acting in concert with the domain-general learning mechanisms embodied in the Rumelhart network.

Differences in frequency of occurrence between basic names and names at other levels certainly contribute to the basic-level advantage in our model but are not necessary to produce a basic-level effect. Indeed, we would suggest that such differences in frequency are not so much causes as effects—that is, the frequency structure of the language reflects the ease with which names come to mind, which in turn arises from the operation of similarity-based facilitation and interference processes. The resulting frequency differences do of course enhance the advantage of basic-level names, as we have seen in these simulations. In a sense, though, we view this frequency effect as secondary to the more fundamental similarity-based generalization process that gives rise to it.

The same principles that explain the overall advantage for the basic level in some of our simulations also provide an account of the relationship between typicality and basic-level effects. Because atypical items are represented as distal to more typical items, they are less susceptible to forces of similarity-based generalization. Hence the system is better able to learn idiosyncratic properties (such as specific names) for such instances, but is also slower to learn the properties they share with their more typical neighbors. We observed this effect in simulation 5.2, which showed that when word frequencies were controlled, specific names were more active on average than were basic names for atypical (but not typical) items, and that the model learned the correct basic name more quickly for typical than for atypical items.

Of course, the particular pattern of acquisition observed in the model depends on the particular distribution of events to which it is exposed during learning. We have investigated the poles of some of the parameters influencing the model's behavior: the frequency with which it encounters names at different levels of specificity, and the degree of similarity structure apparent in the distribution of attributes across different groupings of items in the environment. There are other parameter choices between these poles that we have not yet investigated, which might have greater ecological validity. For example, in all the simulations we have discussed, the model was given a great deal of exposure to properties shared by items in the same global category: properties such as *has skin, can move*, and *has roots*. This choice contributes to the general-to-specific differentiation of concepts investigated in chapters 3 and 4, and as we have seen, it may also influence the degree to which basic-level naming advantages are observed when word frequencies are controlled. One might argue that in the real world, infants and children get little exposure to some of these kinds of properties, and hence that a better choice would be to train the model with fewer such properties. These issues are extremely difficult to adjudicate, and we do not wish to take a strong stand on the matter, although we do note that some properties not included in our training corpus (having visually apparent eyes, for example) are consistently observed in animals but never found in plants (as discussed in chapter 2).

In any case, our simulations have explored an extreme example of what would happen if there were absolutely no coherent covariation of properties at the superordinate level. The *intermediate structure only* condition in simulation 5.3 represents just such a position: no information about global similarity structure was provided in the model's environment in that simulation. We may interpolate from such an extreme simulation to understand how the model might behave under different parameter choices. To the extent that intermediate structure is most apparent in the attribute structure of the environment, the system will show stronger basic-level effects, and will differentiate between intermediate categories more quickly. To the extent that global structure is apparent in the environment, basic-level advantages will be weakened, and the system will take longer to differentiate among intermediate categories. These effects will interact with the frequency with which particular names and properties are encountered in the world, to determine the strength with which the property is activated in a particular semantic task.

Influences of Differential Experience with Objects and Their Properties: Familiarity and Expertise Effects

The Rumelhart model provides a means of situating long-established basic-level phenomena within a broader theoretical framework that also encompasses progressive concept differentiation and the robust preservation of general information in disturbed semantic cognition. Our account of these phenomena suggests that the frequency and similarity structure of one's experience with various objects in the world importantly constrains the semantic representations one acquires, and the pattern of behavior one exhibits in semantic tasks. One implication of this view is that different constellations of experiences should give rise to different semantic representations and different patterns of performance in different individuals. In this section we will consider how semantic task performance varies with differences in the structure of experience, both in the model and in empirical studies. As we will see, the simulations allow us to understand frequency effects in naming during early childhood and in semantic dementia, as well as several interesting phenomena arising in the study of expertise.

Simulation 5.4: Effects of Familiarity on Naming in Development and Dementia

We will begin by considering how the model's naming behavior is influenced by its familiarity with a given concept, and in particular, the robust finding that both children and semantic dementia patients will inappropriately extend familiar category names to semantically related objects (e.g., labeling a picture of a pig with the name *dog*; see Hodges, Graham, and Patterson 1995 for further discussion). We suggest that these behaviors arise as a consequence of principles familiar from the preceding work: children overextend familiar names to related objects as a consequence of similarity-based generalization in early learning, whereas semantic dementia patients misattribute the properties of familiar or typical instances to related objects as a result of the learned mappings between these properties and subregions of the representation space.

To simulate the effect of familiarity, we trained the model with the same corpus of training patterns used in simulation 5.1 (see appendix B, table AB.3), but with the frequencies adjusted so that dog patterns were encountered more frequently than were the other mammal patterns in each epoch of training. Specifically, we conducted three simulation runs, with each dog pattern (e.g., *dog is*, *dog can*, *dog has*, *dog ISA-specific*, *dog ISA-basic*, *dog ISA-general*) appearing equally often (run 1), eight times more often (run 2), or sixteen times more often (run 3) than any other mammal pattern (see appendix A for pattern-frequency tables). Thus in runs 2 and 3, dogs were effectively more "familiar" to the model than were other mammals. In all three runs we ensured that the frequency of bird and fish patterns was equivalent to the total frequency of mammal patterns, and that the frequency of plant patterns was equivalent to the total frequency of animal patterns. Name frequencies were assigned as in simulation 5.1, so that basic names were three times as frequent as general and specific names. Otherwise the network was trained as described in the previous sections.

In figure 5.11, we plot the activations of all the name units for the first 5,000 epochs of training in run 2 (dogs eight times more frequent than other mammals), when the network is queried for the basic name of three items: *goat*, *robin*, and *oak*. Early in learning,

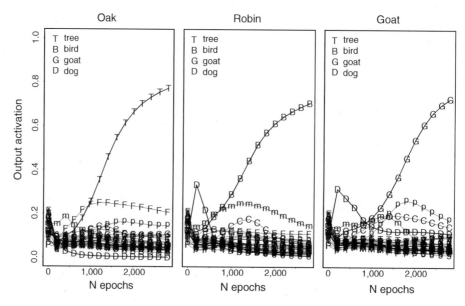

Figure 5.11   Activation of all the name units when the model is probed for its knowledge of basic names, in a network trained with dog patterns eight times as frequent as other mammal patterns in the environment. Early in learning, the network tends to inappropriately activate the name *dog*, especially for related objects.

the model shows a tendency to inappropriately activate the name *dog* for some items. This tendency is most persistent for the most similar concept (*goat*), more transient for the distantly related concept (*robin*), and not present at all for the unrelated concept (*oak*). No other name unit is inappropriately active for these inputs. Thus, like the children in Mervis's study, the network shows a tendency to extend the frequent label *dog* to similar objects during early word learning, but not to dissimilar objects.

The details of the network's tendency to overgeneralize depend on the details of its training experience. For example, the tendency to extend the name *dog* to birds and other nonmammals as well as to other mammals will depend on the degree of differentiation of mammals from nonmammals when naming begins, and this in turn will depend on the details of the similarity relationships between mammals and nonmammals as well as on relative frequencies of exposure to different kinds of information (including name information) about each. Thus, the model's tendency to extend the name *dog* even to robins may be somewhat unrealistic, and may reflect inadequacies of the training corpus. On the other hand, such extension of frequent mammal names to birds does occur in semantic dementia, especially for atypical birds (Hodges et al. 1995), so this aspect of the model's performance may not be completely inappropriate.

To investigate the influence of familiarity on naming in dementia, we damaged the model in the same manner described in chapter 3, and queried it to provide the names of various items using the same strategy described previously. Of particular interest in this simulation is the model's tendency to inappropriately extend the name *dog* to similar objects under damage. For each simulation run, we damaged the network fifty times at each of four levels of severity, and examined its responses when naming the five mammals. Specifically, we were interested in the model's *category-coordinate errors*—for example, how often did the model inappropriately name the pig a *dog, cat, mouse,* or *goat*?

In figure 5.12 we show the number of times each mammal name was given to an incorrect mammal item by the network under damage, when the network has been trained with dogs equally frequently, eight times more frequently, or sixteen times more frequently than other mammals. For example, the line labeled *cat* indicates the number of times the name *cat* was given to either the dog, mouse, goat, or pig. When all mammals appeared equally frequently in the model's training environment, the network overextended the five mammal names to an incorrect mammal with about equal frequency. However, when dogs appeared more often in the training environment, the network was much more likely to inappropriately overextend the name *dog* to a related item than any of the other mammal names.

Because the network is trained so frequently with the input *dog* paired with various relations, it learns to use the name *dog* even before it has successfully differentiated this item from other

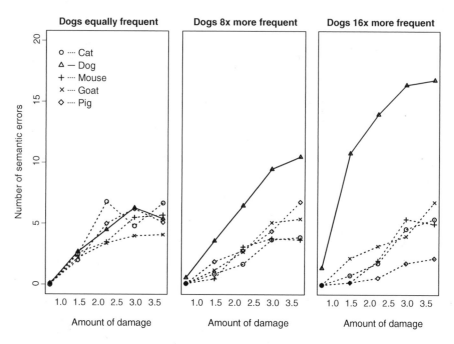

Figure 5.12   The figure shows the number of times each mammal name (*cat*, *dog*, *mouse*, *goat*, or *pig*) was given to an incorrect mammal instance by the network under increasing amounts of damage. For example, the line labeled *cat* indicates the number of times the name *cat* was given to either the dog, mouse, goat, or pig. The model more frequently extends the name *dog* to an incorrect mammal when dogs appear more frequently in the training environment.

animals. Consequently, similarity-based generalization leads the network to overextend the name to other animals early in learning. As the *dog* representation becomes differentiated from the other animals (first from the birds and fish, later from the other mammals), the network grows increasingly able to associate different responses with each animal, and the tendency to overextend the name is gradually eliminated.

The simulation also illustrates that under damage, the model is more likely to incorrectly apply a highly familiar name than a less familiar name to similar items. This tendency is quite clear in semantic dementia, and the model appears to be able to capture it. Exactly why does the model overextend frequent names? To consider this, we refer back to figure 3.9, which shows the distribution of items and predicates in an abstract semantic representation space. When we increase the relative frequency of dog patterns during training as we did in simulation 5.4, the region of semantic space predicated by the name *dog* grows. Consequently, when degradation in the form of noise is added to the system, neighboring items are increasingly likely to fall into this region.

To demonstrate this property of the model, we looked to see how its basic naming response changes as its internal representation state moves further and further away from the *dog* representation. We started by setting the *Representation* units in the model to the learned pattern corresponding to *dog*. We then gradually altered this pattern to make it more and more similar to one of the other learned mammal representations (such as the *cat*). The goal was to determine how far from the *dog* representation the network could get before it ceased to activate the name unit *dog*, and began to activate the name unit corresponding to the other mammal (e.g., *cat*). How does the model's behavior in this respect differ when it is trained with dogs as frequently or more frequently than other mammals?

Figure 5.13 shows what happens as the network's internal state moves from *dog* toward each of the other mammal representations. When the network was trained with all mammals equally frequent, the activation of the *dog* name unit declined with distance from the network's representation of *dog*, while the other mammal's name unit activation increased approximately symmetrically. When the network was trained in an environment with frequent dogs, however, the space to which the label *dog* applies expanded: the activation of *dog* did not decline until the internal representation state was very close to the other mammal's learned representation. It is apparent that the region of semantic space devoted to representing properties of dogs has ballooned outward.

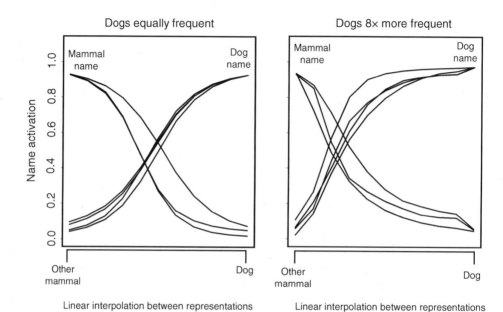

Figure 5.13 Activation of the various mammal name units as the network's internal representation state moves between the learned representation of *dog* and each of the other mammals, when the network is trained with dogs as frequent as other mammals (left), or eight times more frequent than other mammals (right). The lines labeled "Dog name" indicate the activation of the *dog* name unit as the network's representation state moves from the learned representation of *dog* (at the extreme right) toward each of the other four mammals (at the extreme left). The lines labeled "Mammal name" show the activation of the corresponding mammal name unit (e.g., *cat, mouse, goat,* or *pig*) throughout the same trajectory. The *x* axis corresponds to the value of the parameter *p* in the following linear interpolation formula used to create the interpolated representation *R*: $R = pD + (1 - p)T$, where *p* is the mixing proportion, *D* is the representation of *dog*, and *T* is the representation of the other (target) mammal—for example, *cat, mouse,* and so on. The name *dog* extends to a broader range of representation space when the network is trained with dogs more frequent in the environment (right-hand graph).

Simulation 5.5: Domain-Specific Expertise

Next we consider the range of phenomena arising from the study of expertise. Recall that experts prefer to name at the subordinate level in picture-naming tasks (Tanaka and Taylor 1991); verify category membership equally rapidly at the basic and subordinate levels (Tanaka and Taylor 1991; Johnson and Mervis 1997); and differentiate subordinate items to a greater degree in their domain of expertise (Boster and Johnson 1989). Here we will show that in our model, all three of these findings can arise as a simple consequence of more extensive exposure to the items in the expert domain. Increased experience in a domain leads to increased differentiation of item representations within the domain—so that learning and processing the attributes that individuate items within the domain are less influenced by similarity-based interference. We investigated these effects in the model in simulation 5.5.

To create "expert" networks, we manipulated the frequency of fish patterns relative to bird patterns in the training environment. Specifically, we created a bird expert by training a network with eight times more bird than fish patterns in the environment, and a fish expert by training it with eight times more fish than bird patterns. We also ensured that the sum totals of bird and fish patterns together were equivalent in the two training runs (see appendix A for frequency tables). We applied this frequency manipulation to all bird and fish patterns, including names, and assessed the network's naming behavior over the course of learning.

We again applied the Levelt heuristic for selecting the model's naming response, choosing the most specific name active above a threshold of 0.7. Table 5.6 shows the responses of both networks for all the birds and fish after 8,000 epochs of training, at which point they have learned to name all items within their domain of expertise with specific labels. Note that this does not indicate that the network does not know the correct basic name for objects in the domain of expertise—it simply means that both specific and basic names were active above threshold. By contrast, in the

Table 5.6   Naming responses for bird and fish "expert" networks after 8,000 epochs of training

OBJECT	FISH EXPERT	BIRD EXPERT
robin	bird	robin
canary	bird	canary
sparrow	bird	sparrow
penguin	bird	penguin
sunfish	sunfish	fish
salmon	salmon	fish
flounder	flounder	fish
cod	cod	fish

novice domain, both networks label all items with the correct basic name.

Category Verification

We examined the strength of activation of the specific and basic names for all of the birds and fish, to determine how expertise affects the basic-level advantage in category verification in the model. To assess this tendency in the model, we looked at the mean activation of the correct specific and basic names for items within or outside the domain of expertise across the two networks (treating the strength of activation as a model analog of verification time, as prevously discussed). Figure 5.14 shows these data, averaged across the four bird or fish items, at three different points during training. The analysis shows a strong basic-level advantage for items outside a network's domain of expertise: the basic-level name is much more strongly activated than is the specific name. Though not shown in the figure, this advantage persists through to the end of training. Within the domain of expertise, the effect

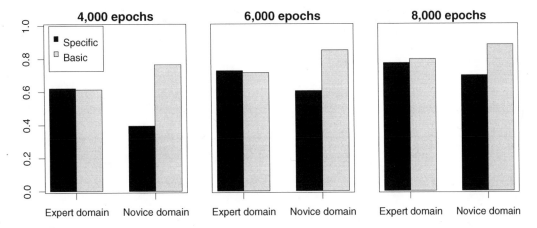

Figure 5.14 Activation of the correct specific (black bars) and basic (gray bars) name units, averaged across bird and fish items, for bird and fish "expert" networks at three points during training. For items outside the domain of expertise, the basic name is much more strongly activated than is the specific name at all points during training. For items within the domain of expertise, this basic-level advantage is eliminated.

is eliminated or greatly attenuated—specific and basic names are activated equally strongly throughout training, even though basic names appear as targets three times more frequently than do specific names in the model's training corpus. Given the assumed relation between activation and verification time, the networks' performance corresponds to a tendency to identify objects most quickly at the basic level in the novice domain, but about equally quickly at the basic and subordinate level in the expert domain.

Differentiation of Subordinate Items

Studies of unconstrained sorting show that experts divide objects in their domain of expertise into a greater number of groups than do novices (Boster and Johnson 1989). To show that the model also differentiates subordinate items to a greater degree in the expert domain, we measured the mean Euclidean distance between

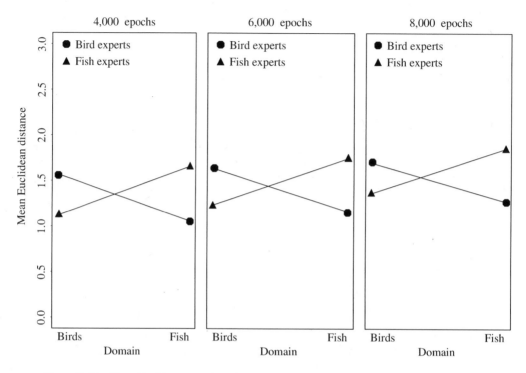

Figure 5.15   Mean Euclidean distance between pairs of *bird* and *fish* exemplars in the two expert networks at three different points during learning. Throughout training there is a greater distance between pairs of items in the expert domain.

internal representations of the various birds and fish in both expert networks, at different points in training. The results are plotted in figure 5.15.

Throughout training, objects in the expert domain are on average further apart from one another in representation space than are items from the novice domain. Thus, for bird experts, the average distance between pairs of bird representations is greater than is the average distance between pairs of fish representations. As learning proceeds, all the internal representations grow further and further apart; however, this difference between expert and novice domains persists through to the end of training.

Discussion

The fact that the networks quickly learned to apply specific labels to items in their domain of expertise is not surprising, since all names in the expert domain were eight times more frequent in the training set than were names at the same level of inclusiveness in the novice domain. Thus, all three levels of naming were learned quickly for objects in the domain of expertise, and the name-selection heuristic ensured that the most specific of these would be chosen as the network's naming response.

The fact that internal representations are better differentiated in the expert domain, however, suggests that these word-frequency choices are only part of the reason the network quickly acquires specific names for frequently encountered items. This tendency also derives from forces of similarity-based facilitation and inter-ference. Because the internal representations of highly familiar objects get pushed further apart in representation space, the net-work encounters less interference when learning specific names for these items, and accrues less benefit from facilitation when learn-ing basic names. Consequently, the network shows little tendency to activate basic name units more strongly than specific name units in the domain of expertise, even though the basic names are three times more frequent than are the specific names. By contrast, in the novice domain, the network does not receive as much pressure to differentiate between objects, and as a consequence the forces of facilitation and interference lead to a strong basic-level advantage for these objects.

In fact, similarity-based generalization is powerful enough to show these effects even when word frequencies in the network are controlled. To demonstrate this, we ran another simulation in which each name appeared equally often in the training environ-ment (as in simulation 5.2), but with either bird or fish patterns eight times more frequent in other relation contexts. The network's naming responses after 8,000 epochs of training are shown in table 5.7. The model again learned to name most items at the speci-fic level in the domain of expertise, and at the basic level in the

Table 5.7 Naming behavior in bird and fish expert networks after 8,000 epochs, when the models are trained with all words equally frequent in the corpus

OBJECT	FISH EXPERT	BIRD EXPERT
robin	bird	bird
canary	bird	canary
sparrow	bird	sparrow
penguin	bird	penguin
sunfish	sunfish	fish
salmon	salmon	fish
flounder	flounder	fish
cod	fish	fish

novice domain. Because the bird and the fish "experts" were exposed to exactly the same distribution of names during training, this effect was not simply due to a greater frequency of names in the expert domain. Rather, it reflects the comparative ease with which specific properties are learned for items whose representations have been strongly differentiated, as a consequence of the frequency with which they are encountered.

These simulations demonstrate that the increased frequency of exposure to items in a particular domain does not simply cause the network to accelerate its learning about object properties. Instead, the network comes to represent such items differently—differentiating them to a greater degree, and consequently devoting a larger semantic subspace to their representation. These differences in representation again have consequences for the ease with which the model learns to complete particular propositions. As the item representations in the expert domain grow further apart, the network is less able to capitalize on similarity-based generalization to learn their basic properties. Effectively, it becomes harder for the network to learn how highly familiar items are similar, and easier to learn how they differ. Of course, these effects also interact with frequency of exposure to particular input-output patterns to determine the rate at which knowledge of individual properties is acquired by the model.

The simulations we have reported here illustrate that some aspects of the expertise effects that have been observed in various experiments could arise simply from greater frequency of exposure to information in the expert domain. However, we do not intend to suggest that experts and novices necessarily receive exposure to exactly the same kinds of information. For example, bird experts tend to focus very particularly on the distinguishing visual markings of particular species of birds (markings that are usually not detectable to the naked eye, but that require binoculars), making them experts in visual identification of particular bird species, while bird novices may have virtually no awareness of many of these distinguishing markings (Tanaka and Taylor 1991). Thus the experience of a bird watcher may be more heavily weighted toward information that distinguishes particular birds, relative to novices, whose experience of various birds may be far more homogeneous. This would tend to increase the differentiation effects we have seen in the above simulation.

Simulation 5.6: Different Kinds of Expertise in the Same Domain

Related to the fact that experts may have different kinds of experiences from novices is the further fact that there can be different kinds of experts, even in the same domain—and these different kinds of experts may come to represent the same familiar objects differently. For example, landscape architects, park maintenance workers, and biologists may sort the same set of trees into different categories—even if the trees in question are equally familiar to each group (Medin, Lynch, and Coley 1997). Such differences, we suggest, may arise from differences in the particular kinds of information to which different types of experts get exposed. For example, landscape architects have good reason to consider how a tree looks in its surroundings, whereas biologists may not care how it looks so much as whether it has certain distingushing biological properties. In the course of their day-to-day interactions with trees, then, these experts may be exposed to different kinds of properties, and as a consequence may acquire different knowledge structures governing their judgments about how trees are similar to one another.

The Rumelhart network offers a means of capturing these effects, because it is trained with different sets of properties for each item, construed as occurring in different situations or contexts. As discussed in chapters 2 and 3, the *Relation* units in the model can be viewed as simplified representations of the different situations in which a set of items may be encountered. Each situation/context calls attention to a different set of the item's properties—for instance, some situations highlight an item's behavior (*can* properies), whereas others highlight its visual appearance (*is* properties)—and the degree to which different items tend to share properties can vary from context to context. Hence, each context specifies its own similarity structure. If just one of these contexts were emphasized in the network's training experience, the similarity structure within that context would have greater overall influence on the representations it acquires. Thus differential exposure to different relation contexts should lead to very different similarity structures over the model's internal representations.

To demonstrate this, we manipulated the frequency with which the model encountered objects in various relation contexts during learning, and examined the resulting representations at the end of training. To create a "visual" network, concerned with the visual properties of objects, we trained the model with *is* patterns eight times as frequent as *can* or *has* patterns. To create a "functional" network, concerned with the behavior of objects, we trained the model with *can* patterns eight times as frequent as *is* or *has* patterns. The actual patterns used in both runs were the same familiar patterns from simulation 5.1 (appendix B, table AB.3)—all that was changed in this simulation were the pattern frequencies (see appendix A). As in simulation 5.1, basic names for all objects were three times more frequent than general or specific names. We trained the model for 12,000 epochs, at which point it had learned to correctly activate all output properties to within 0.1 of their targets.

Figure 5.16 shows hierarchical cluster plots of the learned internal representations for all twenty-one objects, in the networks trained with either *is* or *can* patterns eight times more frequent than other contexts. The visual network learned a different and relatively arbitrary set of similarity relations compared to the functional network.

Both the visual and functional networks ultimately learn to activate the correct output units for all the objects in all relation contexts. Why, then, does the network learn different internal representations for these items? The reason is that, in different contexts, various items have different tendencies to share attributes. A group of objects that share the same *has* and *can* properties do not necessarily have many *is* properties in common. For example, the canary and the daisy, which are very different from one another in other contexts, share the attributes *is yellow* and *is pretty*. Considering only visual attributes (i.e., *is* properties), then, the canary and the daisy are more similar to one another than are the canary and the robin. When the network frequently encounters objects in a context that requires it to activate visual properties (the *is* context), the idiosyncratic similarities that derive from an object's appearance have a greater influence on the learned similarities across internal representations in the network. By contrast, when the network is exposed to objects most often in a context requiring it to activate the object's behavioral properties (the *can* context), the behavioral similarities across objects have the greatest impact on the network's learned internal representations. In this case, the *can* properties align well with our instincts about semantic structure, and with the verbal labels we attribute to objects. That is, objects called *birds* share many behaviors with one another, and few with other objects in the model's environment. Thus, the network learns

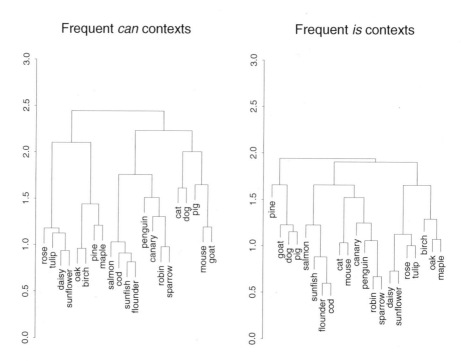

Frequent *can* contexts   Frequent *is* contexts

Figure 5.16   Similarities across learned internal representations for twenty-one items in networks trained with either *is* or *can* contexts eight times more frequent than other contexts. The similarity structure learned depends on the frequency with which the objects are encountered in these contexts. Thus, these different kinds of "expertise" lead the network to form different internal representations for the various objects. The similarity structure revealed in the left-hand plot captures intuitively appealing semantic similarity relations, because objects from the same semantic category tend to share many *can* properties in the model's environment. The similarity structure captured by the right-hand plot is somewhat more arbitrary, revealing the influence of increased exposure to *is* patterns in the network's training regime. In the training environment, *is* properties are not systematically related to an item's semantic category.

to assign representations to these items that emphasize their behavioral similarity to one another, and their distance from other objects, when trained with *can* contexts occurring most frequently. We suggest that the same is true of the experts studied by Medin, Lynch, and Coley (1997): the contexts in which they encounter the objects in their domain of expertise, and the manner in which they are required to interact with these objects, influence the similarity relations they come to represent.

Our simulations have shown that the nature and relative extent of the model's experience with particular items or sets of items have a dramatic effect on its performance. More and more experience leads to more and more conceptual differentiation, gradually eliminating the advantage of basic over subordinate levels of representation. More importantly, different experiences lead to the acquisition of different representations, with experience that emphasizes the appearance of things leading to representations differentiated on the basis of visual information, and with experience that emphasizes the behavior of things leading to representations differentiated on the basis of function.

Of course we do not wish to imply that the particular choices of types of information we have considered here adequately capture all differences in the kinds of information that different kinds of experts can learn. On the contrary, the examples we have chosen are only meant to be illustrative. Our intention has been to suggest that the mechanisms at work in our model provide the engine needed to allow a semantic knowledge system to absorb the particulars of experience in ways that capture certain aspects of the effects of expertise.

Generality of the Observed Simulation Results

All of the simulations in this chapter revolve around the effects of variations in frequency and attribute similarity of training experiences. First we argued that the primacy of the basic level in naming and early overextension of very frequent basic-level names reflect the interplay of these factors, and subsequently we argued that the patterns of performance seen in different types of experts also reflect effects of differences in frequency of exposure to particular items and/or particular types of information about items.

It should be noted that many of the properties we have illustrated in our model are robust and general properties of other models. For example, Schyns (1991) illustrated how a Kohonen network archictecture can exhibit differential degrees of differentiation as a function of varying relative frequency of training, and many of the properties we have discussed have been demonstrated in the model of Rogers et al. (forthcoming), which differs from the Rumelhart network in many details. Other modelers have considered several related phenomena (see, for example, Cree, McRae, and McNorgan 1999; Moss, Tyler, and Devlin 2002; McRae, De Sa, and Seidenberg 1997; Tyler et al. 2000). Thus, we wish to make clear that we are not claiming that the Rumelhart model is uniquely or even ideally suited to capturing these kinds of effects. Rather, we suggest that the properties we have seen in the simulations reported here are robust and fairly general characteristics of a wide range of different connectionist models; the Rumelhart model simply exemplifies the properties of the class of models, indicating that they provide fruitful vehicles for addressing a wide range of different aspects of semantic cognition.

Given these comments, it is our belief that the main determinant of the structure of semantic representations is the frequency and similarity structure of experience. It is true that the encoding of experience depends on perceptual systems that may influence the pattern of similarity and dissimilarity, as discussed extensively in the preceding chapter. It is also true that there are a few domain-general principles of learning and processing that allow experience to shape the representations that arise in the model (see chapter 9 for further discussion). Within these constraints, the specific patterns seen in the model—and, we would argue, humans—are shaped by the characteristics of the learning environment.

6 Category Coherence

To this point we have considered how the mechanisms that support the acquisition and use of semantic knowledge under the PDP theory offer an alternative to the categorization-based mechanisms that are often assumed by more traditional theories of semantic memory. We have focused on demonstrating how the PDP theory might explain a range of empirical phenomena, including classic findings that have typically been interperted within a categorization-based framework (such as "basic-level" phenomena and typicality effects) as well as findings that pose challenges for categorization-based theories, such as those resulting from the study of expertise. We have argued that the PDP theory provides a way of thinking about these phenomena that resolves some of the contradictions facing categorization-based theories, such as the seeming primacy of basic-level category knowledge in some contexts on the one hand, and the progressive differentiation of concepts and greater robustness of general semantic knowledge in dementia on the other.

We are certainly not the first to suggest that categorization-based theories are too limited to provide an adequate basis for understanding semantic knowledge acquisition and semantic task performance, nor are we the first to offer an alternative to the categorization framework. In chapter 1, we noted that limitations of categorization-based models, and the articulation of an alternative theoretical framework, have received wide attention among the proponents of theory-theory. Just as is the case with the categorization framework, there are variations in the positions of theory-theorists and others who adopt related positions; however, to recap what we take to be the main points, adherents of the framework share a commitment to the idea that cognition generally (and semantic cognition in particular) cannot be explained solely with reference to statistical or associative learning processes like those invoked by many categorization-based theories, but must also take into consideration "causal theories" that subserve the interpretation, explanation, and prediction of events in the environment. That is, semantic knowledge does not consist solely in knowing which objects have what properties—equally important (or possibly more important) is knowing something about the causal reasons why certain properties inhere in particular objects, and how a given object will behave (or cause other objects to behave) in different situations.

Accordingly, we discern two broad aims of research in the theory-theory tradition. The first has been to delineate the theoretical challenges faced by categorization-based models (and other so-called associationist theories), by documenting empirical phenomena that are difficult for such models to accommodate without additional constraints and processes. The second has been to demonstrate the special role played by causal knowledge in constraining semantic task performance. In our view, both of these endeavors have been useful in demonstrating the richness and complexity of the semantic cognitive abilities of young children. Many interesting and ingenious experiments have convincingly demonstrated that semantic cognition is in some ways more constrained, and in some ways more flexible, than is suggested by standard categorization-based theories. The studies also show that causal-explanatory information can influence semantic task performance. However, the theory-theory tradition has provided relatively little in the way of a characterization of the actual mechanisms—the representations and processes—that support the behavior exhibited in these experiments. Though theory-theorists agree on the basic tenet that semantic task performance must be constrained to some degree by causal-explanatory knowledge, there is relatively little attention to the precise form in which such knowledge is stored or to the characterization of the processes by which it exerts its influence on knowledge acquisition and task performance. Even when theory-theorists consider explicitly what it means to claim that children's thinking reflects the use of theories (e.g., Gopnik and Wellman 1994; Gopnik and Meltzoff 1997), they often stress abstract structural and functional characteristics of theories, rather than explaining how the content of a theory might be represented, or how theories work to influence semantic task performance.

In this and the next two chapters, we will consider whether the PDP framework can provide an account of the phenomena that have motivated theory-theory. We have already seen that the learning and processing mechanisms embodied in the Rumelhart model "go beyond" the simple tabulation of pairwise object-property correspondences in some respects. For example, the model acquires internal representations of objects that permit it to generalize its knowledge from one item to another. This generalization in turn affects the ease with which the model can acquire new knowledge about object properties. Based on coherent covariation of properties, the model learns to "attend to" some properties more than others. The knowledge stored in the network's weights at a given point in time, and the internal representations that arise from this knowledge, provide constraints on the network's acquisition of new knowledge, and on its performance in semantic tasks—making some properties easier to learn and activate than others.

In these three chapters we will consider further how the principles of knowledge acquisition and semantic task performance familiar from preceding chapters can be extended to explain the particular phenomena studied by theory-theorists. In the present chapter we will review data showing that different groupings of objects and constellations of properties are not all created equal. Some groupings provide a more useful and intuitive basis for knowledge generalization than others; some constellations are easier to learn, induce, and remember than others; and some properties are more "important" for semantic task performance than others. That is, the acquisition of knowledge about object properties, and the similarities existing among different groups of objects, are subject to constraints. According to the theory-theory, these constraints derive from knowledge about the causal mechanisms by which properties inhere in objects. Such causal theories influence which category representations or concepts are stored in memory (Murphy and Medin 1985), how these representations are used to direct semantic inference (Carey 1985), and which attributes are particularly important for representing which concepts (Keil et al. 1998). We will describe simulations with the Rumelhart model designed to show how such constraints might emerge as a consequence of the learning mechanisms familiar from earlier chapters. We will then illustrate how these mechanisms can help to explain data from specific experiments within the theory-theory tradition.

In chapter 7 we will consider evidence that, in addition to being constrained in certain respects, semantic task performance is considerably more flexible than is suggested by categorization-based theories. This flexibility has been documented in semantic induction tasks that require participants to make judgments about the properties of novel objects. Of particular interest are two general findings. First, patterns of induction can change dramatically with development, suggesting that the conceptual structures that direct semantic induction undergo substantial reorganization over time. The reorganization revealed by these studies goes beyond the simple differentiation of a taxonomic hierarchy, and suggests that theories of knowledge acquisition through childhood require a mechanism of representational change that permits fairly extensive restructuring of knowledge. Carey (1985) argues that such restructuring is a consequence of underlying theory change. We will describe simulations illustrating how conceptual reorganization of this kind might result from gradual domain-general learning in the PDP framework. Second, semantic induction tasks have shown that even at relatively young ages children can generalize their knowledge in impressively sophisticated ways. As an example, children seem to know that different kinds of properties extend differently from one kind of object to another. For instance, biological properties of a reference object extend to other objects of the same kind but physical properties tend to extend to objects that share other physical properties with a reference object (thus objects of the same size will tend to weigh about the same). Again, these phenomena have been interpreted as revealing the influence of domain-theories on semantic task performance. We will consider how context-sensitive internal representations such as those acquired by the Rumelhart model might account for such flexibility in generalization of different kinds of properties.

Finally in chapter 8, we will examine evidence suggesting that causal knowledge plays a special role in semantic task performance. We will first evaluate evidence from experiments that attempt to implicate such influences indirectly, by manipulating the causal conditions that give rise to an object's observable properties, and asking participants to make semantic judgments about the object. Such studies demonstrate that causal information can indeed influence the inferences that are drawn about an object, and how the item is construed as similar to other kinds of objects. However, we will suggest that causal knowledge is not different from other kinds of knowledge in this respect, and that it may be represented and processed similarly to knowledge about other kinds of object properties in the PDP framework. We will then consider the most direct evidence that causal-explanatory knowledge is crucial to semantic cognition: people's capacity to provide explicit, articulable explanations of events they have witnessed and of judgments they have made.

At the end of chapter 8 we will come to the question of the relationship between the PDP theory and the theory-theory. Should we see the PDP theory as an implementation of the theory-theory that has been proposed by its various protagonists? Or should we see it as a radical alternative position, one that suggests that talk of theories is extraneous or even misleading? For now we leave further consideration of this issue to the reader, and turn attention to specific phenomena.

Category Coherence

Coherence is a term introduced by Murphy and Medin (1985) to capture the observation that, of the many ways of grouping individual items in the environment, some groupings seem more natural, intuitive, and useful for the purposes of inference than others. For example, objects that share feathers, wings, hollow bones, and the ability to fly seem to "hang together" in a natural grouping—it seems appropriate to refer to items in this set with a single name ("bird"), and to use the grouping as a basis for knowledge generalization. By contrast, other groupings of objects are less intuitive, and less useful for purposes of inductive inference. For instance, the set of objects that are blue prior to the year 2010 and green afterward constitutes a perfectly well-defined class, but it does not seem to be a particularly useful, natural, or intuitive grouping. The question posed by Murphy and Medin (1985) is, how do we decide which groupings form good categories and provide a basis for generalization, and which do not?

A commonsense answer to this question might be that we treat as a category those groups of items that have many properties in common. However, Murphy and Medin (1985) argued that similarity alone is too underconstrained to provide a solution to this problem, as we discussed in chapter 1. They emphasized two general difficulties with the notion that category coherence can be explained solely on the basis of the observed similarities among groups of items.

First, the extent to which any two objects are construed as similar to one another depends on how their properties are weighted. As noted in chapter 1, a zebra and a barber pole may be construed as very similar to one another if the property *has stripes* is given sufficient weight. For a similarity-based account of category coherence to carry any authority, it must explain how some attributes of objects come to be construed as important for the object's representation, while others do not. Moreover, as R. Gelman and Williams (1998) have pointed out, the challenge is not simply to derive a set of feature weightings appropriate to all objects, because the importance of a given attribute can vary from item to item. This observation leads to an apparent circularity from some perspectives: a given object cannot be "categorized" until an appropriate set of feature weights has been determined, but such a set cannot be recovered until the item has been "categorized." Gelman and Williams (1998, 52–53) write:

The difference in the predictive value of color for identifying instances of the categories of cars vs. foods has led some to adopt a theory of concepts that assigns different weights to the different perceptual features for a particular concept. We could say that the weight for color given the concept car approaches 0, and, given the concept food, approaches 1. But this will not do either. As soon as we start to assign different weights to the exact same attributes as a function of concept type, we slip in a decision rule that embeds in it an understanding of the very thing that is to be understood, that is we use our different concepts to decide what weights to assign to the seemingly "same" attributes. If so, then the feature in question cannot belong to the list of independent, content-free, decomposable intensional features. We therefore are back to square one with regard to the question of what leads us to decide that a perceptual attribute is more or less important or more or less similar to ones already learned about.

Murphy and Medin (1985) and others have suggested that the challenge of selecting and weighting features appropriately might be resolved with reference to naive theories about the causal relationship among object properties. That is, certain constellations of properties "hang together" in psychologically natural ways, and are construed as "important" to an object's representation, when they are related to one another in a causal theory. For example, perhaps the reason that wings, feathers, and hollow bones are important for representing birds is that they are causally related to one another in a person's naive theory of flight. In this view, causal domain theories constrain the range of attributes that are considered important or relevant for a given concept. Gelman and Williams (1998, 63) go on to write that "we need an account of why some attributes are noticed and others are not. Why do we think that some things are similar to each other even if they are not perceptually alike on their surfaces? What leads us to select a given input as relevant on one occasion but not on another? Our answer is: our domain-specific knowledge structures, for both cognitive development and adult concept learning."

The second argument that Murphy and Medin (1985) and others (Keil 1991; Gelman and Williams 1998) have marshaled against correlation-based learning accounts of coherence stems from the observation that knowledge about object-property correspondences is not acquired with equal facility for all properties. For example, Keil (1991) has suggested that causal theories render some constellations of attributes easier to "learn, induce, and remember" than others. Recent experiments by Murphy (Murphy and Allopenna 1994; Murphy and Kaplan 2000; Kaplan and Murphy 2000; Murphy 2000; Lin and Murphy 1997) and others (e.g., Rehder and Ross 2001) have shown that prior knowledge can indeed have a dramatic impact on the ease with which new information is acquired. For instance, participants can learn novel categories much more rapidly when the properties that characterize them seem to "go together" naturally (given the participants' existing knowledge base), compared to categories whose properties are more arbitrary and inconsistent with existing knowledge. Such results suggest that new learning does not depend solely on the attribute structure of the categories being learned—rather, the way participants respond to the new category structure is shaped in part by what they already know.

Among the most compelling evidence for theory-induced constraints on knowledge acquisition, according to both Keil (1991) and Murphy and Medin (1985), is the phenomenon of illusory correlations—that is, the propensity for children and adults to believe or propound facts about the world that they cannot have learned directly from observation, because these "facts" are not true. For example, children studied by Carey (1985) appeared to believe that worms have bones—something they did not likely learn directly from experience since it is not accurate. Murphy and

Medin (1985) argued that illusory correlations demonstrate that knowledge acquisition involves more than simple learning about object properties, and that such phenomena reveal the ways causal theories enrich and supplement experience in order to support semantic processing.

The issues raised by Murphy and Medin (1985) posed serious problems for the categorization-based models of the day, and they highlight several important questions that should be addressed by any theory of semantic cognition. Specifically:

1. Why do some sets of objects seem to "hang together" in a psychologically natural way, while others do not?
2. Why are some constellations of properties easier to learn and remember than others?
3. Why do children and adults sometimes draw incorrect inferences about the properties of familiar and unfamiliar objects?
4. Why are some attributes important for categorizing an object, while other are irrelevant?
5. Why might a given property be important for categorizing some objects, but irrelevant for others?

As should be clear from the preceding chapters, the PDP approach offers a means of understanding how the semantic system comes to represent objects with similar sets of properties as similar to one another. We have also seen that the similarity relations represented by the system impose constraints on the ease with which the system acquires new information. For example, recall from simulation 5.3 that the model learned basic-level names most quickly for the items in its environment when basic category exemplars were represented as similar to one another and as distinct from other items, but that this was not true if the exemplars of basic categories were represented as dissimilar to one another, or as similar to other items with different basic names. Here we turn our attention to emphasizing how these aspects of the PDP theory address the issues raised by category coherence: why some properties seem to be more "important" for certain concepts than others, where constraints on learning some constellations of properties come from, why some groupings of items are more likely to foster inductive generalization than others, and where illusory correlations come from. To do this we must explain why coherent constellations of features are easier to "induce and remember" than other kinds of properties, and why groupings of objects that share these coherent properties form psychologically natural categories, whereas other groups of objects that share some particular property do not.

To explicitly address these questions, we will begin with a simulation designed to show that the Rumelhart model is sensitive to coherent structure in its environment. We will see that the model exploits this coherent covariation, grouping the objects into tight clusters based on shared coherent properties. Correspondingly we will see that the model has a much easier time learning and strongly activating the coherent properties of each object—in Keil's words, that coherent properties are easier for the model to "induce and remember."

Simulation 6.1: Category Coherence

The training patterns used for simulation 6.1 are shown in figure 6.1. Note that there are no category labels as such; there are only *is*, *can*, and *has* properties. Each of the items (numbered 1–16 in the figure) is assigned six properties, and each property appears as a target for four items. Hence, all properties are equally frequent, and all items have an equivalent number of attributes. In the figure, the attributes are divided into a group of coherent properties (appearing on the left, labeled with uppercase letters), and a group of incoherent properties (on the right, labeled with lowercase letters). The variation in coherence is evident from the way attributes are distributed across items in the figure. The coherent properties always occur together, whereas the incoherent properties are randomly distributed across items. This structure provides an analog in the model to the coherent clusters of properties described by

	is A	can B	has C	is D	can E	has F	is G	can H	has I	is J	can K	has L	is a	can b	has c	is d	can e	has f	is g	can h	has i	is j	can k	has l
1	1	1	1	0	0	0	0	0	0	0	0	0	1	0	0	0	1	0	0	0	0	0	1	0
2	1	1	1	0	0	0	0	0	0	0	0	0	0	0	0	1	0	0	0	1	1	0	0	0
3	1	1	1	0	0	0	0	0	0	0	0	0	0	0	1	0	1	0	1	0	0	0	0	0
4	1	1	1	0	0	0	0	0	0	0	0	0	0	1	0	0	0	0	0	0	0	1	0	1
5	0	0	0	1	1	1	0	0	0	0	0	0	0	1	0	0	0	0	0	0	1	1	0	0
6	0	0	0	1	1	1	0	0	0	0	0	0	0	0	0	1	1	1	0	0	0	0	0	0
7	0	0	0	1	1	1	0	0	0	0	0	0	0	0	0	1	0	0	0	1	0	0	0	1
8	0	0	0	1	1	1	0	0	0	0	0	0	1	0	1	0	0	0	0	0	0	0	1	0
9	0	0	0	0	0	0	1	1	1	0	0	0	0	0	1	0	0	0	1	1	0	0	0	0
10	0	0	0	0	0	0	1	1	1	0	0	0	0	0	0	1	1	1	0	0	0	0	0	0
11	0	0	0	0	0	0	1	1	1	0	0	0	0	0	0	0	0	0	0	1	1	1	1	0
12	0	0	0	0	0	0	1	1	1	0	0	0	1	1	0	0	0	0	0	0	0	0	0	1
13	0	0	0	0	0	0	0	0	0	1	1	1	0	0	0	1	1	0	0	0	0	0	0	1
14	0	0	0	0	0	0	0	0	0	1	1	1	0	0	0	0	0	0	1	1	1	0	0	0
15	0	0	0	0	0	0	0	0	0	1	1	1	1	1	0	0	0	1	0	0	0	0	0	0
16	0	0	0	0	0	0	0	0	0	1	1	1	0	0	1	0	0	0	0	0	0	1	1	0

Figure 6.1   Training patterns for the model (excluding names) in simulation 6.1. Individual item patterns are labeled 1–16, and the different properties are labeled with letters. Properties on the left (labeled with uppercase letters) are "coherent," in that they always occur together. Properties on the right (labeled with lowercase letters) are not coherent, because they do not co-occur reliably with one another. Every instance has three coherent and three incoherent properties, and every property appears as a target for four items.

Keil (1991). In the real world, such clusters may arise from "homeostatic causal mechanisms," as Boyd (quoted in our discussion of these issues in chapter 1) has suggested. For the model, however, such homeostatic causal mechanisms are not directly accessible; what is accessible is the coherent covariation such mechanisms produce. We have assigned arbitrary labels to the items to avoid any causal associations in the mind of the reader, and thereby to focus attention on the issue at hand, namely, the sensitivity of the model to patterns of coherent covariation. While the covariation of a given set of properties may derive from causal forces in the world, our claim is that it is also reflected in the co-occurrence statistics of the environment, and that if it is, a simple network learning algorithm will readily detect it. Our training environment is constructed accordingly.

We trained the model with patterns consistent with the information in figure 6.1. That is, for the input *item-1 can* the target was *B*, *k*, and for *item-5 is* the target was *D*, *j*. The model was not presented with any names (i.e., *ISA* patterns). In this simulation, we did not use noisy units. Each unit in the model had a trainable bias that was treated the same as all other weights in the network. The network was trained for 18,000 epochs (without momentum) with a learning rate of 0.005, at which point it could activate all the correct output properties above a threshold of 0.7. After every 300 epochs, we queried the network with each item paired with *is*, *can*, and *has* and recorded the activation of the ouput units. We conducted five runs with different initial weights and then averaged the results across them.

In figure 6.2 we show a multidimensional scaling of the model's internal representations of the sixteen items, at three points during learning. As noted, every property occurs equally often in

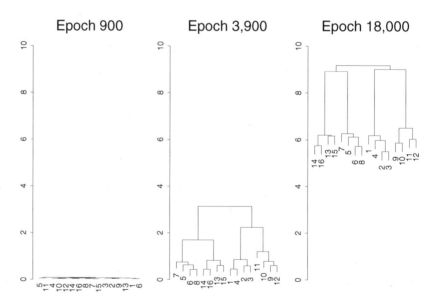

Figure 6.2 Hierarchical cluster analysis of the model's internal representations at three points during learning. Although every property in the training corpus is shared by some grouping of four items, the model organizes its internal representations with respect to shared coherent properties.

the training corpus, in exactly four different items. Thus each property, considered in isolation, might provide some basis for "grouping" a set of four items together in the model's internal representations—for example, considering just the *is-d* property, the model might have reason to "group together" items 3, 6, 10, and 13. However, from the figure it is clear that the model has assigned representations organized primarily by the coherent properties. The network represents as similar those items that have coherent properties in common (such as items 1–4), while the representations of items that share an incoherent property (such as *is-d*) are all quite different from one another. The reason is exactly that explored in previous chapters: because the group of items that share property A also happen to share properties B and C, the model can simultaneously reduce error on all three of these output units simply by representing items 1–4 as similar to one another. By contrast, if the network were to represent the set of items that share property d as similar to one another, it would easily be able to reduce error on the *is-d* output unit, but would have difficulty with all of the other properties, because none of these vary coherently with property d. What matters to the model is not just the propensity for a single attribute to be shared among some set of items, but whether the items that share some particular property also happen to have many other properties in common. Attributes that coherently covary will exert a greater degree of constraint on the model's internal representations.

Coherently covarying properties are also easier for the network to acquire. In figure 6.3, we plot the activation of each item's six attributes (when queried with the appropriate context) throughout training, averaged across the five different training runs. Coherent properties are shown as solid lines, and incoherent properties as dashed lines. The model learns very quickly to strongly activate the coherent properties for all sixteen items, but takes much longer to activate each item's incoherent properties. Because all units were active as targets equally often, and all items appeared in the training environment with equal frequency, this difference is not

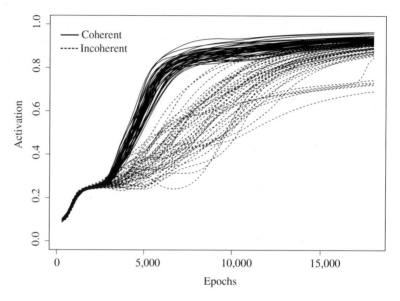

Figure 6.3 Activation of the correct output units for all sixteen items when the network is queried with the corresponding item and context. Coherent properties are shown as solid lines, and incoherent properties as dashed lines. The network quickly learns to activate all of the coherent properties for all of the items, but takes much longer to learn the incoherent properties.

attributable to the simple frequency with which items or properties appear in the environment. The network is sensitive to the structure of the environment that is apparent from the way that coherent sets of attributes covary together across items. For just the same reason that the model showed an advantage for learning "basic" category labels in the *basic structure only* condition of simulation 5.3, it also exhibits an advantage for learning and activating an item's "coherent" attributes.

Coherent Covariation vs. Pairwise Correlation

Our claim that category coherence can arise from sensitivity to coherent patterns of covariation among properties in the environment may seem at odds with recent experiments suggesting that correlational learning alone is insufficient to explain the relevant effects. To the contrary, we believe our account is consistent with the data from many of these studies. The reason is that these experiments have tended to consider just the effects of pairwise feature correlation on semantic task performance, rather than taking into account higher-order patterns of covariation across sets of features.

As an example, consider the following experiment described by Ahn, Marsh, and Luhmann (2002). Participants were provided with verbal descriptions of two exemplars of a familiar category, such as birds. Both items were described as having five properties, three of which were common to all items in the category, and two of which were not. For example, they might be told that bird A

has wings
has feathers
has two legs
lives near the ocean
eats fish

whereas bird B

has wings
lays eggs
has a beak
is white
eats fish

Participants were then asked to judge which of the two items was more typical of its category. The critical manipulation concerned the relationship between the two properties in each list that were not common to all members of the category—in this example, *lives near the ocean* and *eats fish* for bird A, and *is white* and *eats fish* for bird B. These properties were carefully selected to be significantly and equivalently correlated with one another across a large set of known exemplars from the general category, according to attribute-listing norms described by Malt and Smith (1984). For instance for the category of birds, eating fish is strongly and equivalently correlated with both living near the ocean and having a white color, according to Malt and Smith's attribute-listing experiments. However, in Ahn et al.'s (2002) experiment, this correlation was judged spurious for one of the items in the pair (e.g., according to university undergraduates, there is no causal relationship between having a white color and eating fish), whereas in the other case it was judged to result from a causal relationship (e.g., undergraduates believe that some birds eat fish because they live near the ocean). Thus, the pairwise correlations among the five properties were matched across the two items, but for one item, there was a known causal relationship between two properties. The interesting finding was that participants reliably judged the item with the "causally related" attribute pair to be more typical of its category than the item with the spuriously related pair—supporting the idea that more weight or importance is assigned to properties that are causally linked.

According to the authors, this pattern demonstrates that semantic judgments are influenced by knowledge that goes beyond the simple correlation of attributes. Specifically, they suggest that the data reveal the influence of causal knowledge or causal theories on the importance attributed to the different features. However, the simulations above suggest an alternative explanation: perhaps participants weighted the "causally linked" properties more strongly because these covary coherently with many other properties, whereas the other pair of correlated properties do not. For example, "living near the ocean" and "eating fish" together call to mind a set of shorebirds that have many other properties in common: the ability to glide, dive, and swim; a tendency to nest in cliffs; distinctive cries; and so on. In contrast, "having a white color" and "eating fish" could apply to a somewhat more disparate set of birds, sharing a less coherent set of properties—for instance, "being white" and "eating fish" might equally apply to ducks, geese, and swans as to seagulls, terns, and sandpipers. The shorebirds, in addition to sharing the correlated properties used in this example, have many other properties in common that will also covary with eating fish and living near the ocean, and such patterns of coherent covariation across many different properties may serve to boost the importance of "living near the ocean" relative to "having a white color" for these birds.

To illustrate the importance of coherent covariation (as opposed to pairwise correlation) in the model, we replicated simulation 6.1 using a slightly different training corpus. Each item was assigned six coherently covarying attributes and six incoherent attributes, just as described above. Each item was also assigned three pairs of perfectly correlated properties—again, each property occurred the same number of times in different objects. Although the two properties within each pair correlated perfectly with one another, they did not vary systematically with any of the other properties. As before, every feature occurred equally frequently in the training corpus, and every item had exactly the same number of attributes (six coherent, six correlated, and six incoherent).

As in the previous simulation, the network acquired internal representations grouped according to the propensity for objects to share the coherently-covarying attributes. Also as before, this allowed the network to learn these properties more rapidly and to activate them more strongly. Figure 6.4 shows the mean activation of the coherent, correlated, and incoherent properties, averaged across all items for five different simulation runs. The coherent properties are clearly learned most rapidly, and the incoherent ones least rapidly, as before. Pairwise correlation affects learning, but crucially the correlated features that also covary with other features are learned more rapidly than those that are simply correlated with each other and nothing else.

The simulation establishes that the model is sensitive to patterns of coherent covariation over and above patterns of simple pairwise correlation. By virtue of this sensitivity, it may come to weight "causally linked" properties more heavily than spuriously correlated properties in experiments like Ahn, Marsh, and Luhmann 2002. In this view, it is not knowledge about the causal relations

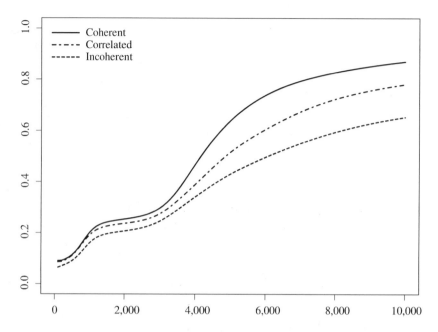

Figure 6.4 Mean activation of coherent, pairwise-correlated, and incoherent properties, averaged across all target properties and items from five different runs of the simulation.

among the linked properties that explains the effect, per se. Rather, the properties that Ahn and colleagues (2002) describe as "causally linked" may simply be properties that, in the participants' experience, covary coherently with many other properties.

Work by Billman and colleagues (e.g., Billman and Knutson 1996; Kersten and Billman 1997) supports the view that human learning is sensitive to coherent covariation. In the paradigmatic experiment, participants were shown drawings of scenes involving unfamiliar animal-like creatures situated in a particular context (Billman and Knutson 1996). Each scene had seven types of attributes, and each type of attribute had three possible values. Participants were instructed to study a series of such drawings for as long as they liked, without any instruction as to how they would later be tested. After the study period, they were shown pairs of novel drawings, and were asked to decide which was "most like the kind of thing you saw before."

The important experimental factor involved a manipulation of the covariance structure of the study items. In both experimental conditions, two of the seven properties (the *test* properties) were strongly correlated with one another across the corpus. However, in the "structured" condition, these properties were also correlated with two other properties (themselves highly correlated), whereas in the contrasting condition (the "isolating" condition) they were not. The interesting result was observed when participants were shown two novel pictures, one including the two pairwise-correlated properties and one not. Participants in the structured condition decided with high likelihood that the drawing with the correlated properties was the same kind of thing as the study items, whereas participants in the "isolating" condition were considerably less likely to do so. In both conditions, the two properties were equally correlated with one another—what differed was whether this pairwise correlation was itself part of a larger pattern of coherent covariation in the study set. When it was, participants were more likely to strongly weight the test properties in the subsequent categorization task.[1]

Discussion of Simulation 6.1

The simulations in this section show that the mechanisms embodied in the Rumelhart model accomplish exactly what Keil (1991) suggests needs to be accomplished in order for categories to be coherent—they make "homeostatic causal clusters" of properties in the environment easier for the model to learn, and easier to induce and remember later. The Rumelhart model does not simply tabulate information about first-order concept-feature correlations —a charge that has sometimes been leveled against similarity-based models. Rather, it relies on the richer array of high-order intracategory and cross-category correlations that capture the non-homogeneity of semantic space described by Boyd (1986; cf. Keil 1991). The clusters of "tight bundles separated by relatively empty spaces" that, in Keil's words, arise from the causal structure of the environment, could well describe the representations discovered by our model. In fact, we can view the learning mechanisms embodied in our model as a means of assimilating knowledge of the "homeostatic causal clusters" that Keil and Boyd suggest exist in the world. Although the system does not acquire explicit representations of causal mechanisms, it is nevertheless sensitive to the coherent structure of the environment produced by such forces. That is, the system adapts its representations to reflect the coherent structure of the environment. Thus, in a sense, the system's representations encode knowledge of the causal mechanisms that produce such structure in the first place.

In summary, according to the theory-theorys category coherence is grounded in a system of implicit theories about the causal forces that give rise to the particular constellations of properties that inhere in different kinds of objects. We have shown that in the PDP framework, categories achieve coherence through the operation of a learning mechanism that is sensitive to the pattern of covariation exhibited among properties of objects in the environment. Can the operation of this mechanism also explain related empirical phenomena that have been argued to implicate causal theories? In the remainder of the chapter we will focus on two such phenomena: *illusory correlations*, or the tendency for children and adults to attest that certain objects and properties co-occur in the world when in fact they do not (Murphy and Medin 1985; Keil 1991); and *feature importance*, or the tendency to weight the same features differently for different kinds of objects in semantic generalization tasks (e.g., Macario 1991; Murphy and Medin 1985).

Simulation 6.2: Illusory Correlations

In chapter 1, we discussed an example of illusory correlations: when explaining why various objects could or could not move up and down a hill by themselves, children would ignore the presence of some features in a picture (e.g., feet on a statue), and would attest to the presence of other features clearly not visible in the picture (e.g., claiming that the echidna has feet; Gelman 1990).[2] Illusory correlations have been interpreted as providing important evidence for the theory-theory, because they appear to pose a problem for simple correlational-learning and categorization-based theories of conceptual representation: if children acquire their semantic knowledge simply by learning which objects have which properties, why should they make these claims, which are clearly in violation of their perceptual experience? Under the theory-theory and related approaches, such inferences reflect the application of knowledge of causal mechanisms. For example, Gelman (1990) suggests that children might be predisposed to attribute motion of animate objects to parts that enable movement. Thus, even when such parts are not directly visible they may fill them in due to the operation of this predisposition.

Actually, as we also noted in chapter 1, a categorization-based theory might explain illusory correlations by relying on a property-inheritance mechanism in a taxonomically organized system. In the study described above, children may categorize unfamiliar objects like the echidna at a general level such as *animal*, then use information stored at this level to attribute to the echidna the typical properties of the class of animals (e.g., feet). Our simulations offer a different explanation: perhaps illusory correlations are caused by the regularizing influence of similarity-based generalization. We investigated this possibility in the next simulation.

The attribution of legs that are not seen readily arises in the Rumelhart network if an object with a coherently covarying property, such as fur, is presented to the network as the basis for finding a representation, using the backprop-to-representation mechanism discussed in chapter 2. Backprop to representation allows the network to derive a representation of the object that can then be used to impute to it other, not actually experienced properties, based on previous experience with patterns of property covariation.

In simulation 6.2, we used a version of the Rumelhart model trained with the same patterns and frequencies described in simulation 5.1. Due to the structure of the training set, the network frequently experienced the covariation of fur with legs and other properties shared by the five land animals during acquisition. We

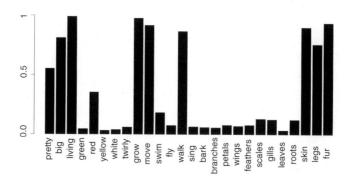

Figure 6.5 Activation of output properties for the representation of an object described only with the property *has fur*, discovered by the network using backprop to representation. The model makes reasonable assumptions about the properties a furry object might have. Like the children in Gelman's (1990) study, it predicts that the object can move and has legs, even though it was not given either of these properties.

stopped learning after 3,000 epochs (well before full mastery of the training set, consistent with the young age of Gelman's participants) and then carried out a simulation of Gelman's (1990) experiment. Specifically, we "showed" the model a novel object analogous to the *echidna*, and used backprop-to-representation to assign the object a new representation, specifying only the single target property *has fur*. Once the model had found an appropriate internal representation, we queried it in the *is*, *can*, and *has* contexts, to determine what other properties it would attribute to the object.

Figure 6.5 shows the activation of the various *is*, *can*, and *has* output units when the model is asked about the echidna. The network made reasonable guesses about the item's other properties, activating properties common to the mammals. Like the children in Gelman's (1990) study, the model inferred that the object can move and that it has legs, even though this information was not given to the model as it derived its internal representation.

The model's behavior results from similarity-based generalization. To activate the property *has fur*, the model must find a representation of the echidna similar to the other items that have fur, namely, the mammals. By virtue of this similarity, the other properties common to mammals generalize to the echidna. Of course, this is exactly the "property-inheritance" mechanism described by Rumelhart and Todd (1993), by which distributed representations can promote the application of stored semantic knowledge to various test items.

The model's tendency to generalize across items that share coherently covarying properties goes beyond simply inferring missing properties; it can actually lead the model to highly inaccurate misattributions, even when repeatedly exposed to the correct information. To demonstrate this in the network, we next looked to see how its knowledge about the irregular properties of objects developed throughout learning. For example, among the plants, the pine tree is the only object that does not have leaves. Thus, the pine stands out as an aberration, lacking one property shared by all those items it otherwise shares many properties with. Conversely, among the animals in the network's environment, the canary is the only one that can sing; given this training corpus, then, this property represents an arbitrary and idiosyncractic property not shared with other similar items. We again trained the network exactly as described in simulation 5.1, and examined its tendency to attribute the property *has leaves* to the pine tree and *can sing* to the canary, after every fifty epochs of training.

In figure 6.6 we show the activation of the *has leaves* and the *can sing* units when the network is probed with the inputs *pine has* and *canary can*, respectively. At epoch 1,500, the network has been presented repeatedly with target information indicating it should turn off the *has leaves* unit when presented with *pine has* as input. Nevertheless, it strongly activates the *has leaves* unit in response to this input. This is clearly an example of an illusory correlation, in that the network attributes to the object a property that, on the basis of its experience, it clearly does not have. Similarly, by epoch 1,500 the network has repeatedly been given target information indicating that the canary can sing. Despite this, it shows no tendency to activate the output *can sing* when asked

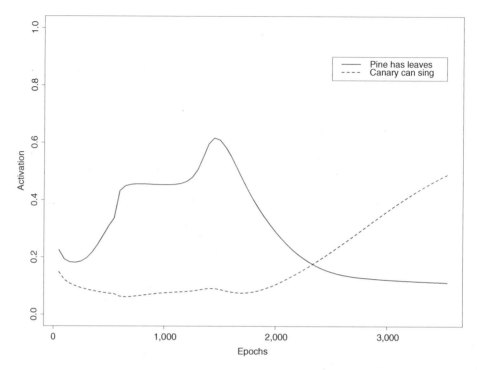

Figure 6.6   The activation of the *has leaves* and *can sing* output units across the first 5,000 epochs of training, when the network is probed with the inputs *pine has* and *canary can*, respectively. At epoch 1,500, the network has been trained 150 times to turn off the *has leaves* unit in response to the input *pine has*, and to turn on the unit *can sing* in response to the input *canary can*. Despite this, the network still activates the *has leaves* unit for the pine tree, and fails to activate the *can sing* unit for the canary.

what a canary can do. It should be noted that by epoch 1,500, the network has no trouble responding to queries about properties that the pine and the canary have in common with their neighbors. For example, the network knows that the pine does not have legs and that the canary can fly. It only has trouble learning about the ways these objects differ from closely related items. The network "creates" a correlation between the pine and the property *has leaves* that does not exist in its environment, and "ignores" the strong correlation that does exist between the canary and the property *can sing*, while learning the other properties of these objects correctly.

Why does the model show these illusory attributions? Early in learning, it assigns similar representations to all the plants, including the pine tree. Because most of the plants have leaves, this property is learned quickly and generalizes to the pine tree by virtue of the covariation of other properties of pine trees with the remaining coherent properties of other trees. Even though the network has been shown repeatedly that the pine tree does not have leaves, such learning is overwhelmed by similarity-based generalization. As the pine differentiates itself from the other plants, these forces diminish. The same influences prevent the network from activating the property *can sing* for the canary until it is sufficiently distinguished from other animals (including other birds), all of which cannot sing. These simulations suggest that we can interpret at least some kinds of illusory correlations as the simple overgeneralization of regular properties. The forces at work are the same as those that lead children (and the network) to overextend familiar names to related items during development.

The Influence of Prior Knowledge on New Learning

From these simulations, it should be clear how existing "background" knowledge can influence the acquisition of information about new concepts, as demonstrated in a series of studies by Murphy and colleagues (Murphy and Allopenna 1994; Murphy and Kaplan 2000; Kaplan and Murphy 2000; Murphy 2000; Lin and Murphy 1997). In a representative experiment, Murphy and Allopenna (1994) taught participants about different categories of unfamiliar vehicles. Each new category was described as having several features, and participants were required to remember which properties were characteristic of which kind of vehicle. In one condition, the categories were "coherent," in that their characteristic properties seemed to naturally go together, given the participants' general background knowledge. For example, participants in this condition might be told that vehicles in category A are typically found in the Arctic, have runners on the front, are wrapped with thick insulation, and have a tank filled with anti-freeze mounted on the back. In the contrasting condition, the new categories were "incoherent," in that their characteristic properties did not naturally seem to go together. For instance, participants in this condition might be told that vehicles in category A are typically found in the jungle, have runners on the front, are wrapped in aluminum foil, and have a tank filled with sand mounted on the back.

In both conditions, participants did not likely have preexisting concepts corresponding directly to the kinds of vehicles in the experiment. However, the basic finding was that participants were much better at learning and remembering a category's properties in the coherent than in the incoherent condition. According to Murphy, the reason is that coherent categories "make sense" given the system of general world knowledge the participants bring with them into the experiment. Knowledge about the cold climate of the Arctic, the difficulty of driving in deep snow, the need for human beings to keep warm, and so on, effectively "explains" the properties in the coherent category, making them easier to remember or reconstruct at test. In contrast, general background knowledge does not help to explain or predict the properties of the incoherent category, and hence such categories are more difficult to master.

From the preceding simulations, it is apparent that the network's state of knowledge at a given point in time will greatly influence the facility with which it learns the properties of new concepts. Specifically, the network will learn a novel concept's properties more rapidly if these properties are generally consistent with patterns of coherent covariation in the network's experience. This effect will be observed even when the particular combination of properties that characterize the new concept is completely novel to the network.

To see this, consider what happens in the model from the previous simulation, after it has been trained, when it encounters two different kinds of novel items. Both items have a combination of properties that the model has never before encountered, but as in

Murphy's experiments, they differ in the extent to which these properties "belong together" given what the network has learned from the training corpus. For example, we might present the network with a new item that has roots, petals, and bark. In the model's training corpus, petals and bark never co-occur, so this item is effectively a new concept to the network; however, roots, petals, and bark all "go together" in the sense that items with these properties are represented fairly similarly by the network (they all fall within the "plant" part of the space), and the property *has roots* covaries coherently with having petals and having bark. If we were to present this item to the trained network, and use backprop to representation to find a suitable representation for it, the network would be able to capitalize on what it already knows to come close to mastering the item's properties, even without any additional learning. That is, it will find a representation partway between the flowers and the trees, which strongly activates *has roots* in the output, and partially activates both *has bark* and *has petals*. The network will not likely be able to fully activate the latter two properties, because they have never occurred together in its experience—hence it will be unable to find an internal representation that simultaneously activates them. The network's preexisting knowledge goes a long way toward accommodating the item's properties, leaving only a little additional work required to fully master the item.

In contrast, we might present the network with a new item that has roots, wings, and gills. Again, these properties have never occurred conjointly in the network's experience, but in this case, the combination of properties completely crosscuts the patterns of coherent covariation in the network's training environment. Not only do wings and gills never occur together in the network's experience, but neither of these co-occurs with roots, and the familiar items that have roots, gills, or wings have very different internal representations. The knowledge stored in the network's weights will not therefore be very useful for simultaneously mastering the new concept's properties—the model will be unable to find an internal representation that strongly activates all three properties. In this sense, new concepts with incoherent sets of attributes will be much more difficult for the system to master.

The model suggests an explicit process whereby the knowledge already stored in the human semantic system can help participants learn about new concepts when their properties are generally consistent with overall patterns of experienced coherent covariation. Total mastery of the new concept's properties will also likely depend to some extent on the complementary fast-learning system in the hippocampus and related structures, even for coherent concepts. But for incoherent categories, acquisition of the new properties will receive little support from the semantic system, and will depend almost entirely on the fast-learning medial temporal lobe system.

Simulation 6.3: Category-Dependent Attribute Weighting

As discussed in chapter 1, several authors (Murphy and Medin 1985; Keil 1991; Gelman and Williams 1998) have emphasized the fact that an individual feature does not always contribute equally toward determining how different objects are similar to one another. Rather, a given feature may be important for discriminating among some kinds of objects but not others. For example, color is important for identifying kinds of food, but not kinds of toys (Macario 1991). The contribution of a particular feature can vary depending on its stimulus context—that is, depending on the other features that make up the stimulus description (Smith and Medin 1981).

We have seen that the model has an advantage for learning and activating the coherent properties of objects, as a consequence of its sensitivity to the correlational structure of the environment. How might these processes explain the apparent differential "importance" of the same attribute when it appears in different objects?

To answer this question, we examined the model's ability to learn and make use of feature dependencies when representing test objects with familiar properties, using backprop to representation to simulate data reported by Macario (1991). Macario (1991) showed children novel objects varying along two dimensions (color and shape). When the children were led to believe the objects were a kind of food, they most often generalized a new fact on the basis of shared color, but when led to believe they were a kind of toy, they more often generalized on the basis of shared shape. Thus, the children appeared to weight color more than shape for food items, but shape more than color for toys.

We wish to show that such feature dependencies come to be captured by the weights in the network after it has been trained. To do this, we added four new output units to the network, standing for the properties *is bright*, *is dull*, *is large*, and *is small*. We assigned these properties to the familiar objects in the network's environment (the plants and animals) in such a way that size but not brightness was important for discriminating between the trees and flowers, and brightness but not size was important for discriminating between the birds and fish. Thus, all the trees were large and all the flowers were small, but a given tree or flower could be either bright or dull, whereas all the birds were bright and all the fish were dull, though a given bird or fish could be either large or small. The brightness attributes, then, covaried coherently with other properties within the animals but not within plants, while the size attributes covaried with other properties in the plants but not animals. The pattern of covariation we have used is not, of course, actually found in plants and animals in the real world; we use it only to illustrate that the model can assign different weights to the same property in different categories. We trained the model for 3,000 epochs, then used backprop to representation to see how it would represent different items varying in size and brightness, given that the items shared a property common to either plants or animals.

We assigned brightness and size attributes to four test items, as shown in table 6.1. In the first simulation run, we also assigned to

Table 6.1   Distribution of attributes across four test objects in simulation 6.3

	BRIGHT	DULL	LARGE	SMALL
Object 1	1	0	1	0
Object 2	1	0	0	1
Object 3	0	1	1	0
Object 4	0	1	0	1

these items an attribute shared by the plants (*has roots*); in the second, we assigned to them an attribute shared by animals (*has skin*). In both runs, we used backprop to representation to derive an internal representation for each item, by backpropagating from the output units corresponding to *bright*, *dull*, *large*, *small*, *roots*, and *skin*. We then examined the similarities among the four test-item representations in each case.

Figure 6.7 shows the results of a hierarchical cluster analysis on the network's internal representations of the four test objects, when they share a property common to plants (left-hand figure) or animals (right-hand figure). When the network is "told" that the objects all have roots like the plants, it groups them on the basis of their size; when told that they all have skin like the animals, it groups them on the basis of their brightness. Moreover, these similarities constrain how the network generalizes new knowledge from one test object to another. When the objects share a property with plants, the model represents them as similar on the basis of their size. In this case, if the model were to learn a new fact about, say, the small bright item, it would be more likely to generalize the property to the small dark item than to the large bright object, precisely because it represents as similar the two small items. The opposite consequence is observed when the test items all share a property with animals—the model is more likely to generalize new

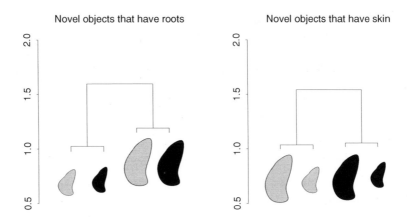

Figure 6.7   Hierarchical cluster analysis of the model's representations of test objects varying in brightness and size, and sharing a property common either to all animals or to all plants. When the objects share a property common to the plants (*has roots*), the network groups them on the basis of their size, which is important for discriminating flowers from trees. However, when the objects share a property common to animals (*has skin*), the network groups them on the basis of their brightness, which is important for discriminating birds from fish in the network. Thus, the network has learned that brightness is "important" for animals, but not for plants.

information on the basis of brightness than size, because in this case it represents as similar those items that share the same brightness values. Like the children in Macario's (1991) experiment, the model represents different similarities among a group of items, and generalizes from one to another differently, depending on the superordinate category to which the items belong. That is, the network seems to "know" that brightness is more important than size for representing animals, but that the reverse is true for plants.

Intuitively, we can understand the model's behavior with reference to the distribution of predicates across representation space. Consider how the network comes to represent an object that is bright and large, compared to one that is bright and small. When the objects both share a property with the plants, such as *has roots*, the network must assign to them representations that lie somewhere within the space spanned by the predicate *has roots*. Within this region, the only objects that are large are the trees, which exhibit coherent covariation of several other properties, whereas the only objects that are small are the flowers, which have their own set of coherent properties, different from those of the trees. Thus the bright-large test object will receive a representation similar to the trees, whereas the bright-small objects will receive a representation similar to the flowers. The property *is bright* does not vary coherently with other properties within the plant domain, and as a consequence, exerts little influence on representations among the plants.

The opposite consequence is observed when the same test objects share a property with animals. In this case, they must receive representations that fall within the region of semantic space spanned by the predicate *has skin*. Within this subspace, all the fish are dull, and all the birds are bright. To activate the property *is bright*, both objects must be represented as similar to the birds. The property *is large* does not vary coherently with other properties in this domain. Thus, both large and small objects fall within the same small region of semantic space (i.e., proximal to the other birds), and hence are represented as similar to one another.

The contribution of size and brightness information to a test object's internal representation depends on other attributes in the stimulus context—specifically, the presence of properties shared by animals or plants, which, in conjunction with size and brightness information, precisely constrain the representation assigned by the network. Thus, the simulation serves as a demonstration that sensitivity to informative attribute conjunctions can be acquired by a domain-general learning mechanism that adapts the model's representations to the statistical structure of the environment. In this view, the importance of an attribute (such as size or brightness) in a particular concept representation derives from its statistical co-occurrence with other attributes and conjunctions of attributes in the environment.

Summary of Findings

As we have seen in several places, the learning mechanisms that subserve knowledge acquisition within our PDP theory give rise to representations that capture the high-order statistical structure of the environment. Items that share several intercorrelated properties with one another, and few with other objects, form "coherent" groupings, in that they are represented as similar to one another, and are likely to foster productive generalization from one to the other. Accordingly, the intercorrelated attributes shared by these groups of objects are "important" for their representation, in two respects. First, such properties are more easily learned and more strongly activated than others. We demonstrated these effects in simulation 6.1, in which the model learned to activate the coherent properties of objects much more rapidly and strongly than their incoherent properties, even when all properties occurred equally frequently in the environment. Second, these properties provide strong constraints on the internal representations the system derives for test items. Because birds are the only kinds of objects likely to have feathers and beaks, the semantic system is constrained to represent objects with feathers and beaks as similar to familiar birds. Other properties such as color and size may be less consistently intercorrelated with one another, and consequently exert less of an influence on the internal representations of objects discovered by the learning algorithm. For example, the set of all things that are red do not have many other properties in common —hence, the system does not represent such groups as similar to one another internally, and the set does not form a coherent category. Additionally, the property *is red* does not provide a systematic constraint on how the system represents a test object, simply because the representations of various things that are red are distributed widely throughout the semantic representation space. Thus when a novel red object is encountered, there are several different regions of the space the system can use to represent the object. Finally, we have seen that the relative "importance" of a particular attribute may be conditioned on the presence or absence of other features that signal what domain or type of object the attribute applies to. The weights that encode the network's knowledge about object-property correspondences are sensitive to domain-specific interdependencies among features. Hence, the contribution of a given stimulus feature to the model's internal representation of the object can depend on the presence or absence of other features in the stimulus.

An important source of information on the development of conceptual knowledge comes from studies of inductive projection. In such studies, children at different ages are asked to answer questions about the properties of novel and familiar objects. In some cases, they may be told a new fact about an item (e.g., "this dinosaur has warm blood"), and then asked whether the fact is true about other kinds of objects (e.g., "Do you think this other kind of dinosaur also has warm blood?"). In other cases, they may simply be asked about properties of presumably unfamiliar things (e.g., previously unfamiliar animals), or about properties of things that may be somewhat familiar but where it is unlikely they have learned directly about the property in question (e.g., "Do you think a worm has a heart?"). In this chapter we will consider results from inductive projection studies. We will focus particularly on Carey's (1985) work demonstrating that patterns of inductive projection can change dramatically between the ages of 3 and 10. For Carey, such changing induction profiles are important in part because she sees them as indicating underlying theory change. She points out that determining whether children at different ages have the same underlying concepts is a nontrivial problem, which may only be solved by considering the "theoretical context" in which the concepts are presumed to be embedded. Carey (1985, 199) writes:

One solution to the problems of identifying the same concepts over successive conceptual systems and of individuating concepts is to analyze them relative to the theories in which they are embedded. Concepts must be identified by the role they play in theories. A concept [in one theory (aus)] is undifferentiated relative to descendents [i.e., successor theories] if it contains features of those descendents, and if the [earlier] theory states neither any relations among those features nor any separate relations among those features and other concepts....

If the above analysis is correct, differentiations must be analyzed relative to the theories in which the differentiating concepts are embedded. Young children represent the concept *animal* and the concept *plant*. They can also form the union *animals and plants* and even know some properties true of animals and plants (e.g., that they grow). Why, then, do we wish to deny them the concept *living thing*? Because as yet they represent no theoretical context in which the concept *living thing* does any work. The coalescences of *animal* and *plant* into the concept *living thing* occurs as part of the knowledge reorganization documented in this monograph.

For Carey, changing patterns of inductive projection provide a key basis on which to diagnose a developing child's theory of causation. In her view, the emergent theory of biology in which the concept *living thing* comes to play a role is itself constituted in part of knowledge about the causal mechanisms that give rise to the shared properties of living things. All living things grow, reproduce, consume nutrients, and eventually die. In Carey's view, 10-year-olds (and adults) realize that all of these properties are consequences of a shared underlying nature. By contrast, she suggests, 4-year-olds conceive of these biological facts as arising from a very different kind of psychological causality of the sort often used to explain aspects of human behavior: something might grow because it "gets the idea" from other things that grow, for example.

The key issues for Carey (1985) are the characterization of children's conceptual knowledge, and in particular the demonstration that conceptual knowledge of living things undergoes a massive reorganization near the end of the first decade of life. In spite of the fact that conceptual reorganization is so central an issue in her work, she has little to say about the mechanisms that lead to change. She does appeal to learning about the biological functions of eating, breathing, growing, and so on, and suggests in several places that the accumulation of such information provides the basis on which theory change might occur. But she does not venture to say much about *how* the accumulation of such information causes conceptual reorganization. She further suggests that given the pervasiveness of the reorganization of conceptual knowledge of living things, it is unlikely that such change could be easily conveyed through a simple instructional sequence. "The burden of the description in this monograph," she states,

is the far-reaching ramifications of the child's conceptual organization— the concepts affected range from individual species, to superordinates such as animal, plant, and living thing, to biological functions such as eating, breathing, and growth, to matters of reproduction and its relation to gender identity, to the nature and function of internal organs, to the relation between mind and brain. A short instructional sequence would hardly change all that. (p. 199)

We see in this quotation and in other places a sense that Carey believes it is the accumulation of a large body of disparate biological knowledge—spanning several domains, including feeding and metabolism, life and death, reproduction, and so on—that leads to theory change. Yet it is a mystery to her that theory change is even possible. (See also Carey and Spelke 1994; Fodor 2000.)

In the present chapter, we will consider the patterns of empirical findings that Carey and others have presented on inductive projection in developing children between the ages of 4 and 10, and we will present simulations indicating how analogs of these patterns may be seen in the behavior of the Rumelhart model as it gradually learns from experience. We will not attempt to simulate the specific patterns of inductive projection seen by Carey and others; rather our focus will be on showing that the different *types* of changes that she points to as indicative of underlying theory change can be seen in the changing patterns of inductive projection, and in the underlying representations, within the model. Like Carey, we will suggest that these kinds of changes arise from the accumulation of knowledge across a very broad range of items and situations, and that they reflect an underlying reorganization of conceptual knowledge structures. However, we will also suggest that the mechanism driving this accumulation and reorganization is akin to that operating in the PDP theory. In this view, conceptual reorganization is influenced partly by the coherent covariation of properties encountered only rarely and across widely varying situations and contexts. It is also influenced by exposure to new information about objects as they are encountered in novel contexts later in life—for example, as children are taught explicit facts about familiar objects in school.

Carey's data, as well as other findings, support the following points about inductive projection over the course of development:

- Patterns of inductive projection evolve over time in development. For example, when told that a human has a certain unfamiliar internal organ (*spleen* for young children or *omentum* for older children and adults), the pattern of projection of this organ to other things becomes progressively narrower with development.

- Patterns of inductive property attribution can be different for different kinds of properties of objects. In older subjects in particular, some properties such as *eats* and *breathes* are distributed fairly evenly across all animals (and are even sometimes attributed to plants), whereas others (such as *thinks*) are much more narrowly attributed. Other studies (Gelman and Markman 1986) indicate that even quite young children can project biological properties differently than physical ones.

- There is a general tendency for patterns of inductive projection to become more specific to the particular type of property over the course of development. For example, Carey notes that the pattern of projection of *spleen* by four-year-old children matches the pattern of projection of eight out of ten other properties that humans have. Six- and ten-year-old children and adults show progressively more differentiated patterns of projection for different types of properties.

- Patterns of inductive projection can coalesce as well as differentiate. For example, adults project biological properties central to living things, such as eating and breathing, to plants as well as animals, something that four-year-old children rarely do, contributing to Carey's suggestion that they treat such properties as biological characteristics shared across exemplars of the acquired concept of living thing.

As we will see in this chapter, the Rumelhart model exhibits all of these phenomena, suggesting that it provides a useful framework for capturing the emergent structured nature of knowledge that leads Carey to attribute theories to children, and also for capturing the processes underlying the organization and reorganization of such knowledge over the course of development.

Inductive Projection

In the model, knowledge about an item independent of its context is encoded in the weights projecting from the *Item* to the *Representation* layer. This knowledge provides a generic, base representation of a concept, and as we have seen in earlier chapters, it can exhibit progressive differentiation over the course of development. However, it is a key point of Carey's work—and one that others in the theory-theory tradition have stressed as well—that knowledge of a concept not only consists of some single static representation, but also of knowledge about how the concept fits in to each of several different subdomains. It is the fact that a concept and its properties fit differently into different conceptual domains—physical, biological, and psychological, to name the three discussed specifically by Carey—that largely motivates Carey's appeals to specific domain theories for each of these domains. Moreover, it is the fact that these patterns change with development that motivates her claim that knowledge undergoes a major reorganization over the course of development.

We have stressed up to now how context-independent concept knowledge evolves in development, but we have not yet considered how concept representations vary across different contexts. The model provides for the possibility of context-dependent representations on the *Hidden* layer, where inputs from the relation units (the *is*, *can*, *has*, and *ISA* units) come together with inputs from the *Representation* layer. This convergence allows the model to capture different similarity relations among the same set of items, depending upon the context in which they are encountered. We now turn to these context-dependent representations to understand how patterns of inductive projection can change over the course of development.

When a new property is associated with a representation in the *Hidden* layer, the likelihood that it will also be activated by a different item will depend both on the input from the *Representation* and from the *Relation* layers. Because different relational contexts emphasize different similarity relations, the model will come to generalize different kinds of features in different ways. Of course it must be acknowledged that the range of contexts provided in the model is highly restricted, and so the extent and nature of context dependency in the model will be likewise highly constrained. Yet we will see that over the course of learning, changes in these context-dependent representations lead to changing patterns of inductive projection, illustrating all of the phenomena itemized above.

We tested the network's generalization of new facts at different points during learning, and looked to see how its behavior differed for *is*, *can*, and *has* properties. First, we will consider what happens when the network is told of new properties for familiar objects, similar to Carey's example of teaching children or adults about an unfamiliar internal organ. We will then consider the more complex situation explored by Gelman and Markman (1986) in which children are taught about properties of unfamiliar objects.

Simulation 7.1: Inductive Projection and Its Differentiation in Development

To explore the model's inductive projection behavior, both as a function of context and of development, we investigated its tendency to project different kinds of newly learned properties from one object to other objects, at two different points during training.

We added a new output unit to the *Attribute* layer to represent a property called *queem*. We trained the model just as described in simulation 6.3, using the same patterns and frequencies described in that section, including the properties *is small, is large, is bright,* and *is dull*. No occurrences of the novel property *queem* occurred during this overall training, which we take as providing the background developmental experience base onto which a test of inductive projection can be introduced. We assessed inductive projection after 500 and 2,500 epochs of this background experience. For this test, we stopped training and taught the network a new fact about the maple tree: either that the *maple can queem,* that the *maple has queem,* or that the *maple is queem*. Recall from chapter 2 that, in a more complete architecture, we would expect this rapid learning to be carried out by the hippocampus, which we believe plays a key role in storing new information without producing interference in the cortical semantic knowledge system (McClelland, McNaughton, and O'Reilly 1995). To simulate this ability in the Rumelhart model, we adjusted only the weights received by the new nonsense property from the *Hidden* layer, so that acquisition of the new fact was tied to the network's representation of *maple* in the given relational context. Adjustments were made to the weights until the unit's activation exceeded 0.9. In each case, when the network had learned the proposition, we stepped through all twenty-one items, each presented with the relation used in training, to see whether the model would activate the new property *queem*.

The results are shown in figure 7.1. Early in learning, the network generalizes the novel property from the maple to all of the plants, regardless of whether it is a *can, has,* or *is* property; there are slight differences in its handling of the *is* property compared to the others, in that it tends also to generalize to some degree to the animals as well. By epoch 2,500, however, the model has learned a much stronger differentiation of the different contexts; the *can* property continues to generalize to all the plants while the *has* properties now generalize only to the other trees. The *is* properties

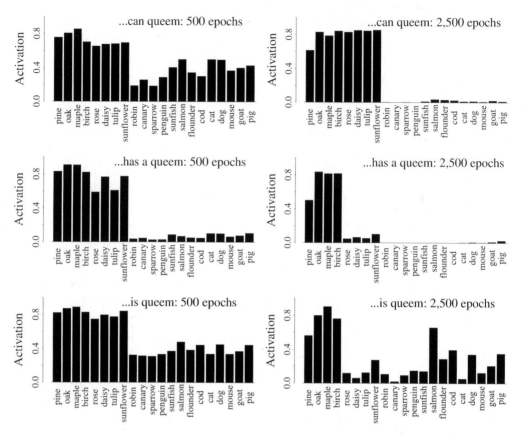

Figure 7.1 Barplot showing the activation of the nonsense property *queem* when the network is queried with various inputs, after it has learned that the maple *can queem*, *has a queem*, or *is queem*. If the network learns the new property after 500 epochs of training, the property generalizes across the entire superordinate category, regardless of the relation context. However, when the network is taught the novel property after 2,500 epochs of training, it shows different patterns of generalization, depending on whether *queem* is understood to be a behavior, a part, or a physical attribute.

also generalize predominantly to the other plants, but not so evenly, and they generalize to some extent to other things (with which the maple happens to share some superficial attributes). Thus, when the network has learned that the *maple is queem*, it shows some tendency to generalize the novel property to items outside the superordinate category; it shows no such tendency when it has been taught that *queem* is a behavior (i.e., a *can* property) or a part (i.e., a *has* property).

The results indicate that the model comes to behave in inductive projection tasks as if it knows that some kinds of properties extend differently than others. Moreover, this knowledge undergoes a developmental progression. The model gradually sorts out that different kinds of properties should be extended in different ways. Just as the network's internal representations of objects in the *Representation* layer adapt during training to the structure of the environment, so too do its context-sensitive representations over the *Hidden* layer. That is, the weights leading from the *Representation* and *Relation* layers into the *Hidden* layer adjust slowly, to capture the different aspects of similarity that exist between the objects in different contexts. Items that share many *can* properties generate similar patterns of activity across units in the *Hidden* layer when the *can* relation unit is activated. However, the same items may generate quite different patterns across these units when one of the other relation units is active in the input.

In figure 7.2, we show a multidimensional scaling of the patterns of activity generated across the *Hidden* units, for the same sixteen items in two different relation contexts, after the model has finished learning. (We excluded the mammal representations from this plot simply to make it less cluttered. They lie between the birds and fish in all three plots.) The plot in the middle shows the learned similarities between patterns for different items in the *Representation* layer. The top plot shows the similarities across *Hidden* units for the same items in the *is* context, whereas the bottom plot shows these similarities in the *can* context. In the *can* context, all the plants receive very similar representations, because

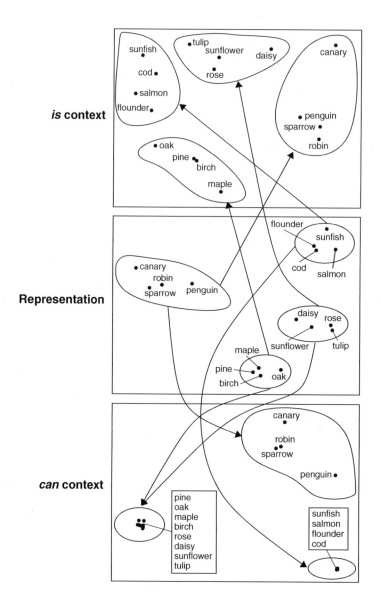

Figure 7.2 Multidimensional scaling showing the similarities represented by the model for objects in different relation contexts. The middle plot shows the similarities among object representations in the *Representation* layer. The top graph shows the similarities among the same objects in the *Hidden* layer, when the *is* relation unit is activated. The bottom graph shows the similarities across these same units when the *can* rela-

they all have exactly the same set of behaviors in the training environment—the only thing a plant can do, as far as the model knows, is grow. As a consequence, the model generalizes new *can* properties from the maple to all of the plants. By contrast, in the *is* context, few properties are shared among objects of the same kind. Thus, the network is pressured to differentiate items in this context, and as a result it shows less of a tendency to generalize newly learned *is* properties.

The other relation contexts not shown in the figure (*has*, *ISA-specific*, *ISA-basic*, *ISA-general*) also remap the similarity relations among the items in the model's environment, in ways that reflect the degree to which the items share properties in the relevant context. Thus, the plants are all represented as similar to one another in the *ISA-general* context, because they all share the same general name, but they are represented as distinct from one another in the *ISA-specific* context, because each has a unique specific name. In the *has* and *ISA-basic* contexts, intermediate clustering structure is represented, because objects from the same intermediate group (e.g., trees, flowers, mammals, birds, and fish) all tend to have the same parts and (with the exception of mammals) the same basic-level name in the model's environment. Thus, these representations turn out to be structured quite similarly to the base representations in the *Representation* layer. Just as for these base representations, the network's representations of objects in a given context depend on the attribute structure of the environment, and in turn these representations constrain how the network learns and generalizes new properties.

Figure 7.2   (continued)
tion unit is activated. The *is* relation context exaggerates differences among related objects—for example, relative to the similarities in the *Representation* layer, the trees are fairly well spread out in the *is* context. Moreover, similarities in object appearances are preserved in these representations—for instance, the canary is as close to the flowers as to the other birds in the *is* context, by virtue of being pretty. By contrast, the *can* context collapses differences among the plants, because in the network's world, all plants can do only one thing: grow.

In summary, we see that in this simulation, the model shows three of the four characteristics of developmental patterns of inductive projection that were itemized above. This can be seen in the model's projection of the property *has queem* from *maple* to other things. It is apparent that the representations and processes that govern the model's induction behavior undergo change over time: the model first extends the property across the entire category of plants, and later restricts its generalization to the category of flowers. Considering the model's projection of different kinds of properties in different ways, we note that after 2,500 epochs of training, the model treats the property *has queem* quite differently from the property *can queem* and somewhat differently from the property *is queem*. Concerning the tendency for patterns of inductive generalization to become more specific, we see clearly that this is true in the model; early on its inductive generalizations of all types of properties are fairly similar, while at 2,500 epochs they become much more strongly differentiated as a function of context. Hence the model captures several aspects of the changes in inductive projection that Carey interprets as indicative of underlying theory change. We have yet to address coalescence, a critical aspect of Carey's findings on conceptual reorganization; we will do so after a further consideration of the differential projection of different kinds of properties, examined in the next simulation.

Simulation 7.2: Differential Projection of Different Kinds of Properties

As a further demonstration of the specificity of inductive projection that can be captured in the model, we conducted a simulation of an experiment described in chapter 1, which shows that children are capable of projecting different kinds of properties in different ways, some of which violate the constraints imposed by the taxonomic hierarchy (Gelman and Markman 1986). In the experiment, children were shown two pictures of novel objects, and were taught their names and a new fact about each. For example, they might be shown a picture of a brontosaurus and a rhinoceros. They would then be told that the first object is called a "dinosaur," which has cold blood, and that the second object is called a "rhinoceros," which has warm blood. In a different condition, the children might see the same objects with the same names, and be told that the dinosaur weighs ten tons whereas the rhinoceros weighs only one ton. The subjects were then shown a picture of a third object (a triceratops), which more closely resembled the rhinoceros. However, the children were told that the triceratops was called a "dinosaur," like the brontosaurus. The authors found that when children had been taught a biological fact about the first two animals (e.g., that one was warm-blooded and the other cold-blooded), they were more likely to use category membership as the basis for generalization, and conclude that the triceratops had cold blood like the brontosaurus. When they had learned a physical property (e.g., that one weighs ten tons and the other weighs only one) they were less systematic, but post hoc analysis showed that they were sensitive to similarity of appearance, generalizing physical properties most strongly across objects that were highly similar in appearance.

Simulating an analog of this experiment with the model required a combination of three steps that we have not previously used together in the same simulation. First, we had to "show" the network two unfamiliar animals—analogs of the brontosaurus and hippopotamus—and allow it to find suitable representations for them using backprop to representation. Next we had to teach the model some new facts about the animals: their names as well as novel properties of two different types. We used *has* properties as analogs to biological properties, and *is* properties as analogs to physical properties. Finally, we had to "show" the network a third animal (analogous to the triceratops) closely resembling the rhinoceros analog, but sharing the same name as the brontosaurus. Of interest, then, is how the network generalizes the newly learned biological and physical properties from the two example animals to the test animal.

To accomplish this, we combined techniques familiar from the simulations above. First, we trained the network with the same patterns and training regime used in simulation 6.3—with the properties *is large* and *is small* reliably differentiating the flowers from the trees, and *is bright* and *is dull* reliably differentiating the birds from the fish. At 3,000 epochs, when the network had not yet completely mastered all of the items, we stopped training and began our simulation of Gelman and Markman's experiment.

We then created analogs of the hippopotamus, brontosaurus, and triceratops triad intended to provide inputs to the model analogous to the information provided to the children. Since the "animals" in the model are not really equivalent to the rhinoceros, and so on, and since we wish to emphasize the abstract correspondence between the characteristics of the model and of the children, we have chosen to designate the items we constructed with the labels *alpha* and *beta* for the two exemplar objects and *tau* for the test object (note that these are not names actually taught to the model, just labels we use to refer to these items in our presentation). We assigned to the alpha the properties *has skin*, *has legs*, *is small*, and *is dull*, and to the beta we gave the properties *has skin*, *has legs*, *is large*, and *is bright*. In the experiment, the triceratops picture was visually more similar to the rhinoceros than to the brontosaurus. To capture this in the model, we assigned to the tau the same visually apparent features as to the alpha (*has skin*, *has legs*, *is small*, and *is dull*).

We "showed" the network the alpha by backpropagating error from all of the relevant output units (*skin*, *legs*, *large*, *small*, *bright*, and *dull*), and using backprop to representation to find a representation that would activate the subset of these properties belonging to alpha (*skin*, *legs*, *small*, *dull*). We then did the same thing for the beta, backpropagating error from the output units *has skin*, *has legs*, *is large*, and *is bright* until the network found a representation that would activate these output units.

When the network had found suitable representations for the new animals on the basis of their familiar properties, we taught it some new facts about each: that the beta *ISA-basic Xyzzyx*, *is ten tons*, and *has cold blood*, and that the alpha *ISA-basic Yatta*, *is one ton*, and *has warm blood*. We added a new output unit to represent each of these properties, and trained the network to activate the appropriate output unit when given either the *beta* or *alpha* representations as input in conjunction with the *ISA-basic*, *is*, or *has* relation. For example, to teach the network that the beta has cold blood, we would set the *Representation* units to the pattern corresponding to the *beta* representation, turn on the *has* unit in the *Context* layer, and then train the network to turn on the output unit corresponding to *cold blood* and turn off the output unit corresponding to *warm blood*. When learning these new properties, the model was permitted to adjust only the weights received by the new property units, just as described for the learning of *queem* properties in simulation 7.1. When the network had finished, it was able to correctly activate both the familiar and novel properties for both the alpha and the beta inputs.

Finally, we had to "show" the network the tau picture and indicate that its basic-level name is the same as that of the beta, but that its appearance is more similar to that of the alpha. To achieve this, we simply backpropagated error from the units that represent the visual properties of the tau (*has skin*, *has legs*, *is small*, *is dull*), as well as from the output unit corresponding to the basic name *Xyzzyx*. Using this error signal, we allowed the network to find a representation for the tau that would activate all of these output units in the appropriate relational context. Thus, the model had to find a representation for the tau consistent with its existing knowledge, which allowed it to activate both the name *Xyzzyx*, which it shares with the beta, and the visual properties, which it shares with the alpha.

Of interest after the network has found such a state is how it generalizes the new facts it has learned about the alpha and the beta to the tau. Note that the model has not been taught either of the novel "biological" (*has*) or "physical" (*is*) properties about the tau—that is, it has not been "told" whether the tau has warm or cold blood, or whether it weighs one or ten tons. To test whether the model has made reasonable inferences about these properties, we queried the network with the *is* and *has* relations, and examined the activation of the new property units.

Table 7.1   Activations of the new property output units when the network is queried for its knowledge of the alpha, beta, and tau

ITEM	ISA		IS		HAS	
	Xyzzyx	*Yatta*	*one ton*	*ten tons*	*cold blood*	*warm blood*
Alpha	0.12	0.93	0.94	0.06	0.03	0.81
Beta	0.93	0.11	0.05	0.94	0.84	0.16
Tau	0.64	0.32	0.61	0.31	0.82	0.14

Note: The activations of *Is one ton/ten tons* and *Has warm blood/cold blood* represent inductive projections of these properties to the tau from the alpha and beta respectively.

In table 7.1 we show the activation of the six new property units (corresponding to the properties *ISA-basic Xyzzyx, ISA-basic Yatta, is one ton, is ten tons, has cold blood,* and *has warm blood*) when the network is queried for its knowledge of the tau. The network activates *Xyzzyx* more than *Yatta*, as it should, since it was trained to do so. More interestingly, the model strongly activates the property *has cold blood*, showing that this biological attribute has generalized from the beta, with which it shares the same basic-level name. However, it also activates the property *is one ton*, showing that the physical property has generalized from the alpha, with which it shares many physical properties. Like Gelman and Markman's subjects, the model seems to know that some kinds of properties (i.e., *is* properties) generalize across things that look the same, but others (i.e., *has* properties) generalize across objects that share the same name.

To correctly activate the properties it shares with the alpha but not the beta—*is small* and *is dull*—the network must find a representation for the tau that is similar to the alpha in the *is* context.

However, to activate the name *Xyzzyx* the network must represent the tau as similar to the beta in the *ISA-basic* context. Because the weights leading from the *Representation* to the *Hidden* layer are already configured to remap the similarities between items depending on the relation context, the network is able to find a pattern of activation across the *Representation* units that satisfies these constraints.

Because the tau and the alpha are represented as similar to one another in the *is* context, all of the *is* properties the network has learned about the alpha generalize to the tau, including the newly acquired ones. Because the tau and the beta are similar to one another in the *ISA-basic* context, the name *Xyzzyx* extends to the tau. But why do the newly learned *has* properties of the beta generalize to the tau?

The reason is that the network has learned to represent the same similarities between objects in the *ISA-basic* and *has* contexts. In the network's training environment, items that share the same basic name also have a strong tendency to share *has* attributes. For example, all of the birds share the properties *has wings* and *has feathers*, whereas all of the fish share the attributes *has scales* and *has gills*. Thus, items that are similar to one another in the *ISA-basic* context are also similar to one another in the *has* context. To name the tau as a *Xyzzyx* the network represents it as similar to the beta in the *ISA-basic* context. The overlapping representations are then used across *Hidden* units when the network is queried with the *has* context, and the network extends the properties of the beta to the tau.

The simulations demonstrate how our model can behave in ways specific to the combined constraints provided both by an item and by its relational context. It also brings out how the model can use the same representations across different contexts when these representations have to do similar work. The system shades its representations for use in different contexts, while exploiting similarity of conceptual representations to afford a basis for inductive projection. As we will see, this tendency to exploit shared structure across contexts may be relevant to cases of reorganization of conceptual representations based on coalescence of information across contexts.

Reorganization and Coalescence

We have not yet seen how the third kind of reorganization described by Carey—coalescence—may also arise in the model. However, the simulations we have discussed suggest at least one property of the model that may give rise to coalescence in the semantic system. Recall from our simulation of bird and fish experts (simulation 5.5) that the network learned different similarities among the same set of items, depending on whether they appeared more frequently in the *is* or the *can* relation context. Thus, the frequency with which the model encounters particular kinds of information can have a great influence on the internal representations it acquires, independent of its knowledge about particular contexts and situations. Although living things may have many properties in common (e.g., they all have DNA, they all breathe, they all grow and die), many of these shared properties are nonobvious (Gelman and Wellman 1991). For example, animate objects may be considered members of the same class by virtue of sharing various internal organs, but these properties are often not apparent in their outward appearance. Properties less diagnostic of an item's ontological status may be readily apparent in the environment. For example, an object's shape, color, texture, parts, and patterns of motion are apparent every time the object is encountered. Information about its insides, its metabolic functions, or other aspects of its behavior may be available only sporadically. Moreover, opportunities for acquiring this information likely change as the child develops—for example, children presumably acquire a great deal of nonobvious biological information when they attend school. Carey herself appears to hold the view that at least part of the reason younger children lack an intuitive biological theory is that they have simply not been exposed to enough information about the correspondences among nonobvious characteristics of plants and animals.

The account of conceptual reorganization consistent with these observations, then, is that as children acquire information about the nonobvious properties of objects, this introduces new constraints that lead to changes in underlying knowledge representations. That is, nonobvious properties provide new information about how apparently unrelated objects (such as mammals, insects, and trees) are in fact quite similar to one another in several respects. This view appears to be very similar to Carey's, but she provides no mechanism whereby the assimilation of this information can actually lead to the relevant underlying change. What we would like to suggest is that the learning mechanisms operating in the Rumelhart model, which should by now be quite familiar, provide just the sort of mechanism needed to allow such representational changes to occur. Indeed we will suggest that these learning mechanisms also provide a way of seeing how reorganization might occur even in cases where the information available to the child remains constant over time (although still in a way differentially accessible). The simulations presented next are intended to illustrate these points.

We wish to demonstrate two different but related points: First, as the availability of different kinds of information in the model's environment changes, its internal representations of objects undergo conceptual reorganization. Second, even if the availability of different kinds of information is held constant, there can be conceptual reorganization if different kinds of information differ in their patterns of availability. We consider the two points in sequence in what follows, beginning with an examination of the effects of changes in availability over development.

Simulation 7.3: Coalescence

Recall that the various items in the model's environment have different propensities to share properties in different contexts—for

example, the various birds all share the same *can* properties but
have quite different *is* properties. We have already seen that when
the model is trained very frequently with *can* properties, it acquires quite different internal representations than it does when
trained with the *is* context most frequent (simulation 5.5). To simulate changes in the availability of different kinds of information in
the model, we varied the extent to which the model is trained with
the *is* properties that denote perceptual attributes such as color and
size.

In simulation 7.3a, we first exposed the network to items in the
is context only. After 500 epochs of training with these patterns,
we examined the similarities acquired by the model. We then continued training, this time exposing the model to all items in all relation contexts, including the *is* context. After a further 500 epochs
training, we again looked at the similarities among the model's internal representations of the same items. This provides a crude
analogy to the situation in which the system is initially exposed to
visual information alone, and only later is exposed to other kinds
of information about objects.

In simulation 7.3b we adopted a more graded approach to
changes in availability of different kinds of information. Throughout training, the network was exposed to all of the various properties (*is*, *can*, *has*, and the three *ISA* contexts). However, we
gradually varied the relative frequency with which different kinds
of information were presented to the network over time. Initially,
can, *has*, and *ISA* properties were presented only once for every
100 presentations of an *is* pattern. After every 10 epochs of training, we increased the frequency with which the *can*, *has*, and *ISA*
patterns appeared by 1; for example, after 20 epochs each *has*
pattern appeared twice for every 100 presentations of an *is* pattern; after 30 epochs, 3 times, and so on. After 1,000 epochs of
training, all patterns appeared equally frequently in the model's
environment.

In simulation 7.3a, where pattern frequencies were held constant
the network was exposed to 768 training trials in each epoch. In

simulation 7.3b, the network was initially trained with each *is* pattern appearing 100 times, and all other patterns appearing once in each epoch. Frequencies were then adjusted every 10 epochs as described above. The order of the trials within each epoch was permuted in all simulations. All units were assigned a fixed bias of −2. As in most of the simulations described previously, the model was trained with a learning rate of 0.005, with noisy hidden units, and without momentum.

In figure 7.3 we show hierarchical cluster plots of the similarity relations among the sixteen items in the model's environment at two different points during training, for both stimulations. Mammal items are excluded to keep the plots simple and clear. The top two cluster plots show the results from simulation 7.3a, after training with just the *is* context (left-hand plot), and after further training with all six relation contexts (right-hand plot). After training with just the superficial *is* properties, the model groups items in ways that do not reflect their underlying semantic relations, but only their *is* properties, which are idiosyncratic and unsystematic. In fact, it groups the sixteen items primarily on the basis of their color, in part because there is somewhat more sharing of color across different objects than most of the other *is* properties that were used. Thus, three items under the leftmost branch are all white (the tulip, penguin, and cod); the four beneath the rightmost node are all yellow (the daisy, canary, sunflower, and sunfish), and so on. Obviously, we do not intend by any means to suggest that color is the basis on which young children actually organize their conceptual representations (or even that daisies, canaries, and sunfish are really all the same color). The patterns of similarity represented in the *is* context in our model do not realistically capture the properties of children's early experience (as discussed in chapter 4), and thus would not be expected to lead to representations like those children actually use. The point of this simulation is simply to illustrate that representations arising on the basis of similarity structure available from the ensemble of early experiences can later be restructured when changes in experience

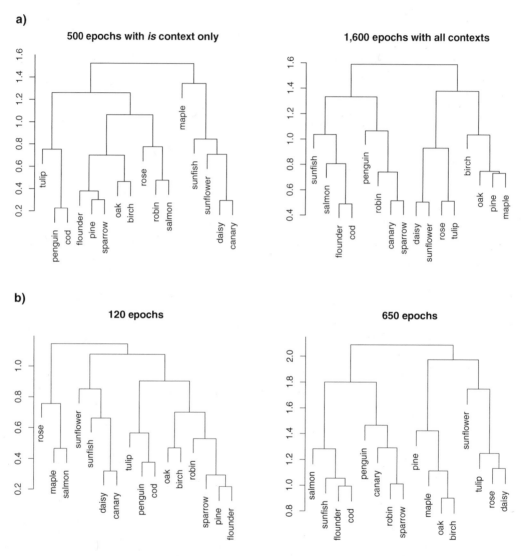

Figure 7.3 Hierarchical cluster plots of the model's internal representations in two simulations that demonstrate conceptual reorganization in the model. Plot (a) shows similarities in the model's representations after 500 epochs of training with items in just the *is* context (left-hand plot), and after 1100 further epochs of training with all six relation contexts (right-hand plot). Plot (b) indicates these similarities when the model is trained with gradually changing context frequencies.

provide information indicative of a different structure. Once the model has been exposed to information about other kinds of object properties, the superficial similarities present in the *is* patterns no longer reflect the overall similarity structure. As a consequence, its internal representations of the sixteen animal and plant items reorganize to capture the very different similarity relations that exist among items that share the same behaviors, parts, and names. Similar results were observed in simulation 7.3b: early in learning the network acquires representations in which items with similar *is* properties (again primarily color) are represented as similar. As the frequency with which other kinds of information increases, this early organization gives way to a scheme in which more appropriate semantic similarity relations are represented.

Figure 7.3 shows that both differentiation and coalescence can occur in the model as a consequence of manipulating the relative availability of different kinds of information in the environment. After training with the *is* context only, or with the *is* context more frequent than others, the model represents the daisy, the sunflower, the canary, and the sunfish as similar to one another and distinct from other items, presumably because they share the same color. After further training with all six contexts, or with these contexts growing more frequent, this early grouping has split apart—these four items are represented as quite distinct from one another with the exception of the two flowers, which remain similar. In contrast, new clusterings of item representations coalesce in the model after further training with all relation contexts. While the four fish were distinct from one another in the earlier representations, they are now represented as quite similar to one another, and as distinct from other items. Thus it is not the case that the later model's representations form a simple superset or subset of the earlier model's representations. Instead, the later model's internal representations find no obvious progenitor in the earlier model's representations. One might go so far as to say that the latter model's conceptual system is *incommensurable* with the earlier model's, capturing a key element of what Carey has suggested characterizes the representational changes that occur during development.

Two Different Aspects of Coalescence   The results of simulations 7.3a and 7.3b should seem fairly obvious, given the sensitivity of the model to similarity structure in its training environment. If networks organize their representations in response to environmental structure, it should not be too surprising that representations reorganize when the structure of the environment changes. Perhaps it will be less obvious, however, that this reorganization represents a coalescence, in two different senses of the word—senses that we think Carey herself intends in using the term to describe conceptual reorganization in childhood. Specifically, Carey (1985) uses the word *coalescence* to refer to the fact that younger children, already in possession of distinct concepts for *plant* and *animal*, later achieve an overarching concept of *living thing* that encompasses these earlier concepts. She also uses the term to suggest that the discovery of this new concept represents a gathering together of knowledge about structure common to plants and animals—structure that may only be apparent across domains that are often treated quite separately (at least in the developmental literature). Such domains might include, for example, what it means for something to be alive versus dead, how reproduction occurs, the use of energy for growth, competition with other species, the nature of biological processes such as eating and breathing, and so on. A general concept like *living thing*, within which different varieties of living things are construed as similar, does a lot of "work" to account for observations across these different contexts. It is precisely this fact that, in Carey's view, ultimately drives the emergence of a naive biology—that is, the coalescence of plant and animal concepts within the general concept *living thing*.

Both of these kinds of coalescence are characteristic of the changes seen in our model. First, the emergence of the conceptual hierarchy of plants (including trees and flowers), and that of animals (including birds and fish), represents a coalescence of these "concepts" out of the earlier representations in which the same items were dispersed across clusters organized primarily by color. But second, and most interestingly, this coalescence of concepts in our model arises precisely because the model is sensitive to shared structure present across different relational contexts. That is, the final representations discovered by the model capture those aspects of structure that are consistent across the individual contexts. The reason is that the model does not treat these contexts as completely distinct from one another. Instead, it derives representations that tend to be rather similar, though not identical, across the different contexts. Units in the *Representation* layer must, of course, use exactly the same representations in different contexts; but importantly the units in the *Hidden* layer also tend to do so, because the same pool of units is used to represent all combinations of item and context. Just as the network tends to represent individual items as similar until learning drives them apart, so too does it treat different contexts as similar initially—providing a basis for learning in one context to influence representation in another. The network learns to produce different outputs in different contexts by differentially adjusting a shared set of underlying representations—those coded by the *Representation* layer. But because the different contexts start out quite similar to one another, common structure apparent across contexts can shape the representations that emerge in both *Representation* and *Hidden* layers. We will return to this aspect of the network in the discussion at the end of this chapter.

We now turn our attention to simulation 7.3c, which will illustrate the importance of sensitivity to cross-contextual structure in our account of conceptual reorganization during development. For this simulation, we did not vary the frequency of different patterns across time at all. Instead we made *is* properties generally more available in the environment by requiring the model always to activate these properties, regardless of which context unit was given in the input. For example, when presented with *robin has* in the input, the model was required to activate all the *is* properties true of robins, as well as all of their *has* properties. Similarly, when presented with *robin can* in the input, the model was again required to activate all of the *is* properties, as well as the *can* properties. Thus the information coded in the *is* patterns in this simulation was more frequently available than the information coded by the other property types. Additionally, the information previously tied to the *is* context was independent of context, while the other property types remained context-dependent. The network had, in this case, a relatively simple job to do in learning which *is* units to activate for a given concept, and it received very frequent teaching input for this task. Conversely it had a relatively complex job to do in learning how to deal with each of the other contexts, since these involved completely nonoverlapping sets of output units for each of the three contexts.

Nevertheless, the network was capable of exploiting the shared structure that existed across these different contexts. The results of the simulation, shown in figure 7.4, are similar to those seen in

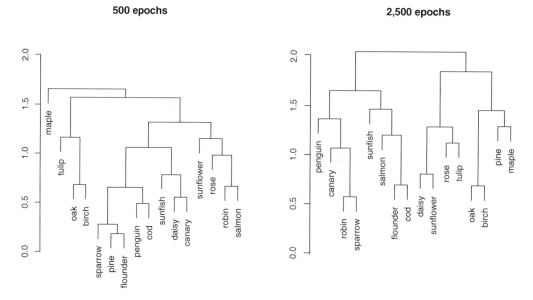

Figure 7.4   Hierarchical cluster plots of the model's internal representations in simulation 7.3c, in which the model is required to activate appropriate *is* properties for all contexts. The model is trained with the same patterns throughout, but its representations undergo a reorganization similar to that seen in simulations 7.3a and 7.3b.

simulations 7.3a and 7.3b. Early on, the dominant influence of superficial similarity (apparent across the *is* properties) is still evident, though less clear cut than in the other simulations. After 500 epochs of training, the model has divided the items into several small clusters that do not correspond well to global semantic categories. These clusters are organized largely, although not completely, by color (e.g., in the rightmost cluster three of the four items are red). Most important for our argument, the representations that emerge later in learning capture more fully the shared structure present across the various other contexts. That is, the pattern of property covariation across the different contexts has coalesced to determine the similarity structure ultimately expressed by the underlying representations.

Global or Context-Sensitive Reorganization?

In discussions with some colleagues, we have found a considerable hesitation to think that adult conceptual representations of living things really do coalesce into an integrated representation of living things across the domains of plants and animals. Rather, they suggest, it is possible to see that animals and plants do share many things in common, while feeling that they are nevertheless fundamentally quite separate kinds of things. These intuitions seem consistent with Carey's views. Within their intuitive biology, she seems to suggest, adults and older children see a coalescence of plants and animals into a common concept of living things, but within other contexts they may see them as quite different things.

Although we have not explicitly offered simulations of these points, we note briefly that our approach offers a range of possibilities with respect to these issues. For example, it seems quite possible that the coalescence of knowledge across one set of contexts (life and death, reproduction, and so on), in giving rise to an intuitive biology, would not completely restructure the underlying representations so long as there remains a different basis for organization, relevant to a different set of contexts. In our view it is quite likely that individuals differ greatly in these respects, depending on the precise nature of their experience with living things. Thus, for some, biological knowledge of the kind Carey describes may become the fundamental organizing framework for knowledge about all living things, whereas for others this kind of knowledge may remain highly context sensitive (e.g., related to "things I learned in school"). These differences would depend heavily on the details of individual experience.

Discussion

The simulations discussed in this chapter demonstrate that PDP models can provide a mechanistic explanation of both the context sensitivity exhibited by children and adults in semantic induction tasks, and the apparent reorganization of conceptual knowledge throughout childhood revealed by the experiments described by Carey and others. According to the PDP theory, semantic induction is mediated by the similarities among distributed internal representations constructed by the semantic system for novel and familiar objects in its environment. These internal representations are conditioned on the system's knowledge about an object's familiar properties and its sensitivity to informative interdependencies among stimulus attributes, as we saw in the last chapter. They are also conditioned on the system's knowledge about the particular context in which the task is performed. The system may represent the same set of items differently, depending on whether it is required to retrieve *is*, *can*, or *has* properties. Context-sensitive projection—the ability to project a new property in different ways depending on the type of information—depends on this capacity to condition internal representations on contextual information. Because different similarity relations are represented in different contexts, the system can show different patterns of induction for different kinds of properties. Thus we agree in part with Carey's (1985) suggestion that any assessment of the child's conceptual structure must take into account the context in which the concepts are being used in a given situation. Carey uses the term "theoretical context," reflecting her view that the use of a concept is theory dependent. While we do not view the knowledge in our networks as constituting a theory per se, different situational contexts do highlight different subsets of an item's properties. In the model, knowledge about these contexts (like all other knowledge) is coded in connection weights and serves to restructure the representation and use of particular items in a way that is reminiscent of the role of "theoretical context" in Carey's framework.

As we have stressed several times, the internal representations constructed by the system depend on the knowledge stored in its weights. These weights change as the system gains more experience in the world; consequently its internal representations change as it learns, and so too does its generalization and induction behavior. We have seen that the different ways representations can change with learning in the Rumelhart network encompass the various kinds of representational change observed through childhood, as inferred by Carey from semantic induction tasks. Like children, the network initially shows a tendency to generalize new facts in more or less the same way, regardless of the kind of information, but later begins to generalize different kinds of facts in different ways. We have seen that the network gradually differentiates its internal representations, making finer and finer distinctions among objects and hence changing the likelihood with which it will generalize from one to another. When superficial "perceptual" properties are more readily available in the environment, the model's internal representations undergo a kind of perceptual-to-conceptual shift, with the network initially representing objects with similar "appearances" as similar regardless of their semantic relatedness, and only later settling on more conceptual representations. That is, the model's representations undergo both differentiation and coalescence, and the model also learns that different kinds of properties generalize differently. Carey (1985) suggests that analogous phenomena observed in child development indicate changes in the child's underlying theories. Interestingly, change of this kind emerges in our model from the very same mechanisms that also promote the coarse-to-fine differentiation of concepts in infancy, the emergence of basic-level advantages and their interaction with typicality, and various aspects of expertise. To our knowledge, our theory is the first to achieve this kind of unification across such a broad range of phenomena in conceptual representation and development.

While it will be clear that we think our simulations are highly relevant to the issues explored by Carey in her book, it may be worth noting that we suspect that Carey, and perhaps many others, will not be entirely convinced that our model fully addresses the issues targeted by her work. In part this reaction may relate to the fact that we have not yet dealt with a central claim of theory-theory, namely, the claim that the knowledge supporting concepts is largely causal in nature. A further and related point is that we have not yet considered how knowledge of the kind acquired by our networks might be used to provide a basis for producing and understanding explanations. We certainly would agree with these points, and indeed, discussion of these specific issues is the main task of chapter 8.

Quite apart from these issues per se, we still suspect that some researchers will hesitate to fully adopt our view that the PDP framework offers a useful guide for understanding knowledge of the sort that theory-theorists concern themselves with. We have some sympathy with such a perspective, for it is clear that the simulations we have presented do not capture the full richness of the content of human conceptual knowledge. The question is where to place the blame for this shortcoming. Does it lie in the fundamental nature of the mechanisms we have described, or does it lie in the impoverished nature of the actual content our network has been asked to learn? Our conjecture is that the problem is primarily of the latter kind. We think (as we shall endeavor to explain in the next chapter) that the simple *is*, *can*, and *has* contexts that we have explored thus far do not do full justice to the range of different kinds of contexts across which we acquire our conceptual knowledge, and we likewise feel that the immediate activation of output units corresponding to particular object properties does not do full justice to the range of outputs or expectations our conceptual representations must be expected to sustain.

On reading these comments, some readers may be tempted to wonder in just what sense we might be offering our PDP theory as a framework for understanding conceptual knowledge and its development, and in just what way we might suppose the simple network models we have explored here provide any kind of useful model for understanding these issues. Our response to this is simple. We suggest that certain characteristics of the model—its ability to exploit shared structure across contexts, its ability to organize and reorganize in response to experience—reflect the operation of core principles and mechanisms afforded by the PDP framework, and that the more complex models that will be needed to capture the full content of human conceptual knowledge will operate by these same principles. The principles govern the behavior of the Rumelhart model as it assimilates the content appearing in its limited training environment, and these behaviors serve to illustrate how we would expect the same core principles to play out in a model capable of assimilating the richer structure present in real experience. Of course the network architecture would need to be adapted for this purpose, but we suggest that any successful model will preserve important aspects of the architecture of the Rumelhart network. After our treatment of causality and related issues in chapter 8, we will return to these issues in chapter 9.

The experimental findings we have considered in the last two chapters demonstrate that the acquisition of semantic knowledge (and performance of semantic tasks) is subject to constraints—some feature constellations are easier to learn than others; some groups of objects support generalization better than others; different kinds of information may generalize in different ways. Under the theory-theory, these constraints are imposed by "naive theories" about the causal forces that explain the co-occurrence of properties in an object concept. Within our model, the ability to capture these constraints arises from the same processes that give rise to the advantage of general over specific information in dementia, the progressive differentiation of concepts in development, the effects of frequency and typicality, the advantage of the basic level, and various other findings. That is, within our network the constraints arise from domain-general learning and experience with the structure present in the training environment coupled with the dynamics of learning that arise from the use of distributed representations. No special invocation of domain-specific theories was required to address these phenomena.

In light of the above, one might be tempted to propose that a PDP network acquiring knowledge under the pressure of experience might provide the underlying mechanisms necessary to embody the knowledge that has led theory-theorists to suggest we use causal domain theories to constrain our semantic cognition. However, in spite of the results of the preceding chapters, the case for this proposition remains, at this point, incomplete. There are additional experimental findings and considerations relating specifically to the idea that at least some of the knowledge governing semantic cognition is causal knowledge, and to the idea that one of the roles of such knowledge is to provide explanations for observed events. The question we address in the present chapter is, could the PDP approach be extended to address these additional findings and considerations? Our approach to this question will be more speculative than the approach we have taken in the preceding sections of this book, since we will not be offering additional simulations. Instead we will give an informal sketch of how these issues might be addressed within the PDP framework.

The work that will be the focus of our attention in this chapter investigates causal knowledge and causal inference across a wide age range, from age 2.5 years to adulthood. We will not be focusing on the large body of research that has arisen on the perception of causality in infancy (Michotte 1963; Piaget 1930; Leslie 1984; Leslie and Keeble 1987; Cohen, Chaput, and Cashon 2002), even though many of the issues that will be considered in this chapter have arisen in this work as well. For instance, some investigators have used evidence from infant looking-time experiments to argue for innate domain-specific mechanisms that detect causal relationships (e.g., Leslie 1995), whereas others have suggested that an early sensitivity to causal interactions might develop through domain-general, experience-dependent perceptual-learning mechanisms (e.g., Cohen et al. 1999, 2002). Our own approach is more similar to the latter perspective, and though we will develop it with reference to data from older children and adults, we expect that our basic account would extend well to the findings in the infant literature.

In the first part of this chapter we will consider the possibility of encompassing within the PDP framework knowledge about the causal origins of an object's observed properties, knowledge about the causal relations among observed properties, and knowledge about an object's causal properties. By "causal properties" we intend something similar to what Wilson and Keil (2000) describe as *causal powers*. They write:

It may seem as though "causal powers" is another name for a property or object, but the real sense seems more one of an interaction between a kind of thing and the world in which it is situated. Thus we can understand and explain something in terms of its causal powers, which means not just listing its properties as sets of things attached to it, but rather listing its *disposition to behave in certain ways in certain situations.* (p. 108; our emphasis)

When we speak about knowledge of an object's causal properties, we mean knowledge about how the object participates in events and what the consequences or sequelae are of that participation. This may broaden the concept a bit beyond the uses of others, but certainly still includes what Wilson and Keil refer to with the term *causal powers.*

According to theory-theory, the knowledge that underlies semantic judgments in many domains is embodied in causal theories, and as a consequence, knowledge about the causal properties of objects, or about the causal relations existing among an object's observed properties, plays an especially important role in constraining semantic cognition. In the classic example, which by now will be very familiar, what gives the properties of having wings and having feathers their central place in our understanding of birds is their causal role in enabling flight. That is, the importance of wings, feathers, and flight for the concept *bird* results from stored knowledge about the causal links among these properties. In search of evidence that such causal knowledge strongly constrains concepts, several researchers have conducted experiments to determine whether semantic judgments are influenced by information about an object's causal powers, or about the causal origins of or relations among its properties. Key experiments described by Keil (1989), the work of Ahn and colleagues (Ahn 1998; Ahn, Marsh, and Luhmann 2002; Ahn et al. 2000, 1995), and studies described by Gopnik (e.g., Gopnik and Sobel 2000; Gopnik 2001), all tend toward the conclusion that semantic judgments are influenced by knowledge about causal origins, causal relations, and causal properties of objects. These results, reviewed below, have often been taken to support the conclusion that causal knowledge is in some way special or privileged, relative to other kinds of knowledge about objects. Moreover, some very recent experiments have found that the causal attributions made by quite young children often accord, at least approximately, with normative theories of optimal inference (Gopnik et al., forthcoming; Sobel, Tenenbaum, and Gopnik 2002)—bolstering the argument for an innate mechanism specialized to discover causal structure.

In the past two chapters, we have shown that the centrality of certain properties for a given concept (such as wings, feathers, and flight for the concept *bird*) might arise from the learning processes at work in our networks. In that account, it was not an appeal to causal links per se, but to the coherent covariation of having wings, feathers, and hollow bones with flying, that gave these properties their central place in our model. Even so, we do not mean to suggest that people are not sensitive to causal processes or that they do not rely on this sensitivity in making semantic judgments. In agreement with other investigators, we believe there is good evidence that even quite young children can and do learn about the causal properties of objects, and that they can use what they have learned about these properties to influence other aspects of their semantic cognition. However, we also believe that such knowledge need not be considered different or separate from other types of semantic knowledge, nor should it be construed as incompatible with a PDP approach to semantic knowledge representation. Rather, we will suggest that knowledge about the causal properties of objects may be similar to knowledge about other properties of objects—it may be acquired through domain-general learning principles sensitive to the structure of the environment (in this case, sequential structure), just as is knowledge about the appearance, parts, movements, and names of objects. In turn, causal properties of objects may be particularly important for representing some kinds of objects for the same reason that other properties such as color or shape are important for other kinds of objects:

causal properties may vary consistently with what certain kinds of things are called, with aspects of their physical structure, and with other regularities that arise from experience with them. We will review the experiments cited above, which specifically point to the role of causal knowledge in governing semantic cognition, and we will explain how models like those from previous chapters could be extended to address the data from these studies. We will also discuss briefly how the general-purpose mechanisms in the PDP account relate to those employed in normative theories of optimal inference, as discussed by Gopnik and colleagues (e.g., Gopnik et al., forthcoming).

In the second part of the chapter, we will consider a related issue that has been raised by some of the champions of theory-theory: the ability to provide explanations for events, and the tendency to seek explanations and find them satisfying or useful when we experience events that may be unusual or surprising. Some investigators (e.g., Gopnik and Wellman 1994) have suggested that one of the primary functions of a theory is to provide a basis for explaining observed events, while others (e.g., Gelman 1990) have relied on children's explanations of their semantic judgments to support their claims about the nature of the domain knowledge that underlies their judgments and decisions. But the relationship between the "causal knowledge" that people exhibit implicitly in their behavior, and the explicit verbal explanations they can provide if asked, is murky at best (Wilson and Keil 2000). Classic studies by Nisbett and Wilson (1977) demonstrated that people rarely have accurate knowledge of the factors influencing their decisions in a range of cognitive tasks, suggesting that the explanations children and adults provide for their semantic judgments may not transparently reveal the true mechanisms giving rise to their behavior. More recent work by Keil (Keil, forthcoming; Wilson and Keil 2000) suggests that, appearances to the contrary, overt explanatory knowledge for many everyday phenomena rarely runs very deep in normal adults. From such experiments, it is not clear how the ability (when present) to provide overt and detailed explanations relates to the mechanisms that support everyday semantic task performance.

We accept that under some conditions people can offer explanations of observed events, and that they can also sometimes provide explanations for their judgments and decisions in semantic tasks, but we provide a somewhat different perspective on how these explanations relate to the judgments and decisions themselves. Specifically, we consider the explanations that people hear to be among the sources of information that drive the development of semantic representations, and we consider the explanations people generate to be among outputs that their semantic knowledge allows them to produce. Thus we consider explanations to influence and to be influenced by the representations we form of objects and events, but we do not view them as having any privileged or special status, just as with names.

We have no illusions that we will convince all skeptics that the PDP framework can be extended successfully to address the effects of causal knowledge on semantic cognition or to capture all aspects of people's explanations. What we do hope is that the chapter serves to indicate the general stance a PDP approach to the phenomena under consideration might take, and to provide a prospectus for the future research that will obviously be necessary to establish whether indeed this approach might be successful.

The Role of Causal Properties of Objects in Semantic Cognition

As noted, there is substantial support for the view that causal knowledge plays a role in semantic cognition. Generally the aim of the relevant studies has been to demonstrate that participants make different semantic judgments about a given item, depending on their knowledge about the causal forces that give rise to the item's properties, or about the item's own causal powers. In some cases, the relevant causal information is relayed to participants through verbal statements about sequences of events (e.g., Ahn 1998; Ahn et al. 2000; Keil 1989; Springer and Keil 1991). In others, participants directly observe sequences of events, and make their own inferences about causal forces (e.g., Gopnik and Sobel 2000). Using such methods, it has been convincingly shown that semantic task performance can be influenced by at least three different kinds of causal knowledge: knowledge about the forces that give rise to an object's observed properties, knowledge about the causal relations among an object's observed properties, and knowledge about an object's causal powers (i.e., its participation in observed event sequences). We will first review the experiments documenting these phenomena, and will then consider how the PDP approach might extend to explain them.

The Importance of Knowledge about Causal Origins

Keil's studies of children's reactions to object transformations provide a particularly well-known example of the methodology described above (see Keil 1989). In a representative experiment, children were told about a raccoon who underwent some event that resulted in its looking like a skunk. Children in different conditions of the experiment heard different stories about the nature of the change. In one story the raccoon was wearing a costume. In another, it was given an injection by scientists when it was a baby, so that when it grew up it looked like a skunk. Other causal stories varied in the degree to which the mechanism of change could be construed as biological. In all cases, the children were asked whether the raccoon was still a raccoon, or whether it had become a skunk. Young children were willing to accept that the change in appearance signaled a change in kind, regardless of the mechanism by which the change was induced. However, older children were willing to accept that some kinds of transformations (such as the injection) might result in a change of kind, but did not accept other transformations (such as the costume) as leading to a kind change. Thus, for older children, the willingness to accept a change in kind depended on the particular causal mechanism from which the object's appearance was said to have arisen.

Such studies indicate that the judgments about "kind" drawn from a stimulus object are sensitive to information about the causal forces that give rise to the stimulus's properties. When children of sufficient age are shown a picture of a skunk and are told it is a raccoon in a costume, they draw one set of conclusions about what kind of thing it is (i.e., that it is "really" a raccoon), but when shown the same picture with a different sequence of events they draw a different conclusion (i.e., when given the injection story, many decide that it has "really" become a skunk). Thus, the causes of the animal's appearance, and not just its appearance itself, influence children's semantic cognition.

The Importance of Knowledge about Causal Relations among Attributes

Using methods similar to Keil's, Ahn and colleagues (Ahn 1998; Ahn et al. 2000) have demonstrated that both children and adults are apt to weight "cause" properties more heavily than "effect" properties when categorizing novel objects. In one experiment, two groups of college undergraduates were told stories about a new kind of orchid discovered in Central Africa called *Coryanthes*. Both groups were told that 80 percent of Coryanthes have *Eucalyptol* in their flowers, and that 80 percent attract male bees. However, the groups were given different stories about the causal relations between these properties. Group A was told:

Because Coryanthes have Eucalyptol in their flowers, Coryanthes tend to attract orchid male bees; Eucalyptol, which has a strong smell of Eucalyptus, tends to be attractive to most male bees.

Group B was told:

Because Coryanthes tend to attract orchid male bees, they usually have Eucalyptol in their flowers; while orchid male bees are collecting nectar from Coryanthes, they tend to leave Eucalyptol obtained from other flowers in Coryanthes.

Thus, both groups were given the same information about the novel object's properties. What varied was the story about the causal mechanism linking the two properties: in the first story, the property *has Eucalyptol* was understood to cause the property *attracts male bees*, whereas the reverse was true in the second story. Participants were then asked the following two questions:

1. Suppose a flower in Central Africa has Eucalyptol, but does not attract orchid male bees. How likely is it that this flower is a Coryanthes?
2. Suppose a flower in Central Africa attracts orchid male bees, but does not have Eucalyptol in the flower. How likely is it that this flower is a Coryanthes?

Participants judged that the flower was more likely to be a Coryanthes when it shared whichever property had been described as "causal" in the story they heard: *has Eucalyptol* for group A, and *attracts male bees* for group B. Because the design of the experiment was counterbalanced, and participants in both groups were provided with the same information about the likelihood of Coryanthes having the two properties, Ahn (1998) argued that the pattern cannot have arisen from the participants' prior knowledge about the domain, nor from the explicit covariation information provided in the story. Instead, the data provide evidence that adults are predisposed to treat "causally central" properties as being more important or informative for making category judgments. Further experiments using similar methods have revealed similar effects in 7- to 9-year-old children (Ahn et al. 2000).

These and other studies conducted by Ahn and her colleagues (Ahn et al. 1995; Ahn and Kalish 2000; Ahn, Marsh, and Luhmann 2002) again suggest that the way attributes are interpreted and used to determine category membership and typicality depends on explicit knowledge about the causal relationships that hold between them. Not all pairwise correlations contribute equally to determining an item's conceptual status—instead, the importance accorded a given correlation can vary, depending on one's knowledge about the causal relations among the properties themselves.

The Importance of Knowledge about an Object's Causal Powers

Both in Ahn's work and in Keil's transformation studies, the participants' causal knowledge was tapped by providing them with explicit descriptions of the sequence of events from which an object's properties were understood to have arisen. Another means of assessing the influence of causal knowledge on semantic task performance is to demonstrate the apparent causal properties of particular kinds of objects in (staged) events, and to probe the consequences of these demonstrations for the child's semantic judgments. Gopnik and Sobel (2000) have used this method to demonstrate that the semantic induction behavior of young children (ages 3–4) depends on their knowledge about the causal powers of objects. In this experiment, participants watched an experimenter placing colored blocks on a box sitting on a table. The blocks varied in shape and color, and they also varied with respect to their apparent effect on the box's behavior: for some blocks, called *effective blocks*, the machine would light up and play music when the block was placed on top of it; for others, called *ineffective blocks*, nothing happened when the block was placed on the box. Gopnik and colleagues demonstrated these effects to children, and explored the consequences.

Two results are of particular interest. First, children appeared to use information about a block's causal properties, rather than its shape or its color, to govern decisions about which blocks were the same kind of thing. For example, after seeing that a green block and a black block caused the machine to produce music, whereas another green block and another black block did not, children tended to extend a label (*blicket*) applied to an effective block to the other effective block regardless of the difference in color. In general, after observing their causal properties, children were likely to ignore color and shape similarities, but generalized a newly learned label on the basis of shared effectiveness.

Second, Gopnik and Sobel were able to show that mere association of a block with the occurrence of flashing and music from the box was not sufficient to cause children to assign the same name to two different blocks. To show this, Gopnik and Sobel ran another condition in which the blocks did not make contact with the machine, but were instead waved a few inches above it. With two blocks, the experimenter simultaneously touched the top of the box with a finger, and flashing and music occurred. With the other two blocks, the experimenter placed the finger near but not on the box and there was no flashing or music. In this condition, children tended to extend a label given to one block that had been associated with flashing and music to another block of the same shape or color, rather than to another block that was associated with flashing and music. The authors suggested that this was because the scenario did not induce the children to perceive the blocks as causing the flashing—the children appear to have attributed that to the finger in this case.

These experiments support the idea that knowledge about the causal properties of objects can influence a number of aspects of semantic cognition, including whether objects are perceived as the same "kind" of thing (and hence given the same name), and what properties are attributed to a given object in a particular semantic task. Objects that have very different appearances may be treated as similar to one another, and may foster inductive generalization from one to the other, when they are seen to cause the same observed consequences. The experiments also suggest that the attribution of causal properties is a subtle judgment dependent on more than the mere contiguity of an object with an outcome. In other descriptions of this work, Gopnik (2001) has noted that some children tried to open blocks that appear to cause the box to flash and make music, perhaps suspecting that the effective blocks might have something inside them that allowed them to influence the machine. Thus it appears that when perceptually distinct objects are shown to have similar causal properties, observers may expect them to have certain unobservable internal properties in common, as if children had some idea of how the blocks might have caused flashing and music, and wanted to gain further information relevant to their idea (for example, some children might have suspected that the effective blocks contained magnets that affected the box).

Conformity to Normative Theories of Causal Inference

Finally we consider recent work presented by Gopnik, Sobel, and their collaborators (Gopnik et al., forthcoming; Sobel, Tenenbaum, and Gopnik 2002) in support of their view that children rely on a special mechanism for causal reasoning that derives correct results in accordance with a normative theory of optimal causal inference, often dubbed *Bayes nets* (Spirtes, Glymour, and Scheines 1993, 2001). Bayes nets are graph structures that encode causal relationships and that provide a framework for a formal theory of causal inference (Pearl 2000; Glymour 2001). Several studies have been carried out indicating that even quite young children (down to 30 months of age) are capable of behaving, albeit not always perfectly, in accordance with the normative Bayes net theory. In one of these studies (Sobel, Tenenbaum, and Gopnik 2002), each child witnesses a situation in which two novel blocks (A and B) are placed simultaneously on the blicket detector, which then proceeds to flash and make music. The child has previously seen some objects but not others activate the blicket detector, and is engaged in determining which blocks are blickets and which are not. The witnessed event indicates that at least one, and possibly both, of the objects is a blicket. Interest focuses on the effects of the next event, when object A is placed on the blicket detector alone. In one condition, the detector flashes and makes music; in another, nothing happens. Even relatively young children appear to use the information from the second event to draw conclusions about the causal powers of object B. If A alone fails to activate the blicket detector, they nearly always (94 percent of trials) call B a blicket. If A alone does activate the blicket detector, they are much less likely to call B a blicket (34 percent of trials). Thus the children appear to be inferring something about object B from an event in which only object A appears.

These and related findings are taken to be problematic for what Gopnik et al. (forthcoming) call "the causal Rescorla-Wagner" model (a model with some connectionist-network-like characteristics), and supportive of the view that young children are endowed with a special mechanism for causal inference. Gopnik et al. (forthcoming) propose that this mechanism is domain general, in the sense that it applies to causal inference in a wide range of domains, and in that sense their views have some compatibility with our approach. However, two aspects of their claims (Gopnik et al., forthcoming) set their view apart from ours. They suggest that (1) the mechanism is an innate cognitive module constrained to produce inferences that are consistent with the principles of the normative Bayes net theory, and (2) it is applicable only to causal rather than to other kinds of semantic knowledge. Thus, it is important to consider whether the findings they use in support of their view can be accommodated in our approach, where causal knowledge and inference making are treated as part of a general mechanism for semantic cognition.

Toward a PDP Account of Causal Knowledge and Causal Inference

Under the theory-theory, "theories" about causal mechanisms (and/or about valid rules of causal inference) give rise to the effects of interest in each of the studies reviewed above. We suggest that PDP networks that learn from exposure to event sequences and verbal narratives about such event sequences would be capable of learning about the causal properties of objects from exposure to sequences in which these objects play a causal role. We will also suggest that such networks would also be capable of using such causal properties to influence labeling and other aspects of their semantic cognition, and would even learn from experience how to attribute causality based on experience with situations like those arising in Gopnik et al.'s experiments with events providing ambiguous causal information.

To understand how the PDP approach might be extended to address these issues, we rely on a generalization of the Rumelhart model. In that model, representations of items are acquired through experience with the set of attribute values that occur on the output units when the item is presented as a part of an input that includes the item in each of several relation contexts. More generally, we suggest, as illustrated in figure 8.1, representations of

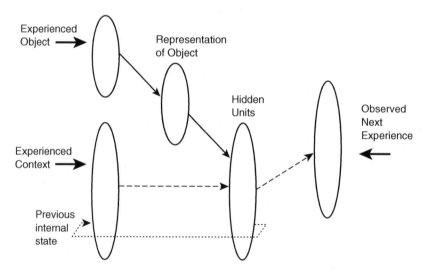

Figure 8.1   A sketch of a network architecture of the sort we envision will be necessary to capture the acquisition of causal knowledge from event sequences. The diagram is intended to suggest a general correspondence with the architecture of the Rumelhart network, in which a concept is experienced in a particular relational context and the legal completions of the propositions are to be predicted. Here, far more generally, we imagine an experienced object perceived in some context, and the task is to predict subsequent experience. Included as part of the context in which this prediction is made is a delayed copy (indicated by dotted arrow from hidden units back to the context) of the preceding internal state of the network. Dashed forward arrows are used in some places to indicate projections that may include recurrent connections.

items are acquired through experience with the entire range of sequelae of an item's occurrence in a wide range of different contexts. Let us call an occurrence of an item with other items an *event*. The "contextual" information co-occurring with the item includes other simultaneously present aspects of the context or situation, together with a representation of prior events that may be maintained internally to influence the interpretation of the current event. In this view, events can include inputs in one or more modalities, including vision, touch, natural sounds, and so on. Similarly, the entire set of sequelae of an occurrence of an item (as an element of an event) includes experience in all modalities (sights, sounds, tactile experiences occurring subsequent to an event, and so on).

The network illustrated in figure 8.1 is similar to networks that have been used in many other studies to investigate how PDP models may extract structure from exposure to event sequences (Elman 1990; Cleeremans, Servan-Schreiber, and McClelland 1989; Munakata et al. 1997). Generally speaking, such models have been applied to information arriving within a single domain (such as vision or language) at a given time. The diagram shown in figure 8.2 suggests how a common internal representation may underlie the interpretation of experience itself and of verbal utterances that may contain covarying information about a given experience. This elaborated architecture captures the idea that semantic representation integrates all aspects of experience, including experienced utterances. Note that learning from listening to other people talk (e.g., listening to one person respond to a question posed by another) could lead the network to discover weights that essentially allow it, too, to produce appropriate responses to questions (see McClelland, St. John, and Taraban 1989; St. John and McClelland 1990; St. John 1992). This characteristic is similar to that of a very wide range of PDP models, including the Rumelhart model. The model is trained by giving it input-output pairs that can be construed as situation-outcome (or current-state/next-state) pairs, and learning is driven by the effort to predict the output (or series

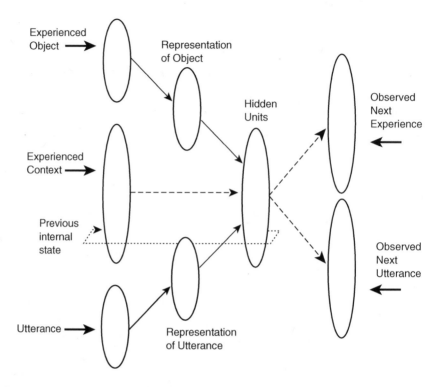

Figure 8.2   A sketch of the architecture shown previously in figure 8.1 but with additional inputs and outputs to illustrate how verbal information could be interfaced with the same network. The architecture allows for experience to influence the interpretation and prediction of language, and language to influence the interpretation and prediction of experience.

of subsequent outputs) given the input (possibly including past inputs). Once trained, the outputs to given inputs are used as the basis for overt responses, including overt predictions of subsequent events, naming responses, and so on.[1]

A key feature of the results of the learning that occurs in such networks is that the representation assigned to a given item is affected not only by the immediate sequelae of the items' appearance at a particular time, but also by observed outcomes at later times. A number of proposals have been offered for how learning may be sensitive to observations that arise at later times. Some algorithms directly and explicitly permit future consequences to shape an item's immediate representation by allowing error to propagate backward not only through the layers of a network but also through time (e.g., Williams and Zipser 1989), so that the weight changes that determine how the item will be represented are partially determined by inputs coming later in time. Perhaps more surprisingly, however, a similar influence of future consequences on immediate representation may also be observed in algorithms that do not pass error information forward or backward in time. For example, some proposals rely on the fact that information relevant for making remote predictions is also often relevant for making more local predictions, so that it tends to be retained even in simple recurrent networks that do not rely on backpropagation through time (Elman 1990; Cleeremans, Servan-Schreiber, and McClelland 1989). Other proposals (e.g., temporal-difference learning, Sutton 1988) rely on methods that make the current internal state similar to the next state—so that, with repetition, earlier and earlier states acquire similarity to particular future states, and thereby come to represent the expected future outcome. For now we do not take a position on exactly which of these proposals is used by the brain—we only suggest that some such mechanism operates to allow the weights in the semantic system to encode information about the later implications of current inputs.

A further property of learning in these networks is that it can be highly sensitive to temporal context: the expectations generated by an item occurring within an event are strongly conditioned by other events in the sequence. For example, in St. John's (1992) work on story comprehension, if a named individual has been placed in the role of a waiter greeting and seating guests early in an event sequence characterizing a visit to a restaurant, then the model will expect this individual to be the one who brings the food and the check, not to be the one who eats the food or pays for it.

With these thoughts in mind let us return to a consideration of the experiments reviewed above, beginning with Keil's transformation studies. We suggest that a learning mechanism like the one we have sketched could provide the basis for children coming to appreciate that an object, even if wearing a very convincing costume, is still the thing it was before it started to wear the costume. Children are likely to have had considerable experience with event sequences involving costumes and disguises. Those of us who have been parents or caregivers to young children may recall how terrifying such costumes and disguises can be for children when they are very young, perhaps because at that point the children do not yet have an acquired appreciation that the costumes only create a temporary change in appearance. But after a child repeatedly witnesses and/or participates in various kinds of costume events (including those related to Halloween, and so on), he or she apparently comes to appreciate that the visible surface properties of animate things can be strikingly but also reversibly affected, and that many other properties remain unchanged. A child can dress as Dracula and a friend as ET or vice versa, but other sources of information (especially for the costumed child personally) will indicate that many of the costumed individual's properties are maintained throughout. Furthermore, both the costumed child and the friend will revert to their prior appearance when they take their costumes off.

Such experiences, we suggest, will cause the child to learn to maintain an internal representation of a costumed individual that retains the properties the person had before they put on the costume, rather than the properties known to be possessed by the things they appear to be while they are wearing the costume. In addition to this direct learning from experiences with individuals in costumes, we also suggest that verbal inputs in the form of statements that are made by others during costume-wearing events and/or stories, movies, and so on about costume-wearing events will contribute to the acquisition of knowledge about costumes. Verbal inputs from others in the course of events in which he or others are wearing costumes (e.g., "Don't you look scary in your Dracula costume, Johnny," or "That's only your friend Sally dressed up like ET'') would help a child learn what it means to say that someone is in a costume and thereby be able to use linguistic as well as visual input to influence their representation of an individual in a costume. Such learning would allow children in Keil's experiment to represent the object pictured as a raccoon even if it looks exactly like a skunk, as long as they are told that in fact it was a raccoon until it put on a skunk constume. Note that we do not suggest that children will need to have had experience specifically with raccoons in skunk costumes, but only that they will need to have had experience with other animate objects in costumes, because we would expect them to generalize across different types of animals, due to their having similar underlying representations. Similarly, children may not need to have direct experience with sequences in which animals are given injections in order to draw conclusions from the story in which the raccoon that received an injection "grew up into" a skunk. Perhaps they will think the raccoon is now "really" a skunk because animals often transform naturally from one apparent "kind" to another as they grow up, the transformation of caterpillars into butterflies and tadpoles into frogs being two clear examples. From this kind of general knowledge about animals, older children may accept that the animal that began life as a raccoon but that "grows up into" a skunk has become a skunk, just as the animal that begins life as a caterpillar and grows up into a butterfly has really become a butterfly.

Similarly, it seems to us that the participants in Ahn's (1998) study likely capitalize on general knowledge they have acquired about the familiar objects described in the stories (such as flowers and bees) in making their categorization decisions. In the example experiment described above, participants were told about a new kind of orchid called a *Coryanthes*, which was likely to attract bees and also likely to contain a substance in its flowers called *Eucalyptol*. Although the participants probably did not know the words *Coryanthes* or *Eucalyptol*, they did likely have considerable knowledge about the properties of flowers, including knowledge about what kinds of properties are generally important for determining a flower's species, gleaned through the kinds of mechanisms discussed in earlier chapters. It is possible, then, that their category judgments resulted in part from inferences about the Coryanthes supported by this knowledge store.

For example, when told that the Coryanthes attracts bees because it has Eucalyptol in its petals, participants were free to make inferences about where the Eucalyptol came from. A reasonable inference (from knowledge about other flowers) might be that Eucalyptol is a chemical produced by the Coryanthes to attract bees. Because they know that flowers from the same species are likely to produce the same chemicals (again from general knowledge about other flowers), they might conclude that having Eucalyptol is more important to being a Coryanthes than is attracting bees. Participants in the contrasting condition were explicitly told that Eucalyptol is not produced by the plant, but is deposited in its petals by the insects it attracts. In this case, they are free to draw inferences about why the Coryanthes might attract bees. Perhaps they infer that the Coryanthes, like many flowers, produces a scent that draws the bees. Again, on the basis of their general knowledge about the "important" properties of flowers, the participants are likely to conclude that attracting bees by producing a certain scent is crucial to being a Coryanthes, whereas having Eucalyptol in their petals is not.

Under this account of Ahn's data, it is not knowledge about direction of causality per se that is directly responsible for the participants' category judgments. Instead, these judgments are driven by the complete constellation of inferences the participants feel licensed to draw about the Coryanthes's likely properties and causal powers, given all they know about flowers and bees generally, and what they have learned about the Coryanthes in particular. The judgments may reflect, not special sensitivity to information about the direction of causation, but a sophisticated form of generalization akin to that operating under the PDP approach.

To see this, imagine the following alternative to Ahn's example:

Scientists have found a new kind of orchid called Coryanthes growing next to a smelting plant in Central Africa. Eighty percent of Coryanthes have smelting ashes in their petals, and 80 percent are picked by factory workers.

EXPLANATION A: The reason Coryanthes have smelting ashes in their petals is because they are picked by factory workers. The workers have ashes on their clothing that fall into the petals.

EXPLANATION B: The reason Coryanthes are picked by factory workers is because they have smelting ashes in their petals. The smelting ashes kill the flowers, and the factory workers have to remove all the dead ones.

In this case, the direction of causality between "having smelting ashes" and "getting picked by factory workers" is manipulated exactly as in Ahn's experiment. However, it seems unlikely to us that participants in either condition will judge one of these properties to be more important than the other for being a Coryanthes. Given what they know about flowers, ashes, and factory workers, participants are likely to infer that neither property is especially important for determining the species of flower.

Thus we would suggest that, in both Ahn's experiments and the hypothetical alternative proposed above, people's judgments will be governed simply by whatever inferences they are inclined to draw about the objects in the story, coupled with their knowledge about which kinds of properties are "important" for which kinds of objects. Both the inferences themselves as well as the weighting of inferred properties arise from the general system of knowledge participants have gleaned through their encounters with like objects and events. Among the range of inferences that might be relevant to a given categorization decision are inferences about causal properties and relations, but we suggest that there is no need to accord any special status to these inferences over others, or to propose special mechanisms to account for the apparent salience of causal information. Just as the children in Keil's transformation studies may be drawing on their general knowledge about costumes, or the way objects can change appearance without changing identity, so too may the adults and children in Ahn's experiments be drawing on their general knowledge about the properties (causal or otherwise) of the objects and events described in her stories.

Of course we understand that some readers may remain to be convinced that this kind of story about the influence of causal knowledge on semantic cognition could ever work in practice. A convincing case will require a simulation illustrating that an actual model can learn all that we claim from experiences with events and their verbal descriptions. While we cannot allay all such concerns, we can at least point to simulations that have been carried out to address related issues. Here we will focus on a simulation designed to explain a phenomenon that has some features in common with the "costume" experiments described by Keil and reviewed above.

This simulation addresses knowledge about the continued existence of objects even when they are out of view. When an object A moves in front of another object B, object B disappears from view —a situation analogous to that in which a costume C is put on by an individual D, so that the individual no longer looks like itself even though it actually remains the same inside. In the case of object permanence, we know that object B is "still there" despite appearances to the contrary; and in the case of a costume, we know that despite appearances it is still individual D standing in front of us, even though the costume replaces D's visible attributes with what might be a very different set of properties. Munakata et al. (1997) demonstrated how a very simple recurrent network could learn to maintain representations of objects that are no longer visible from simple event sequences involving objects hidden by occluders. The essential element of the simulated event sequences was that objects hidden by the occluder became visible again when the occluder moved away. To correctly predict that this would occur, the network learned to maintain a representation of the object during the part of the event sequence when it was hidden by the occluder. That is, Munakata et al.'s model learned to maintain a consistent internal representation of the hidden object during the period of occlusion, even though the model's inputs during this period did not indicate that the occluded object was still present in the environment. Hence the model was able to condition its internal representation of a current input on knowledge about the prior state of the environment. Although of course costumes provide far more complex situations than this, we suggest that this simulation illustrates the fundamental property required for a system to employ knowledge about an item's prior status in order to maintain a consistent internal representation of the item when it is subjected to certain transformations, rather than treating it as having been fundamentally transformed by the alteration. We believe that similar processes may also underlie acquisition and use of knowledge about the consequences of more complicated transformations, such as those in the other conditions of Keil's experiment, and in Ahn's studies of adults.

We now turn to a consideration of the studies on the role of causal powers in naming, since these studies introduce some additional elements (Gopnik and Sobel 2000). First, let us consider the basic issue of sensitivity to the apparent causal properties of objects. Again, by causal properties of an object we simply refer to the sequelae of the object's participation in an event sequence. A large number of studies have investigated the capacity of simple recurrent networks to learn about such sequelae. A basic finding (Servan-Schreiber, Cleeremans, and McClelland 1991) is that such networks become progressively more and more sensitive to the sequential dependencies in a time series (such as a series of letters generated by a transition network grammar of the kind studied by Reber 1969 and others). Likewise as we have already suggested, simulations by St. John (1992) used an architecture similar to that in figure 8.1 to process simple stories based on everyday event sequences such as trips to a restaurant. Among the issues St. John addressed was the ability of his network to learn to anticipate the likely sequelae of going to a restaurant, ordering food, and so on. St. John's networks were able to learn to infer the likely consequences of such actions, assigning individual participants to particular roles in the sequences as suggested above.

We consider the kinds of situations investigated by Gopnik and Sobel (2000) to reflect the operation of mechanisms similar to those at work in the simulations just mentioned. The children in Gopnik's experiment may not have had much experience with blocks that produce music when they are placed on certain boxes—but no doubt they have had experience with other kinds of objects with specific causal properties. Keys, switches, fasteners, bank cards, batteries, openers, remote controls, and many other objects in everyday use have specific causal powers of this type. Furthermore, many of these objects can be quite variable in shape or other aspects of their appearance, yet can be quite consistent in their functions. We suggest that people learn to represent such objects (and, indeed, all other types of objects) from exposure to event sequences in which these objects interact with others and particular consequences ensue. Furthermore, we suggest that people learn that such objects generally have names that depend on these causal properties rather than their appearance, because they hear such names consistently applied to any object that has a particular causal property regardless of variations in its appearance.

Thus, we view the situation in Gopnik and Sobel's experiment as strictly analogous to the situation in the Macario (1991) experiment described in chapter 7. Macario found that children tend to treat items as the same kind of food if they have the same color, regardless of their shape, but treat items as the same kind of toy when they have the same shape, regardless of their color. Similarly, Gopnik and Sobel found that subjects treat items as the same kind of thing when they share the same causal properties, regardless of their shape or color. Based on this analogy, we suggest that one could simulate Gopnik and Sobel's findings in the following way. First, one could train a network like the one in figure 8.1 to predict the outcome of event sequences involving different kinds of items, just as the Rumelhart network is trained to predict the properties of objects occurring in ensembles of item-relation-attribute triples.

We suggest that this training would lead the network to derive quite different representations for tools and implements relative to animals or plants, in that representations of the former would be strongly constrained by an object's causal properties rather than (for example) its shape or color. The reason is that tools and implements of the same "kind" give rise to similar outcomes for various event conditions even though they may vary in shape and color. For example, telephones come in many shapes, sizes, and colors, but are used in similar contexts to achieve similar ends, and hence are construed as the same "kind" of thing.

After training, one could use backprop to representation to derive internal representations for novel objects with particular shapes, colors, and causal powers. In the case of tools and implements, we would expect the model to assign similar representations to items with shared causal properties (regardless of shape or color), and hence we would further expect that a name associated with a particular novel tool would generalize to other objects with similar causal properties, and not to objects with similar color or shape. We should also add that if there are consistent relationships between aspects of the internal structure of objects and their causal properties, such a network will be sensitive to this regularity and will tend to expect certain internal parts to be present when objects have particular causal properties.

As we have noted, there is a further element of the Gopnik and Sobel experiments that should not be neglected in any effort to offer an account of their findings. This is the fact that children appear to attribute causal properties to the blocks they used only when the specific scenario suggested a causal influence of the block (block placed on box that flashes and makes music versus waved above box while experimenter touches it). Can network models of the kind we have proposed provide a mechanism that captures this aspect of children's cognition? We believe they can. The key to this ability, we suggest, is the fact that networks should be able to acquire knowledge of what sorts of actions can produce particular kinds of events. Events involving contact are more likely to produce a response in a machine than events involving just waving something near the object (although of course such effects are by no means impossible in the present world of remote control devices and coded electronic sensors). We expect networks to be able to learn about such matters from observing event sequences, and from this to come to attribute causal power to the object making contact (the finger in Gopnik and Sobel's experiment) rather than the one simply waved over an object (the block).

While the specific scenario just discussed has not yet been simulated, there is an existing model that illustrates how a network can learn from experience to attribute the "cause" of an event to one aspect of a situation and not another, as children do in the Gopnik and Sobel experiment. In this model, Rogers and Griffin (2001) trained a simple recurrent network on event sequences including a number of different objects defined by their patterns of movement (trajectories through time). Among the objects were some that moved along the ground (bottom rows of units in the simulated input array) but that would jump over an obstacle placed in front of them. Thus, the trajectory of motion could be predicted from the identity of the object (as seen in the first few frames of motion) and from the presence of obstacles. Next the network was "habituated" to novel event sequences, in two different conditions. In one condition, the network was exposed to a new object that moved along the ground and then jumped over an obstacle. In another condition, the new object moved along the ground and then jumped at the same place as in the first condition, but in this case the obstacle was presented in a different location, out of the way of the animal's path of motion, so the jumping could not be attributed to the obstacle. After both habituation conditions, the networks were tested with two conditions in which no obstacle was present. In test condition A, the new object simply moved along the ground according to its characteristic "gait," without jumping. In condition B, the new object moved along the ground and then jumped at the same position where jumping had occurred during training. The results were straightfoward. After habituation with the obstacle present in the location where the jump occurred, the network effectively attributed the jump to the presence of the obstacle—so that when the obstacle was absent at test, it expected the object to move along the ground. Its predictions matched with its observations in test condition A (where the object stays on the ground), but not B (where it jumps). Thus, the network habituated with an obstacle present exhibited "surprise" in condition B, as judged by the mismatch between its predictions and the observed event. However, after habituation with the obstacle in an out-of-the-way location, the network effectively attributed the jumping, not to the presence of the obstacle, but to a characteristic of the object, and so in this case its expectations were reversed. In this condition, the network expected the object to jump when it reached the point where it had always jumped during habituation, and hence was "surprised" in condition A, when the object failed to jump.

By the behavior of the network used in the Rogers and Griffin simulation, it would appear that when the obstacle was present at the location of the jump, the network attributed the jumping to the obstacle, not to an intrinsic tendency of the object to jump at that location. But when the obstacle was placed at an out-of-the-way location, the network attributed the tendency to jump to the object. We see this situation as closely analogous to the situation in the Gopnik and Sobel experiment. When a likely cause for some event is present, the event is attributed to that cause (in this case, jumping is attributed to the obstacle; in Gopnik and Sobel, the box's flashing when the object is waved above it is attributed to the experimenter's finger touching the box). When this likely cause is absent, however, the event is attributed to some intrinsic property of the object. Jumping at the specified point is attributed to the object, when the obstacle is out of position to occasion the jump. Similarly, in Gopnik and Sobel, the flashing of the box is attributed to the block when the block is placed on the box (no other likely cause is provided in that condition of the experiment).

We now turn to the recent findings of Sobel, Tenenbaum, and Gopnik (2002) on children's ability to use information about the causal efficacy of one object to adjust their estimate of the causal efficacy of another, in line with the normative Bayes net theory of causal inference. Recall that in these experiments, children witnessed an event in which two objects (A and B) are placed on the blicket detector and it becomes active. Children who witnessed a subsequent event in which A alone does not activate the detector were very likely to then call B a blicket (and to use it when asked to "make the machine go"). Other children who saw that A alone did activate the detector were much less likely to call B a blicket or to use it to make the machine go.

At issue in this study (and others like it) is whether the experiments implicate a special mechanism innately prespecified to make causal inferences, as proposed by Gopnik et al. (forthcoming), or whether domain-general mechanisms also used for noncausal aspects of semantic cognition might provide a sufficient basis for performance in this task. In what follows we suggest that the general-purpose mechanisms and processes we have been relying on throughout this book may be sufficient. The account we offer here is not entirely speculative, since relevant simulations have now been carried out.[2] We offer it as an example of a particular type of account, the details of which have been chosen to bring out the similarity with earlier simulations that were themselves designed to address issues outside the domain of causality.

What we want to suggest is that the backpropagation-to-representation mechanism employed extensively throughout this book could also be used to address the representation of an object's causal powers. We will develop our proposal in stages, beginning with a simpler experiment used as the pretest condition in Sobel, Tenenbaum, and Gopnik 2002. Here the child is shown a range of blocks, some of which are effective and are labeled "blickets," and others that are not effective and so are not blickets. Whether a block is a blicket or not cannot be determined by its appearance alone. When first observing a new block being placed on the machine, we assume the child uses a network like the one shown in figure 8.1 to make an implicit prediction about what will happen next. Such a network, with weights shaped by the child's prior experiences with various objects, would not lead the child to anticipate that the block will cause the box to flash and make music. If, however, the block does activate the detector, this mismatch between observed and expected outcomes would lead to the backpropagation of error information—provoking a change in the child's representation of the block, so that in subsequent trials, the child expects the box to flash and make music when the block is placed on it. That is, if the block sets off the detector, the unexpected event leads the child to assign a causal power to the block. If the detector is not activated, no causal power is assigned.

Now we confront the more complex situation in which the child witnesses two events, one in which blocks A and B are both placed on the detector and it becomes activated, and one in which only block A is placed on the detector. For this case, we assume that the child relies on both events to assign representations to both blocks. This could be done just as described for the single block above, with the proviso that the backprop-to-representation process is interleaved across the two events, so that the network must find representations for each of the two blocks that account simultaneously for both of the witnessed events. This iterative, interleaved process is one that we have relied on elsewhere in the book, where different types of properties were used to assign an appropriate internal representation to a novel object—for instance, when internal representations were assigned to objects with the same appearance properties (*is tall*, *is bright*) but different parts (*has roots*, *has skin*) in chapter 6 (see simulation 6.3).

The iterative, interleaved process we propose will assign a very different representation to block B, which appears only in the compound event, depending on the outcome of the event involving only block A. Consider first the case where block A is not effective by itself. Here the representation assigned to block A by the iterative process will have to be that of an ordinary, ineffective block—otherwise, the network would incorrectly predict that A alone will set off the detector. Thus to account for the compound event, the backpropagation-to-representation process will assign a full measure of causal efficacy to block B. Now consider the case where A is effective by itself. Here, the process must come to represent A as a fully effective block, since otherwise the network would not fully predict activation by A alone. Consequently, there will be far less pressure to assign a high degree of causal efficacy to B—the causal power assigned to A will, in the compound event, account for much of the error that drives the iterative process. Some causal potency may still get attributed to B, depending in part on prior experiences with other blocks in related situations.

As previously stated, this account is intended to illustrate one way a domain-general error-driven mechanism of the sort we have relied on throughout this book could come to assign the appropriate degree of causal efficacy to objects. We are not committed to the particular details of this illustration, but we are committed to one of its essential properties: specifically, it does not rely on a specialized mechanism that is biologically preprogrammed especially for the formulation of causal inferences. Instead, the crucial ingredient of our account is the iterative adjustment of object representations to simultaneously account for multiple observed events.

The procedure we have described appears to be closely related to several of the procedures researchers in the Bayes net community have proposed as the basis for assigning causal efficacies (Danks 2003; Glymour 2001). Thus, it is not our intention to suggest that our connectionist approach is at odds with the Bayes net framework, as explored by these and other investigators. Indeed, we have no doubt that children (and adults) can sometimes make inferences that conform with normative theories of causal inference. Our point is to indicate that this conformity need not reflect the operation of a preprogrammed mechanism specialized to detect causal structure (e.g., Gopnik et al., forthcoming). Instead it could arise from a very general purpose mechanism—one that adjusts representations based on discrepancies between expected and observed events—that plays a role in addressing noncausal as well as causal aspects of semantic cognition.

The Basis of Explanations

In the experiments described above, the "causal theories" thought to underlie the child's behavior are inferred by the experimenter, and no attempt is made to ask the child to articulate the content of the theory. Indeed in many cases, the children in these experiments may not be able to verbally state the causal principles thought to be contained in their implicit theories. For example, the children in Keil's experiments may not be able to articulate any details of the mechanism by which the scientist's injection transforms a skunk into a raccoon. Rather, the interest of Keil's work lies in the fact that children draw one conclusion under one set of conditions (e.g., that the thing that looks like a skunk really is a skunk), and a different conclusion (e.g., that the thing that looks like a skunk really is a raccoon) under a different set of conditions. By examining which conditions support which conclusions at different ages, the experimenter can "diagnose" (in Carey's words; see Carey 1985) the state of the presumed underlying theories that constrain task performance, even though children may be unable to explicitly articulate (and may even be unaware of holding) said theory. That is, the presence of an underlying causal theory is inferred whenever the children *behave as though* they hold such a theory.

In this and the preceding chapters, we have endeavored to show that a PDP network also can "behave as though" it has a theory in model analogs of some of the tasks used to test children. It can behave as though it knows that brightness, but not size, is important for representing animals, and that size, but not brightness, is important for representing plants. It can behave as though it knows that sets of objects that share wings, feathers, and flight make a "good" category that supports induction, whereas groups of objects that share the same color do not. It can even behave as though it knows that things with certain biological properties in common should share the same name, whereas things with similar appearances need not. Like children, a PDP network can condition the judgments it makes in a particular semantic task on its knowledge of both the stimulus attributes and the particular situational or relational context. We have further suggested how PDP models might be extended to accommodate other empirical findings (such as those described by Keil, Ahn, and Gopnik) in which the conditioning information relates to an object's causal properties or causal relationships to other objects.

Based on the above, it appears that network models like the ones we have considered may play many of the roles that theory-theorists have attributed to naive theories. Indeed, the main evidence used to support theory-theory stems from tasks in which underlying theories are "diagnosed" from observed behaviors, and we feel that the PDP framework is well suited to capturing these phenomena. However, some theory-theorists have suggested that the theories children and adults hold are manifest not only in their judgments and decisions in these sorts of tasks, but also in the explanations they give for these judgments and decisions. It is certainly an empirical fact that people can and do often provide verbal explanations for their judgments in semantic tasks, and furthermore, many authors writing in the theory-theory literature have used such overt explanations to support their conclusions (e.g., Massey and Gelman 1988) and/or have suggested that part of theory-theory's appeal is that it offers a framework for understanding such explanations (e.g., Murphy and Medin 1985; Carey 1985; Gopnik and Meltzoff 1997; Keil et al. 1998).

Do overt explanations reveal the operation of underlying theories in semantic task performance? If they do not, what is the basis of overt explanations? In thinking about these questions, let us consider a specific concrete case, Massey and Gelman's (1988) study of children's judgments and explanations about whether various objects can go up and down a hill by themselves. As we have previously mentioned, children in this study are shown pictures of various objects and are asked to say if the object pictured could go up (or down) a hill by itself, then to explain why or why not. Children were very accurate in judging whether a range of living and nonliving things could go up and down a hill by themselves. Massey and Gelman examined the explanations given and found that they fell into several types, including "category membership" explanations ("It can go by itself because it is an animal"), "parts enabling movement" explanations ("It can't move because it doesn't have feet"), and "agent" explanations ("You have to carry it down").[3] What are we to make of these explanations, and what relationship do they bear to the processes people use for producing their semantic judgments?

We will contrast two different approaches to these issues. According to the first, children decide whether something can go up or down a hill by itself by consulting principles that are represented as propositions. In the course of doing so they derive or retrieve other propositions. These propositions can be viewed as providing the basis for their overt explanations. Thus a child in the Massey and Gelman experiment might look at a stimulus picture, decide it is an animal, and then retrieve the propositions encoding their causal knowledge, which might include the information that animals are able to move on their own because they have parts that enable movement. When asked to generate an explanation for the judgment that the pictured animal can move on its own, the child might then report on the propositional content they retrieved in determining that it can do so. This approach might be used to account for the fact that their explanations include statements like "it can move because it is an animal" or "it can move because it has legs."

According to the second approach, the knowledge people use both to make judgments and to provide explanations in semantic tasks is inchoate. By *inchoate*, we mean that the knowledge is built into the apparatus that carries out the process of generating outputs, such that it causes people to behave in certain ways, but is expressly not available for readout as such. In this view, the explicit generation or activation of propositional statements is not an essential intermediary in the process of producing a semantic judgment; instead, judgments and explanations are just examples of the different outputs that the inchoate knowledge can support. The ability to make explanatory statements may arise from some of the same experiences that also give rise to the intuitive judgments that they are offered to explain, but the internal generation of the explanatory statement is not thought of as part of the causal chain leading to the judgment. Again, the idea is that the judgment and the behavioral response are two possible responses supported by a common mechanism, with neither the judgment nor the behavior causally dependent one on the other.

Before we consider the relative merits of these two approaches, it may be worth noting that it is not so clear where most theory-theorists (and others who have argued that semantic judgments rely on knowledge of domain principles) fall with respect to these issues. Researchers often explain children's judgments and explanations with reference to principles that are spelled out in propositional terms, and sometimes even claim that children "reason" with these principles as though they were entertained explicitly (cf. Spelke et al. 1992). Other theorists (e.g., Murphy and Medin 1985) have taken a relatively open stance on this issue, suggesting that some of the content of domain theories is held in explicitly propositional form, but also allowing that some of the knowledge may be implicit. Furthermore, we have already seen that many of the researchers in this tradition are often interested in demonstrating that children behave as though they are using particular principles, and it is not clear that they are always intending to argue that the principles are held in explicit form or are consulted as such in generating judgments and expectations. Some theory-theorists (e.g., Gopnik and Wellman 1994) attribute both judgments and overt explanations to the theories they claim children have, but at the same time choose to call those theories "implicit," and there is little discussion of exactly in what form the knowledge is held or what the relation is between the implicit knowledge and the overt explanations that children actually produce. Indeed some researchers go so far as to state that the principles embodied in children's domain knowledge may be wired into the machinery of processing in ways that seem completely consistent with our view that the knowledge is essentially inchoate. Gelman's (1990) discussion of children's initial knowledge of the basis for animate and inanimate movement is a clear case in point. She states the initial domain principles that she believes children hold in terms of propositions. For example, she suggests that children's initial knowledge about animate movement includes the principle that, in order for an animate object to move, it must have parts that enable movement. She relies on the verbal explanations that children give (e.g., the fact that they often mention parts enabling movement) as support for this view. However, she also clearly states the belief that initial domain knowledge is embodied in the processing machinery, and gives an example of a (real, not artificial) neural network in the barn owl (Knudsen 1983) that embodies the principle that visual and auditory signals both provide information about a single and unitary external physical space. How knowledge initially embodied in this kind of form can result in the overt explanations children give in the Massey and Gelman (1988) experiment is not addressed. In summary, it looks to us as though many researchers working in the theory theory tradition do not have, and indeed do not make it a primary goal to develop, an account of the mechanisms that generate either judgments or explanations (though see Keil and Wilson 2000 for a collection of interesting essays about how one might begin such an enterprise). Even where statements about actual mechanisms are made, as in the case of Gelman (1990), little or nothing is said about how such knowledge could ever lead to an overt explanation.

It might be supposed that the mere fact that people (children and adults) can give explanations for at least some of their semantic judgments would serve as support for the view that they consult propositions (specifically, the ones conveyed in their explanations) in the process of producing their overt judgments. However, a large body of research provides convincing evidence that people's explanations of their overt judgments and decisions may have little to do with the factors that actually gave rise to them.

Nisbett and Wilson (1977) reviewed studies in domains as various as social cognition, perception, and problem solving, all asking participants to explain why they behaved as they did in the experimental task. In one study, subjects were shown four identical pairs of stockings. They were asked to decide which was of the best quality, and then they were asked to explain their decision. The authors found a very strong effect of position on the results, with participants preferring the rightmost stocking to the leftmost stocking by a ratio of 4:1. However, when asked to explain their decisions, participants referred to properties of the stocking such as its weave, texture and color. When asked whether its position in the line-up had any influence on their decision, participants strongly denied the possibility. In another study conducted by Maier (1931; cf. Nisbett and Wilson 1977), participants were faced with the task of tying together two ropes that were hanging from the ceiling. The ropes were too far apart for the participants to grasp both when they were hanging straight down; in order to accomplish the task, they had to use one of a set of implements in the room. Each time the participant succeeded, Maier asked her to try again to solve the problem in a different way. There were several possible solutions, but one proved especially difficult. After the volunteers had been stumped for several minutes, Maier (who was in the room) batted at one of the ropes, apparently absentmindedly, to start it swinging. He reported that, within 45 seconds of this action, most participants siezed upon the difficult solution: tying a heavy object to one rope, swinging it like a pendulum, and then running over to the second rope in time to catch the first as it swung back. Though the cue reliably brought the solution to mind across subjects, no subject was "aware" of it doing so—that is, subjects did not mention Maier's action at all when asked to explain how they hit upon the answer. When pressed, some subjects eventually made reference to the cue, but were in fact more likely to mention other "cues" during the session that did not reliably lead them to discover the solution.

More recently, Keil (Wilson and Keil 2000; Keil, forthcoming) has shown that the explanations offered by adults for a variety of common phenomena are suprisingly impoverished, even for domains in which participants confidently attest to having competent causal knowledge. In these experiments, college students often assert that they have a thorough understanding of the workings of some common object (such as a toilet); but are unable to construct a coherent articulation of this knowledge when pressed to provide a detailed explanation—missing "not just a few arbitrary details, but critical causal mechanisms" (Wilson and Keil 2000, 99). The participants were selected at random from an undergraduate population—hence there is no reason to suspect that their explanatory or conceptual knowledge about the items in the experiment was especially impoverished relative to the general population.

Data from these and similar experiments demonstrate how difficult it is to disentangle the relationships among the verbal explanations that people provide for their judgments, the processes that underlie these judgments, and the causal/explanatory knowledge people hold about a given phenomenon. In particular, it seems that the explicit, articulated explanations people provide in these tasks do not always transparently reveal the factors that actually govern their responses; and the confidence with which people proffer explanations does not accurately reflect their understanding of a given concept or domain.

One of the conclusions that Nisbett and Wilson reach in their discussion of people's explanations is that they are post hoc rationalizations based on a priori theories about their own behavior, that have nothing at all to do with the basis for the actual judgments and decisions. In cases where there is a correspondence between these explanations and the factors that actually govern their behavior, this is seen essentially as a coincidence. While the clear lack of correspondence in some cases seems to provide some support for this view, there are many other circumstances in which there is actually fairly good correspondence between judgments and explanations. For example in his work with children's judgments of the role of weight and distance in Inhelder and Piaget's balance scale task, Siegler (Siegler 1976, 1997; Siegler and Stern 1998) documents a fairly good (though not perfect) correspondence between the pattern of children's judgments of which side of a balance will go down and the content of their verbal explanations. The data suggest more of a correspondence than we feel can be fully attributed to coincidence, and so in our own approach we favor an idea already discussed to some extent in considering Keil's transformation studies, that both judgments and explanations draw on overlapping knowledge, gained through experiences in which there is some coherent covariation between observations and explanations.

In our view, providing an explanation is simply another kind of semantic task, and the statements that people generate in their verbal explanations are generated using the same connection-governed activation processes as are other kinds of outputs. We suggest that a model of the kind sketched in figure 8.2 could provide the necessary mechanism for this. For example, the explanation for some witnessed event would require the generation of a verbal response to a verbally presented question, while the network was holding "in mind" as context a representation of the witnessed event itself. The ability to generate such an explanation would depend heavily on prior experience with other related situations, including cases in which explanations had been given for similar events by others. The network would learn to generate explanations as part of the process of anticipating the explanations others might give after witnessing such events. On this view, learning based on the mismatch between predicted and witnessed explanations provides a basis for the acquisition of connection weights that would support the generation of the network's own explanations. As we have already suggested, once the network had learned to generate appropriate predictions, these outputs could support overt explanation responses when the network itself is probed. In this way explanations would depend on the inchoate, connection-based knowledge derived from experience with prior events.

Knowledge derived from the events themselves, as well as knowledge derived from the explanations provided by others, would be expected to influence performance under this approach. For example, consider again the explanations children give for their judgments that objects can go up and down a hill by themselves in the Massey and Gelman (1988) study. Children may tend to explain that the object can (or cannot) go up the hill by itself because it does (or does not) have feet, partly because the property of having (movable) feet is in the child's experience consistently shared by animals that move by themselves on the ground, and partly because the property of having feet or similarly represented parts may have been mentioned in other episodes of "explaining" the movement of animate objects that the child may have witnessed or participated in. Our account depends on the idea that the particular task context of explanation is one that children often encounter (indeed, by asking "why" they often place themselves in such a context), and we suggest that they learn a great deal about what consitututes a reasonable explanation from such situations.

Clearly the sketch we have given here does not provide anything like a complete account of verbal explanation. We intend it to simply illustrate some initial ideas about how the inchoate knowledge stored in a PDP network might give rise to the ability to provide verbal explanations. To make a convincing case for this account, further simulation work of the kind we have suggested will have to be carried out. One of the challenges that will have to be addressed is to explain exactly why some statements and not others are offered when children are asked to provide overt explanations. Why do children refer to the fact that an object is an animal, or to the fact that it has movement enabling parts (even when these are not visible) in their explanations that an object can move up or down a hill by itself? While this is a challenge for our PDP approach, we would like to point out that other approaches to explanations face similar challenges. Children's explanations do sometimes refer to information that is relevant to the child's decision, but they also often leave other important information out. The child who says that an object can move because it is an animal does not really tell us what it is that enables the animal to move, and the child who mentions that the echidna has feet does not tell us how he knows this. Thus any theory, whether it is based as ours is on inchoate knowledge or as others may be on the idea that knowledge is more explicit, has a great deal of work to do before it can claim to provide an explanation for the particular patterns in children's explanations.

Why Do We Find Explanations Useful or Satisfying?

There is one final issue regarding the role of explanations that may be worth considering. This is the idea developed by Gopnik and colleagues (Gopnik and Wellman 1994; Gopnik and Meltzoff 1997) that children actually seek explanations, and find it satisfying to have an explanation for witnessed events. Indeed, Gopnik and Meltzoff (1997) have gone so far as to suggest that a good explanation is like an orgasm in that it is intrinsically pleasurable and rewarding. They appear to be suggesting that we are biologically prepared to find explanations satisfying, just as we are biologically prepared to find orgasms satisfying. Evolution has provided for this because a good explanation increases our understanding, and understanding itself promotes fitness.

We certainly agree that explanations can be useful. We suggest that their utility lies in their ability to transform an event that appears arbitrary or unpredictable into one that seems far less so. Explanations may fill in the missing steps in a chain of observations—steps that make the observations less mysterious because they can be understood as arising from event sequences that themselves seem familiar, and therefore provide a basis for expecting the observed endpoints. Thus, if a child arrives at a friend's house and is surprised when a vampire opens the door, an appropriate explanation ("Look, your friend Billy is wearing a Dracula costume!") may ameliorate the surprise. Of course, understanding the explanation presupposes just the sort of familiarity with costumes and verbal discussions of costumes that we have suggested might underlie children's state of knowledge at a certain point in development, such that someone or something observed in a particular type of costume is understood to be "really" the same thing it was before it put the costume on. That is, the explanation must bridge between the surprising event and the system of knowledge that supports the child's ability to understand, in a way that allows the child to render the surprising event predictable. We would expect networks like the one in figure 8.2 to be able to learn to use explanations in this way, if the training includes events (sometimes with steps missing from the experienced event sequences) that are accompanied by others' explanations.

More speculatively, we would go on to suggest that it is the property of rendering an otherwise arbitrary and surprising sequence of observations more familiar that makes explanations seem not only useful, but also "satisfying." Consider for example Gopnik's (2001) observation that children in the Gopnik and Sobel (2000) experiment, who have been shown that some blocks ("blickets") cause a box to flash and produce music, will often try to examine the blickets to see if they can figure out what is inside them. Discovering that the blickets contained metal parts (perhaps a whole electronic circuit) might render their effectiveness less surprising, since other objects that contain such parts often have effects on other objects (for example, remote control devices).

What we are suggesting is the idea that children (and adults) may seek explanations to render surprising events and observations less surprising. Such "explanations" may or may not be truly causal explanations, in the sense of describing an actual mechanistic process in sufficient detail to make clear exactly how the result actually occurs. Instead they may simply allude to familiar scenarios within which events similar to the ones observed have previously been observed to occur. Thus, finding that an object has metal parts in it might not really provide anything like a full explanation of how it produces its effect, but it might make it less surprising that the "blickets" produce the effect whereas other apparently identical objects do not.

Obviously a great deal more could be said about the nature and role of explanations than we have said about them here. Our main aim has been to provide some initial thoughts about how the knowledge in a PDP network could be used to give explanations as well as other kinds of overt responses and to suggest why explanations may be useful even if the underlying knowledge a person holds is completely inchoate.

Comparison of the PDP Approach with Theory-Based Approaches

In this and several preceding chapters, we have shown or at least suggested how a PDP approach could address many of the findings and considerations that have been raised by protagonists of theory based approaches. As we hope our presentation has made clear, we find the phenomena themselves quite interesting. They demonstrate clearly that adults and even young children can be quite sophisticated in their semantic cognition. We often find ourselves in agreement with some of the claims of theory-based approaches. For example, we agree with theory theorists that the knowledge that governs our semantic cognition is more than a mere list of the properties of objects—it is clear to us that our semantic knowledge includes knowledge of how objects interact with other objects, of what properties of objects give rise to their other properties, and so on. We have enumerated in table 8.1 a list of several points of agreement between our position and the position of theory theorists. In addition, there are several points of disagreement and contrast that are also enumerated in the table. Here we focus on these in an attempt to bring out just what we feel the key differences are between our approach and aspects of the theory-theory point of view, at least as espoused by some of its protagonists.

Table 8.1   A comparison of the PDP approach and theory-based approaches

---

Points of agreement with theory approaches

A1.   We agree that people possess knowledge about the relations between objects—knowledge that goes beyond what is stored "inside the concept"—and that such knowledge constrains their interpretation of new information and affects their semantic cognition.

A2.   We agree that people are sensitive to the causal properties of objects, and that they can use knowledge about causal properties to perform various semantic tasks, such as naming or attribution of other types of properties (like attributing internal properties to an object that can cause another object to flash and produce music).

A3.   We agree that people's knowledge of objects and of their interactions with one another is subject to change and can undergo reorganization with development.

A4.   We agree that people can often give explanations, and that the knowledge underlying such explanations is influenced by knowledge derived from other forms of experience. We also believe that explanations provided by others influence the knowledge used to interpret inputs arising from observation of events.

Points of disagreement

D1.   We do not agree with those theory-theorists who suggest that one can infer innate domain-specific knowledge from semantic task performance that exhibits domain specificity. We do not wish to suggest that initial knowledge (or constraints on such knowledge) never play a role; we only suggest that such a role is not necessary for the emergence of domain-specific knowledge that constrains the further interpretation of experience.

D2.   We do not agree with those theory-theorists who take the view that causal knowledge is privileged or special. Instead we suggest that sensitivity to causal properties arises from the same general-purpose learning mechanisms that lead to sensitivity to other kinds of properties.

Contrasts between the theory approach and the PDP approach as frameworks for exploring semantic cognition and its development

C1.   Few theory-theorists actually discuss the details of the representation and use of the naive domain theories they postulate, and even fewer discuss the mechanisms whereby such knowledge changes as a result of experience. In contrast, the PDP approach provides explicit mechanisms for the representation, use, and acquisition of the knowledge underlying semantic task performance.

C2.   Even if often unintended, the idea that intuitive domain knowledge consists of a "theory" may tend to bring with it certain characteristics of actual scientific theories that may be undesirable. Specifically, real scientific theories typically contain explicit propositional statements of the principles of the theory and explicit, traceable procedures for deriving new statements that constitute results and predictions of the theory. According to the PDP approach, the tendency to think of intuitive domain knowledge in this way is misleading and counterproductive.

Table 8.1   (continued)

C3. In the PDP approach, the knowledge underlying semantic task performance is an ensemble of continuous quantities that change with experience according to a domain-general learning rule. The knowledge evolves gradually, providing the basis for gradual change, and is subject to graceful degradation, accounting for patterns of breakdown under damage.

Even though we have made this point before, it is probably worth noting as we proceed into this discussion that we are contrasting the PDP approach with a conception of a theory-based approach that is more of a prototype, or perhaps even an archetype, than a real theory held by any individual investigator. In particular, we note that several important contributors to the relevant discussions expressly do not endorse all of the properties we attribute to some version of the theory approach. For instance, Gopnik (Gopnik and Wellman 1994; Gopnik and Meltzoff 1997), a major proponent of theory-theory, considers the possibility that theorylike knowledge may be acquired using a domain-general mechanism, albeit one that may be especially attuned to the detection of causal relations (Gopnik et al., forthcoming). Also, Murphy (2002) eschews the theory approach in favor of what he calls the "knowledge approach," even though he was one of the early protagonists of theory-based approaches (Murphy and Medin 1985), and he expresses doubt about domain specificity, innateness of domain knowledge—even that causal knowledge plays a special role in semantic cognition.

In any case, we now consider those points of contrast between our approach and some versions of the theory approach. The first lies in the question of whether the knowledge that underlies semantic task performance necessarily depends on initial (i.e., innate) principles that provide the seed or skeleton on which the development of semantic cognition depends. Many researchers in the theory-theory and related traditions appear to favor the view that some initial principles are necessary to serve as a base for further elaboration of conceptual knowledge. However, the argument for innateness sometimes rests on little more than the suggestion that known learning procedures appear to be inadequate to explain the acquisition of the semantic cognitive abilities children are seen to possess (Keil 1994). Even the very simple networks that we have employed can acquire domain-specific behaviors similar to those that, according to some theory-theorists, arise from naive domain theories. On this basis, we believe there is little reason to infer from the presence of domain specificity in children that domain theories or domain-specific constraints leading to such theories are innate.

To be clear, we do not reject the idea that there may be some initial constraints on aspects of learning or development; indeed, such constraints can have survival value, and are likely to be selected by evolution. We are inclined to accept, for example, the idea that animals may be endowed with an initial bias to link taste with sickness but not with electric shock (Garcia and Koelling 1966). We also think it likely that the mechanisms of vision (and other modalities of perception) have evolved to facilitate, among other things, the representation of external three-dimensional space (including the unity of external space as signaled by auditory and visual inputs) and the segregation of the perceptual world into objects, and we do not doubt that processing in other perceptual modalities exploits some forms of initial bias. Where we appear to differ from many theory-theorists is in our feeling that, for many aspects of semantic knowledge, there is no clear reason at present to rely so heavily upon the invocation of initial domain-specific principles. Mechanisms exist that can learn to behave in domain-specific ways based on experience, without the need for initial domain-specific commitments.

A second point of possible disagreement with some researchers working in the theory theory tradition lies in the question of whether the fundamental basis of our semantic knowledge is causal. We see knowledge about causal properties as one among many kinds of knowledge, and we certainly agree that children learn about and rely on the causal properties of certain kinds of objects as part of their semantic cognition. What we do not accept is the need to attribute special status to causal knowledge. Furthermore, we do not believe that causal knowledge necessarily carries with it any real appreciation of mechanism. For us causal knowledge instead constitutes the expectations we derive for the distribution of possible sequelae in particular sequences of events. It may also be useful to extend the definition of causal knowledge to include knowledge about which of an object's properties give rise to the observed sequelae, and, where available, to knowledge of the (often unobserved) sequences of events through which the sequelae arise. Also, we fully accept that words like *cause* are part of language and that these words when used can influence how we think about event sequences—possibly leading us on some occasions to assign greater centrality to events that are described as causing other events rather than being caused by them. While accepting all of this, we do not think such knowledge necessarily represents any real understanding of the mechanism involved (as the experiments described in Keil and Wilson 2000 appear to demonstrate), and we do not think it has any privileged status.

As indicated in table 8.1, there are several further points of contrast between the PDP approach and some versions of theory theory. In brief, theory-theory has what we believe is an important and related set of weaknesses, at least as it has been developed up to now. In particular, theory-theory is for the most part noncommittal about the nature of the representations and processes that underlie semantic task performance and the development of semantic abilities. For example, the most systematic statement of theory-theory (Gopnik and Wellman 1994; Gopnik and Meltzoff 1997) contains no specification of actual mechanisms for the representation, use, and acquisition of the knowledge that underlies semantic task performance. Instead the authors point to functions that scientific theories have and argue that the analogy between children's knowledge and scientific theories is useful since children's knowledge appears to subserve similar functions. The subsequent effort by Gopnik et al. (forthcoming) to characterize children's inferences as conforming to normative rules of inference as captured by the Bayes net formalism does not really alter this. The authors are bringing an explicit formal theory to the characterization of children's inferences in various causal reasoning tasks. However, while they have an explicit theory of the responses a child makes, this theory does not claim that the child has an explicit theory. Indeed, Gopnik et al. (forthcoming) eschew any commitment to the nature of the actual mechanism supporting children's inference, considering several possibilities.

Lack of commitment, of course, can be a virtue in cases where such commitments would be premature. In the absence of such commitments, the theory remains underspecified. But there is an additional difficulty. Without a more mechanistic specification, the analogy to explicit scientific theories brings with it a tendency to attribute properties of such theories to naive domain knowledge, whether such attribution is intended or not. In our view, this tendency may be misleading and counterproductive, since these are just the properties we assert naturalistic human semantic knowledge does not actually have.

Real scientific theories are explicit constructions, developed as vehicles for sharing among a community of scientists a set of tools for deriving results (such as predictions and explanations) using explicit, overtly specified procedures that leave a trace of their application through a series of intermediate steps from premises to conclusion. As far as we can tell, few theory-theorists would actually wish to claim that these properties of real scientific theories are also characteristic of the intuitive domain knowledge that underlies the performance of children or adults in naturalistic semantic tasks. We suspect, however, that these aspects of real scientific theories occasionally filter into the thinking of researchers, and may cloud these intuitions in some cases. For example, Spelke et al. (1992) speak of children reasoning from principles stated in propositional form. The idea that children reason from such principles may sometimes provide a useful basis for deriving predictions for experiments, whether or not anyone actually believes that the principle is held in explicit form, and enters into a reasoning process containing explicit steps justified by explicit appeals to specified rules of inference. But it may also bring along with it additional implications that then misdirect thinking, particularly thinking about the possibility of learning or change. For example, the notion that a theory contains explicit principles and/or rules carries with it the tendency to suppose that there must be a mechanism that constructs such principles and/or rules. Yet it is easy to show that the set of possible principles/rules that might be constructed is demonstrably underdetermined by actual evidence, thereby motivating suggestions that there must be initial domain constraints guiding at least the range of possible principles that might be entertained (cf. Chomsky 1980; Keil 1989). However, if no such principles or rules actually form the basis of semantic task performance, it would only be misleading to consider the difficulties that would arise in attempting to induce them. By proposing that learning occurs through the gradual adaptation of connection weights driven by a simple experience-dependent learning process, the PDP approach avoids these pitfalls and allows us to revisit with fresh eyes the possibility that structure can be induced from experience.

In claiming that children's intuitive domain knowledge is not the same as a scientific theory, we do not wish to deny that children are like scientists in many ways. We do not disagree with the many parallels that Gopnik and Meltzoff (1997) see between the activity of children and scientists. For example, children, like scientists, seek to explain observed events and predict future events, and seek to test their explanations and predictions through experiment. Furthermore, we would argue that most scientists, like most children, rely heavily on implicit knowledge as the basis for their insights and discoveries. Where we see the activity of scientists differing from that of children (and everyday adult behavior) is precisely in the goal many scientists have of formulating a rigorous scientific theory: something that can be made explicit and shared among the members of a scientific community.

With these observations in mind, we are now in a position to consider the relationship between the PDP approach to semantic cognition and theory-based approaches. One possible stance some might wish to take would be to suggest that the parallel distributed processing framework should be viewed simply as an implementation of a version of the theory theory—one that simply fills in the missing implementational details. This suggestion had some initial appeal even to us, since we have shown that many aspects of performance that have been taken as evidence for naive domain theories can be captured in our simple connectionist networks. However, we have come to feel that such a conclusion would be misleading, since the representations and processes used within PDP networks are quite different from the devices provided by explicit scientific theories. While the knowledge in PDP networks may be theorylike in some ways, it is expressly not explicit in the way it would need to be in order to constitute a theory by our definition.

One might protest that most researchers working in the theory-based tradition never really meant to suggest that naive domain theories are explicit in this way, and that we should simply adopt a definition of the word *theory* that leaves out this reliance on explicitness. In response to this we would simply say that we prefer to avoid the notion that children's naive domain knowledge constitutes a theory, because we suspect that many people associate explicitness with the concept of a theory, and may as a result become confused by this term. Our model, which does not make use of any explicit formalization to generate predictions, explanations, and so on, is theorylike in some but not all ways. It would only confuse the issues if we treated the model as an embodiment of the kind of knowledge that constitutes a theory.

In summary, although the idea has considerable appeal, we feel that on balance it may be better not to view people's naive, implicit knowledge in a given semantic domain as a theory. This conclusion appears to be largely consistent with Murphy's position (Murphy 2002). Like Murphy, we are convinced that knowledge does play a role in semantic cognitive activities. Our further suggestion is that the PDP approach may provide a useful framework for capturing the acquisition, representation, and use of that knowledge to guide many aspects of semantic cognition.

9 Core Principles, General Issues, and Future Directions

Over the course of the preceding chapters we have presented our case for the PDP approach to semantic cognition. While there will doubtless remain many critics, we hope we have shown that these ideas go at least part way toward capturing several aspects of human semantic cognition within an integrated computational framework. In this final chapter, we will consider some of the fundamental principles at work under the PDP theory and several general issues and open questions. Among the issues we will consider is the role of initial constraints and architecture: Are there innate modules for many different adaptive specializations, as some have claimed? Or is there some design principle that must be respected in a successful model of semantic cognition, as others have suggested? We will also consider the relationship between our approach and Bayesian approaches, how we view thinking and reasoning in PDP systems, and how our theory might be implemented in the brain. As we go along we will point out several of the opportunities we see for the future development and application of the theory.

Core Principles

Predictive Error-Driven Learning

Our current work grows in part out of a long-standing effort to apply the parallel distributed processing framework to aspects of cognitive development (McClelland 1989, 1994a; Munakata and McClelland 2003). A key principle stressed in this work has been the principle of predictive error-driven learning, or as stated in McClelland (1994a, 62):

Adjust each parameter of the mind in proportion to the extent that its adjustment will reduce the discrepancy between predicted and observed events.

Predictive error-driven learning is the engine that drives knowledge acquisition and representational change in many PDP models of cognitive development, including an early model (McClelland 1989) of children's understanding of balance scales (Inhelder and Piaget 1958; Siegler 1976); several simple recurrent network models that address the acquisition of grammatical structure from experience with language (Elman 1990, 1991; Rohde and Plaut 1999); models of object permanence in infancy (Munakata et al. 1997; Mareschal, Plunkett, and Harris 1999); and the recent work of Rogers and Griffin (2001) on infants' expectations about apparent goal-directed action. In influential PDP models of semantic memory, such as the original (Hinton 1981) semantic network described in chapter 2, knowledge acquisition can also be understood as arising from predictive error-driven learning. Hinton's network was effectively trained to predict the complete form of a proposition from a subset of its constituents, and this basic idea is captured in simplified form in the feed-forward models used by Hinton (1989), Rumelhart (1990), and ourselves throughout this book. In all of these cases, developmental change arises from the adjustment of connection weights to reduce a discrepancy between observed and predicted completions of a proposition.

It is clear that not all semantic information comes in the form of three-term propositions, and throughout the book we have sought to indicate how the properties exhibited by the Rumelhart model would arise in other situations, also involving predictive error-driven learning. In chapter 4 we suggested how prediction error might be used to drive learning in a generalization of the Rumelhart model applied to the experience of preverbal infants, in which the input is viewed as capturing a visual representation of the object in a particular situational context, and the output is viewed as capturing the network's predictions about other attributes that might subsequently be observed. Some situations cause others to produce spoken names for objects, and so predictions of the object's name should be activated; others lead to actions executed by the object itself and call forth predictions of what the object might do. Although the training corpus we have used must surely be viewed as drastically simplifying these contexts and corresponding expectations, the network learns by using the same predictive, error-driven learning process we believe is utilized in the naturalistic case. In chapter 8 we indicated how similar principles might extend to networks that anticipate the sequelae arising from the observed participation of items in events, and verbal statements about events, so that representations of objects can be shaped by all aspects of their participation in experience. Thus, in brief, the models we have explored throughout this book, and many earlier investigations, have used predictive error-driven learning as the main force driving the development of internal representations and of context-specific outputs.

In emphasizing this, we do not mean to suggest that the interesting properties of our models could only arise from error-correcting learning, nor that such properties could not arise from other types of learning methods, such as Hebbian or "associative" learning rules, including competitive learning models and Kohonen networks (Linsker 1986; Miller, Keller, and Stryker 1989; Schyns 1991; Miikkulainen 1993). We are more than open to the possibility that these methods might produce similar results, or that such alternative methods might co-exist in the brain together with predictive error driven learning, as proposed by O'Reilly (1996). Whether the use of an explicitly error-driven learning algorithm is required or not is currently an open question; the issue is complex, and we do not see a clear resolution. There are, however, two points that can be made about this issue. First, we believe that one very important aspect of the knowledge we have about different kinds of things concerns knowledge of the implications they hold for future events. Predictive error-correcting learning provides one mechanism for acquiring such knowledge. Second, there are known learning mechanisms that effectively carry out predictive error-driven learning, without explicitly or directly implementing the principle using backpropagation. Thus, we do not assert that predictive error-driven learning is the sole force at work, and we do not assert that such learning need be implemented using backpropagation. We do suggest that some form of predictive error-driven learning does play a role in the gradual discovery of structure in experience that takes place during cognitive development.

Sensitivity to Coherent Covariation

As emphasized in several chapters through the book, the models we have considered are strongly sensitive to patterns of coherent covariation amongst the properties that characterize different items and contexts; and we propose that this too be viewed as an important principle at work in semantic cognition:

Coherent covariation of properties across items and contexts drives conceptual differentiation and determines what properties are central and what properties are incidental to different concepts.

In predictive error-driven models with distributed internal representations, patterns of coherent covariation determine which conceptual distinctions are learned, and the strengths of these patterns (as reflected in the lengths of the corresponding eigenvectors, discussed in chapter 3) determine when they are discovered. In what follows we review briefly the effects of coherent covariation on learning and representation in models of this kind, based largely on the results reported in earlier chapters of this book. Whether all aspects of the way such models respond to coherent covariation can also be captured by other models remains to be investigated.

In several chapters we have seen how coherent covariation of properties can lead to the progressive differentiation of individual item representations into successively finer-grained clusters. Such clusters are the network equivalent of semantic categories, in that items within clusters exert strong mutual influences on each other's representations and support generalization from one to another. Coherent covariation also determines which properties of objects are treated as "important" in the network: those properties that covary coherently with many others are learned more rapidly and exert greater constraint on representation than other properties that tend not to covary with others. On the basis of these findings we have proposed that coherent covariation may be a potent contributor to semantic cognition in human children and adults, just as in our networks.

The notion that concepts are strongly constrained by the coherent covariation of ensembles of properties in experience does not appear to be very prominent in the literature. The idea that semantic cognition may depend in some way on detection of feature correlations is certainly very widespread, but for the most part others have focused on various examples of pairwise correlations. To our knowledge, only Billman (Billman and Knutson 1996), whose work we discussed in chapter 6, has paid specific attention to higher order covariation as a possible force in the emergence of category structure from experience. From the simulations we have described, it seems clear that sensitivity to coherent covariation deserves greater consideration than it has heretofore received, as a potential contributing factor to many aspects of semantic task performance and conceptual development.

In the world, patterns of covariation can be both domain and property-type specific. The principles that organize plants into subcategories differ from those that organize animals, artifacts, or actions into subcategories. Different types of properties, and/or properties relevant in different contexts, may covary with other properties in different ways, and will exhibit different patterns of domain specificity. Size and weight tend to covary across all physical objects, for example, whereas movement-enabling parts (e.g., wings) covary with overall patterns of object motion (e.g., flying) only for restricted subsets of objects. Our models condition their sensitivity to patterns of co-variation by both domain and context, and we suggest that the same is true of children—that the patterns of domain-specific responding apparent in children's semantic judgments emerge from the sensitivity of a general learning mechanism to coherent covariation (as discussed extensively in chapters 6 and 7). Importantly, our models are sensitive to coherent structure, not only within an experience, but also across different experiences and contexts. The ability to extract structure across multiple experiences is crucial to human semantic cognition, because individual experiences only provide exposure to a subset of an object's properties. In discussing the coalescence of the concept *living thing* over development, Carey (1985) emphasized the fragmentary nature of children's exposure to the shared (we would say, coherently covarying) properties of plants and animals. She suggested that, ultimately, an understanding of what it means to be a living thing depends on the coalescence of information across these disparate domains, situations and contexts. Our networks can discover the underlying coherent covariation of properties across contexts, and on this basis we suggest that the mechanisms of learning they employ should be viewed as viable candidate mechanisms for the coalescence and reoganization processes seen in child development.

We also suggest that sensitivity to coherent covariation is a key reason why causal properties of objects—or more generally, the sequelae of their participation in events—are central to their representation and to the judgments we make about their other properties. Objects such as remote control devices have internal properties (internal electronics, push-buttons, batteries) that covary with their causal properties, with the circumstances in which they function properly, and with what they are called; and as with many other artifacts, their surface markings and general shape can vary quite independently of their function (consider the wide variation in the appearance of telephones, radios, and clocks). Causal properties also covary with verbal statements about objects, such as descriptions of their purpose or explanations of how they work. Thus, we suggest, the central role of causal properties in object concepts does not require any special sensitivity to causality per se, but rather flows from a more general sensitivity to coherent covariation.

The flip side of this is that we need not always appeal to causality to explain perceived coherence of a category or perceived centrality of a property. Much empirical work in the theory-theory tradition has aimed at documenting the degree to which semantic task performance and knowledge acquisition is subject to constraints: some categories are easier to learn than others; some properties are more important for a given concept than others; some correlations are more readily noticed and acquired than others. Though in some cases it may seem natural to view these constraints as arising from underlying causal theories, other cases seem less suited to such an account. For example, in discussing the possibility that color is a more central property for polar bears than for washing machines, Keil et al. (1998, 18–19) write, "'White' is causally central to polar bears because the property is closely linked to survival in snow-covered environments. Any other color would impair a polar bear's ability to hunt. The causal mechanisms (evolutionary in this case) underlying the color of the polar bear explain why whiteness is a typical property." In fact it is not at all clear that the perceived importance of color for the concept *polar bear* flows from an implicit or explicit causal theory. We suspect that even fairly young children will judge that being white is more important for polar bears than for washing machines, but we doubt that children know much about the adaptive value of camoflage, or the evolutionary pressures under which polar bears have developed white fur. To explain the importance of color for the concept *polar bear* with reference to such causal theories seems a bridge too far in this case.

Similarly, the effects of existing knowledge on new category learning documented by Murphy and Allopenna (1994) are not always easily viewed as reflecting specifically causal knowledge. As discussed in chapter 6, the authors have shown in a series of studies that it is easier to learn novel categories defined by sets of properties that seem naturally to "go together" than categories defined by arbitrary sets of properties. The preexisting knowledge that supports this effect may encompass specifically casual knowledge, but likely reflects other kinds of knowledge as well (Murphy 2002). For this reason, Murphy eschews an appeal to causal theories in favor of what he calls the "knowledge approach" to conceptual representation and learning.

Such a view is broadly consistent with our own approach, in which both the outputs generated by a network at a given point in time, as well as the representations formed on the basis of new information, are determined by the current configuration of weights throughout the system. The weights in turn reflect the totality of knowledge the network has thus far accumulated; hence semantic task performance and new learning are both constrained by preexisting knowledge, as in Murphy's thinking. Since causal knowledge is engrained in the same weights that encode other forms of knowledge, this approach allows us to understand coherence effects both when they seem to flow from causal relations and when they do not.

Similarity-Based Distributed Representation

One of the starting points of our efforts has been a commitment to the idea that internal representations are distributed. This is a key principle of our general approach toward modeling cognition:

Use similarity-based distributed representations to promote generalization and sensitivity to patterns of coherent covariation.

The defining property of distributed representations is that the same units participate in representing many different items, with each individual representation consisting of a particular pattern of activity across the set. Hinton (1981) first articulated the advantages of this scheme, and the appeal to distributed representation has since become a feature of the PDP approach that separates it from other some other connectionist efforts (Hinton, McClelland,

and Rumelhart 1986). A key feature of distributed representations important for many of the phenomena we have addressed is that what is known about one item tends to transfer to other items with similar representations. In our models, we do use localist input and output units, but these never communicate with each other directly. The influences that localist units exert on one another are always mediated by one or two intervening distributed representations.

A specific property of the Rumelhart model, very important to the way that it functions, is that the network is initialized with very small random connection weights—so that all items initially receive nearly identical distributed representations. The important consequence of this choice is that at first, whatever the network learns about any item tends to transfer to all other items. This allows for rapid acquisition and complete generalization of information that is applicable to all kinds of things; but it also induces in the network a profound initial insensitivity to the properties that individuate particular items. Different items are treated as effectively the same until considerable evidence accumulates to indicate how they should be distinguished, based on patterns of coherent covariation. After each wave of differentiation, there remains a tendency to treat those items not yet distinguished as very similar. In general, this property of the network imposes a very strong tendency to generalize, instead of capturing idiosyncratic differences between items.[1]

Convergence of Influences on Representations and Connection Weights

An additional important aspect of the models we have considered is that the very same sets of hidden units are used for the representation and processing of all aspects of every item, and the representations over these units reflect the convergence of all types of information. This characteristic of the network enhances its sensitivity to coherent covariation of properties across different contexts. To bring out the importance of this, we consider the actual

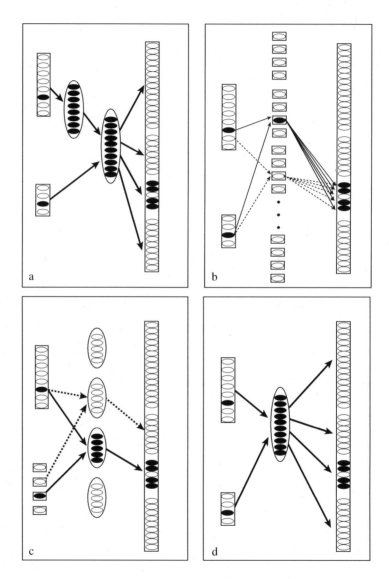

Figure 9.1   Four alternative feed-forward architectures for mapping from localist *Item* and *Context* inputs to sets of output properties. Thick arrows in (a), (c), and (d) indicate full connectivity among units in the sending layer to those in the receiving layer; thin arrows in (b) indicate individual connections. The shading of units indicates how activation spreads forward given the input *canary can*. (a) The Rumelhart network architecture, in which all items first map to a single context-independent hidden

architecture of the Rumelhart network alongside three hypothetical variants of the architecture. In the Rumelhart network (figure 9.1a), one and the same pool of *Representation* units is used to form representations for all items, regardless of the different contexts in which they occur. A second pool of hidden units then conjoins the item and context input, with all units in the pool participating equally in the representation of all items and contexts. In the first variation we consider (figure 9.1b), a separate, localist unit is used for each item-relation conjunction, with no distributed representations used anywhere. In the second variation (figure 9.1c), there are separate pools of hidden units for each relation. In the third variation (figure 9.1d), there is a single pool of hidden units mediating between the localist item and relation inputs and the various groups of output units. As with the Rumelhart model, all variants use a feed-forward activation process, and learn via the back-propagation of error.

How would learning and generalization differ across these network variants? The network with dedicated units for each item-relation pair (panel b in the figure) will exhibit no generalization whatsoever, and will be completely insensitive to coherent co-variation of properties—learning about each item-relation pair will proceed completely independently of every other item-relation

Figure 9.1   (continued)
layer, then converge with context inputs in a second hidden layer. The first layer of hidden units receives error signals filtered through the second, convergent representation; hence the architecture constrains the network to find context-independent representations of individual items that are sensitive to coherent covariation of properties across different contexts. (b) Separate localist representations for every possible conjunction of item and context. Only connections for *canary can* (solid arrows) and *salmon can* (dotted arrows) are shown. In this case the model will not generalize and will not be sensitive to coherent covariation. (c) Separate pools for different contexts. Only connections for the *can* (solid) and *is* (dotted) contexts are shown. Here the model will generalize within context, but will not be sensitive to coherent covariation across contexts. (d) A single hidden layer. In this case the model is not constrained to find context-independent representations for individual items; hence it may divide up the representation space as in (c), so that the model is insensitive to cross-context covariation.

pair. This system would perhaps be able to learn very quickly, but its inability to generalize would be a serious liability. As Marr (1971) noted, no situation ever repeats itself exactly, so that any system, to function as a memory, must exhibit at least a modest ability to generalise. Otherwise, a model that represents all item-context conjunctions locally might learn very rapidly from prior experience, but in a way that would be of little use for future behavior. A system with a better form of generalization is required. Of course the pure form of this model can be softened—particularly if distributed representations were used for the inputs, to capture graded similarity relationships between novel and familiar patterns. Such a scheme might then allow some sort of similarity-based generalization of what is learned about one item to other items with similar input representations.[2]

The network with pools of units dedicated to each different type of relation (panel c) will fare a little better—it will be able to exploit coherent covariation of attributes across different concepts within each relation type. If having wings and feathers tend to go together, this covariation will boost learning of both properties, since they are treated in the model as being of the same type. Items that share wings and feathers will, accordingly, receive similar representations in this context. But what has been learned about an item in one relational context will not influence how the item is represented or processed in another. Learning in different contexts will affect different arrays of weights in this formulation, so that information about the coherent covariation of different property types (e.g., having wings and the ability to fly) will be lost. The ability to exploit coherent covariation of properties across contexts and items requires the use of a single pool of units for the representation of all items in all contexts.

The network with but a single pool of hidden units (panel d) does have this property, and so one might expect it to exhibit behaviors similar to those of the Rumelhart network. In fact, we have run some basic simulations comparing this architecture to the Rumelhart network. Although this network still exhibits progressive differentiation, the effect is much weaker, and overall the learning process is accelerated. It is not fully clear why the effect is weaker. One possibility is that, through learning, different hidden units tend to become fairly specialized to represent different types of relations—just as they are specified to do by the architecture of the network in panel c—so that the error signals propagating back from internal representations for different contexts are not fully convergent. Although such a "division of labor" could happen in the Rumelhart network in the second hidden layer, it cannot happen in the first, since the units there do not receive inputs from context and so must find item representations that are generally suited to all contexts.

This discussion should serve to indicate how the architecture of the Rumelhart network favors the development of internal representations that are highly sensitive to coherent covariation of attributes across different items and contexts. First, all inputs converge on the second hidden layer, so that the same bank of units participates in the representation of all experiences. As a consequence, the network is initially pressured to generalize across all items and contexts, and therefore becomes sensitive to the coherent covariation of properties observed in different items and situations. Second, all of the individual item inputs converge on the first hidden layer, which is insensitive to context—hence the model is initially pressured to generalize across all items, regardless of the context. This design choice effectively prevents the network, via the learning process, from coming to treat the same item completely differently in different contexts. That is, the architecture of the Rumelhart network prevents the model from learning internal representations like those in panels b and c of the Figure. It is by virtue of this architecture that the model is simultaneously able to shade its internal representations of a given item depending on the context; but also to exhibit sensitivity to common structure existing across contexts.

It may also be worth noting that the connections from the *Relation* input units to the convergent *Hidden* units, like all weights in the network, start out very small and random, so that initially all contexts are treated similarly (just as all items are initially treated similarly). As a consequence, learning initially generalizes across all contexts—in order for the network to treat the various relations differently, it must learn to differentiate them. As we saw in chapter 7, the *can* and *is* contexts, because they capture slightly different aspects of structure than the two other contexts, eventually become differentiated from these, but since the *ISA* and *has* contexts have common structure, they share similar representations. Sharing representations across contexts has all the same advantages and disadvantages as sharing representations across concepts. To the extent that there is common structure, shared representations promote generalization; to the extent that there is unique structure, some differentiation is required. Such differentiation occurs only as needed, fostering the greatest possible degree of generalization across contexts.

In short, exploitation of common structure in these models— their sensitivity to coherent covariation of properties within and across contexts—depends on the use of overlapping distributed representations, in which information from all items and contexts converges to affect the same set of units and connections. We state the idea here as what we will henceforth call *the convergence principle*:

Organize the processing and representation of the objects of thought so that all different sorts of information about all objects, in all contexts, converge on the same units and connections.

As we have seen, adherence to this principle facilitates the extraction of representations that are sensitive to coherent covariation of properties both within and, crucially, across different items and contexts—representations that end up capturing the structure most useful to semantic task performance. It is precisely because the Rumelhart model has such a convergent organization that it exhibits the behaviours of interest: although different items have their own input weights, all items share the weights forward from the representation units, and these are affected by experiences with all items in all contexts. Furthermore, because all individual item inputs converge on a shared pool of hidden units prior to merging with the context inputs, the model is effectively prevented from coming to violate the convergence principle through the learning process. The architecture makes it extremely unlikely that the network will acquire completely different representations for items in different contexts.

Many other networks, such as the encoder network model shown in figure 9.2a, also adhere to this principle. In this model, each different type of information about an object (its form, its color, how it moves, what it sounds like, what actions we take on it, what

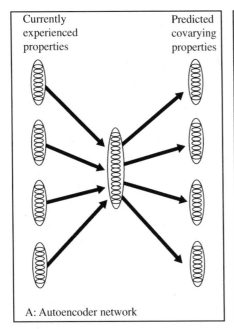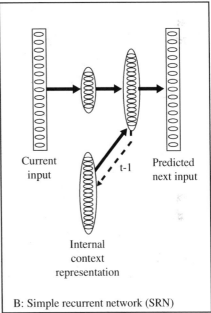

Figure 9.2   Encoder and SRN networks, illustrating how both exhibit the principle of convergent representation. Note that in both cases, all inputs ultimately project through a single representation, providing a point of convergence that allows all experiences to influence weight changes throughout the network.

its function is, the sound of the word for it) is represented on a distinct pool of units; however, each of these communicates only indirectly with the others, via a single common set of hidden units. The hidden units code a single distributed representation that mediates all of the pairwise relationships, and provides a way of capturing the coherent covariation among them. Note that direct connections between the various pools of units would not allow the network to be sensistive to coherent covariation.

The encoder network shown in figure 9.2a is lacking in that it has no provision for conditioning by context. This is a limitation, since the ability to condition expectations appropriately to the context is a fundamental requirement for any reasonable model of cognitive information processing. Another example of a network that does take context into account, while at the same time adhering to the convergence principle, is the simple recurrent network (SRN; Elman 1990) shown in figure 9.2b. In the SRN, only one item at a given time is coded in the input, but the same item may occur in many different temporal contexts. The current item's representation is instantiated across one pool of units (often hidden units; e.g., see Elman 1990), and a representation of the context—actually a copy of the network's previous internal state—is instantiated across another. The connection weights that code the current item's representation are shaped by the item's appearance across all other contexts. To the extent that the item provokes consistent and similar patterns of activity through the net across all contexts, it will exert coherent influences on the weights that encode the input, and to the extent that other items appear in similar contexts, or share similar predecessors and successors, they will be assigned a similar representation. Crucially, these effects arise because changes to the weights projecting out from the input, as well as those projecting out from the context, are filtered through the shared pool of hidden units that participate in the representation of both item and context.

We review these other architectures to make it clear that the convergence principle plays an important role in many different networks, and to indicate that the Rumelhart model is not unique in satisfying it. It is our suggestion that the successes of the model in accounting for aspects of semantic cognition depend, not on the particular details of the Rumelhart network per se, but on the design principle it embodies: specifically, that all relevant experience converges on the same set of units and weights.

Gradual, Structure-Sensitive Learning

The models we have presented rely on the principle of gradual, structure-sensitive learning:

Adjust the weights on the connections slowly, over the course of many experiences sampled from a cognitive domain, so that they will be sensitive to the overall structure of experience.

The simulations we have presented adhere to this principle using repeated sweeps through the same fixed set of training examples, which we view as a providing an extreme simplification of real experience. We see real experience as analogous to learning in a stochastic training environment, in which individual experiences correspond to samples (with replacement) from a distribution that reflects the underlying statistical properties of objects and events in the world (McClelland, McNaughton, and O'Reilly 1995). Some of these statistical properties may be fairly strong and of fairly low order, but others are much subtler and very infrequently encountered. Learning results from minute updates to the connection weights with each sample, with the ultimate aim of finding weights that optimize the network's performance (where performance is quantified in terms of the average prediction error; White 1989). The environment so characterised favours slow learning, for several reasons. Connectionist learning algorithms like backpropagation move connection weights in a direction that tends to reduce the prediction error, but the sampling process introduces noise in the estimation of the gradient, and gradual learning is important to help smooth out this noise. In addition, there is a possibility that weight changes that are too large will actually overshoot the optimal configuration, and lead to an increase rather than a decrease in error. Also, making large adjustments to connection weights to accommodate one or a few idiosyncratic or atypical experiences can destroy much of the knowledge that may have been encoded into the system based on previous experiences. For all these reasons, McClelland and colleagues (1995) argued that it is important for learning to be slow in the semantic system.

The use of a very gradual structure-sensitive learning process in connectionist networks has further appeal in light of the very gradual process of cognitive development. A child at age 10 may have a completely different representation of living things than she had at age 4, but as Carey (1985) notes, this change is not one that occurs over night. The developmental trajectory can involve periods of relative acceleration and deceleration, and key experiences can lead to fairly rapid progress if the mind is ready (Siegler and Klahr 1982), but overall, cognitive development is a very gradual and temporally extended process. These features motivated the early explorations of connectionist models of development described in McClelland (1989), and they continue to form a key part of our overall conception of the nature of cognitive development.

Activation-Based Representation of Novel Objects

A corollary of the gradual, structure-sensitive learning principle is the following activation-based representation principle:

Use a pattern of activation constrained by prior semantic learning to represent a novel object, to avoid disturbing the knowledge that has built up gradually in connections.

If learning in the semantic system is an inherently gradual and incremental process, then such learning cannot mediate the human ability to immediately use new information obtained from one or a few experiences. We suggest that such abilities arise instead from the semantic system's ability to construct useful internal representations of new items and experiences—instantiated as patterns of activity across the same units that process all other items and events—from the knowledge that has accumulated in its weights from past experience.

In several places throughout this book, we have implemented this principle using a process we termed *backpropagation to representation*: we used the mismatch between the model's output and information provided by the environment to allow for the rapid assignment of a representation to a novel object based on exposure to the object's observed properties. The technique iterates between a forward propagation of activation and a backward propagation of error to assign the new representation based on a single experience. Activations and error signals both depend upon the configuration of weights that store the network's knowledge, so that the process effectively allows the network to find a suitable representation of an item from input specifying its properties, based on the network's current knowledge. The representations so assigned are not stored in connection weights within the semantic system—instead we have suggested that they are used directly as the basis for judging semantic similarity and making inferences about the object's unobserved properties and behaviors in other situations.

Rumelhart (1990) used essentially the same process to show how his network could infer, from the category name assigned to a new object ("A sparrow is a bird"), what other properties the object would be likely to have. To our knowledge, however, this approach has not been used to address other aspects of semantic cognition.[3]

What is important about this approach is that it allows the knowledge gradually acquired in the course of development to influence how new information is interpreted. The same result can, of course, be achieved using forward-going connection weights, if the new information is provided as input rather than as target activations for the output units (as explored in chapter 4), or via return connections in a bidirectionally connected network. In any of these cases, the representation assigned to a novel experience reflects, not just the specific sensory information apparent from the environment, but an interpretation of that information based what has been learned from prior experience. As a result of this prior experience, certain aspects of the input may be ignored, and others emphasized; and the representation may be portable to new contexts where it can be used to predict how the object will behave in other situations, again based on knowledge previously encoded in the connection weights. Based on these points, we feel that the direct use of activation-based representations to support semantic task performance is an important but often neglected feature of the paradigm. We envision several potential future applications of the approach, including an application to backward blocking, as discussed in chapter 8.

Once the semantic system has derived a representation for a new object or experience, we must provide for its retrival at a later time. As noted in several places through the book, we believe that this ability depends on a separate fast-learning memory system, thought to be located in the medial temporal lobes, which complements the slower-learning neocortical knowledge system our networks are intended to model. The fast-learning system, we have suggested, binds together the various patterns of activation that arise elsewhere in the brain when a particular input in processed. Such patterns might include information about the directly experienced properties of individual objects (or persons) and the contexts in which they are encountered, in addition to the semantic representations derived by the neocortical system for these items and contexts. On this view, when someone encounters (say) an unfamiliar bird and is told what it is called, the semantic representation assigned on the basis of this experience is associated with the name and the context of its occurrence, via rapid changes in the fast-learning system (which then provides a substrate for subsequent retrieval). Off-line reactivation of the information through this substrate, or repeated encounters with the same information across other experiences, would allow the association to be gradually acquired by the slow-learning semantic system, as discussed in detail in McClelland, McNaughton, and O'Reilly 1995.

This is not the place to revisit the extensive body of experimental findings on amnesia that is consistent with this approach. However, it may be useful to mention that the complementary learning mechanisms outlined above can provide a basis for understanding the phenomenon of "fast mapping," in which children appear to be able to learn new names (and other conceptually important information about an object) from a single encounter (Carey and Bartlett 1978; Bloom 2000). It is now becoming clear that what children learn in such studies depends on their cognitive abilities at the time of learning, and this is consistent with our view that what is learned by the fast-learning system is not the raw experience, but the experience as represented after it has been processed through the existing knowledge system (i.e., connection weights). It remains for the future to apply our approach to the interesting body of findings that have emerged in these and other studies of relatively rapid learning in children.

Perspectives on General Issues in the Study of Cognition

The approach to semantic cognition that we have put forward offers a particular perspective on a range of general issues facing theories in all aspects of human cognition. Here we discuss several of these issues, indicating where there is a need for future research to further the effort to address them.

Modularity and Nativism

Many leading theoretical contributors in cognitive (neuro)science (Chomsky 1985; Marr 1982; Fodor 1983; Pinker 1991) have argued over the years that human cognitive functions may have a modular organization. In the position taken by Fodor, each module performs a limited range of cognitive operations based on information to which it has privileged access; and these computations are impervious to influence from other modules. However, Fodor does suggest that strict modularity may be restricted to relatively peripheral input-output mechanisms, including visual form recognition, auditory word recognition, and receptive and productive syntactic processes. Thinking and reasoning, by contrast, are considered open-ended processes that must have access to all types of information (Fodor 1983). Other researchers (e.g., Keil 1991; Carey and Spelke 1994) argue not so much for modularity, but for innate domain specificity, starting from the view that different cognitive domains (the domain of sentient, animate beings versus the domain of inanimate physical objects, for example) operate according to their own principles. What can the PDP approach to semantic cognition contribute to the discussion of these issues?

First of all, it should be noted that it is not difficult to build domain-specific constraints and a prior "preparation" to exploit certain relationships into a real or simulated neural network. Gelman (1990) has specifically pointed to this possibility in suggesting how certain forms of associative learning might be prepared in advance by evolution. For example, to provide for a unitary representation of space based on both auditory and visual information, it is only necessary to arrange things so that the neurons coding auditory spatial cues project directly to those that represent positions in visual space (Knudsen 1983). Even if the details of the correspondence must then be learned from covariation in the activations that arise from experience, the system has been prepared to learn the right association by the convergent projections provided by evolution. More generally, the initial pattern of connectivity in a neural network can be easily arranged so that representations of particular cues (e.g., taste) project directly to particular outcomes (e.g., nausea), thereby making the prepared cue-outcome association easier to learn than some other relation which must mediated by indirect connections (such as the association between the shape, color, or "noisiness" of a food and subsequent sickness; see Garcia, Ervin, and Koelling 1966).

We are happy to accept these particular cases as examples of biological preparation for certain forms of learning, and we would not venture to doubt that basic sensorimotor, motivational, and survival-related functions are strongly prepared by evolution. The appeal of fat and sugar versus salt, the connection between fear and certain facial expressions, the tendency to experience strong stimuli as noxious and to withdraw from them—these are certainly all either prewired or strongly prepared. Yet we have clearly been reluctant throughout this book to accept that, in general, human semantic cognition is prepared in this way. Instead we have argued that domain-general mechanisms can discover the sorts of domain-specific principles that are evident in the behavior of young children. The tendency of young children to treat movement-enabling parts as relevant to the self-motion of animate objects, to treat color and texture but not shape as relevant to identification of foods, or to treat causal properties but not color or shape as relevant to the identification of artifacts, could all arise from domain-general learning processes, in our view. Of course we cannot claim to have proven our case—all we have shown is that a domain-general learning mechanism could produce these effects. Even so, these demonstrations lead us to ask: Why should we suppose that prior preparation is necessary, if a domain-general processing and learning mechanism can capture the relevant behavioral evidence?

Many cognitive scientists appear to hold that semantic cognition and "thinking" involve general-purpose mechanisms—mechanisms that apply to all types of content more or less equivalently. Indeed, in spite of his modular stance regarding input and output, Fodor (2000) eschews current evolutionary psychological approaches in which the mind consists of a large number of special-purpose mechanisms, each adapted to a particular evolutionary problem faced by our ancestors. Together with others (Marcus 2001; Anderson 1983; Newell 1990), Fodor appears to favor a general-purpose architecture for thinking and reasoning. However, all of these authors have adopted a different approach from ours in their thinking about what the fundamental characteristics of such an architecture must be. In particular, all those mentioned have suggested that the general-purpose mechanism must be a symbol processing apparatus—an apparatus that manipulates symbols according to rules.

Especially in the writings of Fodor and Marcus, the appeal to a symbolic processing system is motivated by the contention that human cognition is regular, productive, and systematic. For these authors, systematicity and productivity suggest "syntactic" (Fodor and Pylyshyn 1988) or "algebraic" (Marcus 2001) rules. By contrast, connectionists like ourselves have argued that most of cognition is only quasi-systematic: regularities virtually always coexist with exceptions; exceptions themselves are rarely perfectly exceptional, but exhibit degrees of consistency with one another and with so-called regular items; and performance in many cognitive tasks is subject to content and context dependencies. These graded degrees of systematicity belie the black-and-white distinction between "regular" and "exceptional" items often required to explain human behavior with reference to symbolic, rule-based mechanisms (e.g., Pinker 1991; Pinker and Ullman 2002).

A criticism that Fodor and Marcus have leveled against connectionist models is that they are not systematic enough; but we would argue that the problem they are pointing to is architecture dependent. In particular, connectionist networks that do not adhere to the convergence principle are likely to be insufficiently sensitive to regularities across different items and contexts. For example, consider the fact that the Seidenberg and McClelland (1989) model of single-word reading failed to generalize sufficiently well to nonwords (Besner et al. 1990). The reason for this failure, according to the analysis in Plaut et al. 1996, was that the same letter was processed by different weights and units when it occured in different contexts. When a different architecture was employed, in which the same letter was always processed by the same units and connections (albeit with other units around them to represent the within-word context), the model's ability to read nonwords improved to a level commensurate with human performance. Plaut,

McClelland, and Seidenberg (1995) considered three alternative ways of ensuring that a given letter is processed through the same weights and units, all of which produced similarly positive results; and yet another method was used to achieve the same effect in the NETTALK model of Sejnowski and Rosenberg (1987).

Correspondingly, the failures of certain connectionist models to generalize appropriately, which have been strongly emphasized by Marcus, may be viewed as resulting from network architectures that violate the convergence principle. Such failures are observed when a network is constructed so that novel test items get processed by units and connections that have not previously been affected by the training experience, or have been affected in a manner that is insensitive to the coherent covariation of representational elements across all items and contexts. Unlike Marcus, we do not see these failings as reflecting a fundamental shortcoming of connectionist models; we see them instead as object lessons in what will happen when the convergence constraint is violated.

In summary, we have suggested that there are important design principles that must be respected by any network that might be proposed as a mechanism for extracting semantic structure from experience. Specifically, it must be designed in accordance with the convergence principle. Conformity to this principle is likely to be selected for by evolution. Ironically, this selection pressure appears to work at least to some degree against the kind of modularity espoused by many evolutionary psychologists. It requires that different kinds of information be brought together, rather than kept apart, to fully exploit the coherent covariation of different kinds of properties across different kinds of objects, in different situations and contexts.

Thinking and Reasoning

As is often the case with PDP models, we suspect that our models will arouse in some readers a feeling that there's some crucial element of cognition that is missing. Even those who feel generally favorable toward our approach may have a sense that there is something to human conceptual abilities that goes beyond implicit prediction and pattern completion. Do we really think this is all there is to semantic cognition? What about "thinking"?

A similar question arose during the early phases of investigation into parallel distributed processing, and it was discussed both in Hinton's (1981) paper on semantic cognition and in the chapter of the PDP books on schemata and sequential thought processes by Rumelhart et al. (1986a). In brief, the suggestion was that temporally extended acts of cognition—what we would in everyday language call "thinking"—involves the repeated querying of the PDP system: taking the output of one prediction or pattern completion cycle and using that as the input for the next. One can view Hamlet's famous ruminations on death ("to die; to sleep—to sleep, perchance to dream") or any other temporally extended thought process in this way.

Rumelhart illustrated the basic idea with a mental simulation of a game of tic-tac-toe, in which a network trained to generate the next move from a given board position simply applied its successive predictions to its own inputs, starting with an empty board. Hinton used a similar idea to suggest how one might discover the identity of someone's grandfather from stored propositions about fathers: One could simply complete the proposition "John's father is _____" and from the result construct a new probe for the father of John's father. Though such applications raise interesting questions about how the appropriate inferences are "strung together" to create useful "reasoning" sequences, the basic idea should be clear: the sequential application of successive internal acts of pattern completion would effectively constitute a "train of thought."

A slightly more general idea is that thinking is a kind of mental simulation, not only encompassing internally formulated propositions or sequences of discrete game-board configurations, but also including a more continuous playing out of imagined experience. This perspective is closely related to Barsalou's proposals (Barsalou et al. 2003), and seems to us to be quite a natural way of thinking about thinking in a PDP framework.

Two further comments may be warranted in this context. First, as Hinton (1981) noted, the results of successive application of the pattern-completion cycle can give rise to new "discoveries," which themselves can then serve as training experiences. Carey (personal communication, June 2002) described her daughter as once having noticed something similar about plants and animals. She may have noticed, for example, that both start out very small and grow bigger over time, eventually reaching a stable adult form and size. Such noticing might depend in part on prior connection-based learning, allowing the child to envision a common growth process for both plants and animals. Once it has occurred, the results could be used as part of the training experience for the PDP network. If stored initially in the hippocampus and occasionally played back to the semantic processing mechanism, such events could influence semantic learning and conceptual development, providing further learning opportunities and possibly contributing to new insights.

Such processes might provide a connectionist's take on the process of "analytic thought" discussed in Carey and Spelke 1994. Presumably such thought processes are often undertaken with a purpose, perhaps requiring maintenance of goals and intermediate results in some active form. Many researchers have suggested that these functions depend on the prefrontal cortex, and lesions to prefrontal cortex certainly disrupt sequential thought processes. Several connectionist models have been introduced indicating how maintained representations of tasks and goals can be used to influence processing in other parts of the cognitive system (e.g., Cohen and Servan-Schreiber 1992; Munakata 1997).

Relationship between PDP Models and Bayesian Approaches

Over the last several years there has been considerable interest in the idea that various aspects of human cognition can be characterized as a process of Bayesian inference. Since the influential work of Anderson (1990), many investigators have now adopted Bayesian approaches in categorization (Anderson and Matessa 1992), memory (Shiffrin and Steyvers 1997; McClelland and Chappell 1998), inductive projection of attributes from one kind of thing to another (Heit 1998), "logical" reasoning as revealed in the Wason selection task (Oaksford and Chater 1994, 1996), and many other domains (see the various papers in Oaksford and Chater 1998). Most recently, Gopnik et al. (forthcoming) have suggested that young children conform to principles attested by Bayesian approaches for updating probabilistic estimates of causal influences in causal Bayes networks (Pearl 1988; Glymour 2001), as discussed in chapter 8.

What is the relationship between these ideas and the approach we have taken here? One perspective might be that they are distinct alternative frameworks for thinking about human cognition. However, in our view, Bayesian approaches are not replacements for connectionist models nor for symbolic frameworks—rather, they provide a useful descriptive framework that can be complementary to these other, more mechanistic approaches. Indeed Bayesian approaches are often cast largely at Marr's (1982) computational level—specifying, for example, a normative theory for inference from evidence under uncertainty. It is a further matter to provide a model at what Marr called the algorithmic level, which specifies the processes and representations that support the Bayesian computation. Connectionist models are cast at this algorithmic level, rather than the computational level, and are thus not in any way inconsistent with normative Bayesian approaches. In some cases, researchers working within a Bayesian framework specify algorithms, but in these instances it is important to distinguish between the algorithms used to calculate normative or Bayes-optimal probabilities, and algorithms that are specifically proposed as models of the way these calculations are performed by people. Anderson (1990), Shiffrin and Steyvers (1997), and McClelland and Chappell (1998) all provide explicit process models that implement Bayesian calculations, whereas Glymour (2001) discusses algorithms that can compute normatively correct causal inferences and remains agnostic about how they might actually be computed by human beings.

It is worth understanding that many connectionist models were either designed to be, or were later discovered to be, implementations of Bayesian inference processes (McClelland 1998). For example, the Boltzmann machine (Hinton and Sejnowski 1986) and Harmony theory (Smolensky 1986), two related connectionist models that receive far less attention than they deserve, are general-purpose frameworks for deriving optimal (Bayesian) inferences from input information, guided by knowledge built into connection weights; and the stochastic version of the interactive activation model (McClelland 1991; Movellan and McClelland 2001) has this property also. The backpropagation algorithm implements a Bayes optimal process in the sense that it learns connection weights that maximize the probability of the output given the input (subject to certain assumptions about the characteristics of the variability that perturbs the observed input-output patterns), as several authors pointed out in the early 1990's (MacKay 1992; Rumelhart et al. 1995).

In general, we believe that connectionist models are highly compatible with Bayesian approaches. Bayesian approaches largely address Marr's computational level, whereas our models are tied more closely to the level he described as algorithmic, where the representations and processes that implement the constraints addressed at the computational level are specified.

There is one important point of difference between our connectionist approach and most of the process models we are aware of that derive from a Bayesian formulation. Unlike the highly distributed connectionist models that are the focus of our own work, the Bayesian models generally operate with a set of explicitly enumerated alternative hypotheses. For example, in Bayesian theories of categorization, an item is assigned a posterior probability of having come from each of several possible categories, and each category specifies a probability distribution for the features or attributes of all of its members. In our own approach there are no such categories, but rather each item is represented in a continuous space in which items are clustered and/or differentiated to varying degrees. We hold that the use of distributed representations has desirable computational consequences, and it will be interesting to explore further how they might be encompassed within a Bayesian framework.

Semantic Cognition in the Brain

The models described in this book provide an abstract theory about the representation and processing of semantic information. Here we briefly consider how the semantic system might be instantiated in the brain, beginning with the idea reviewed above, that knowledge acquisition and representation depends upon two complementary learning sytems. We associate the slow-learning, semantic/conceptual system that has been the focus of our modeling effort here with the neocortex; and place the complementary, fast learning system needed for the rapid initial acquisition of new information (semantic or otherwise) in the medial temporal regions of the brain (McClelland, McNaughton, and O'Reilly 1995). This assignment is, of course, consistent with the fact that lesions to the medial temporal lobe can produce a profound deficit in the acquisition of new semantic information, while leaving the semantic and conceptual knowledge of the world built up over the course of a lifetime of experience apparently unaffected (Squire 1992).

The basis of semantic cognition in the neocoretex has been the focus of a great deal of recent research using a variety of methodologies. Investigations of semantic impairment folowing brain damage, and functional imaging studies of healthy adults, both support the general conclusion that semantic processing is widely distributed across many brain regions. One widely held view is that the act of bringing to mind any particular type of information about an object evokes a pattern of neural activity in the same part or parts of the brain that represent that type of information directly during perception (Barsalou et al. 2003; Damasio 1989; Martin et al. 1995; Martin and Chao 2001; Warrington and Shallice 1984). There are now many studies that support this idea. For example, the brain areas that become active when thinking about actions associated with an object are near those directly involved in executing the action (Martin et al. 1995). The same appears to be true for the movements and colors of objects (Martin et al. 1995), the sounds that objects make (Kellenbach, Brett, and Patterson 2001), and emotional valence (Rolls 2000).

While in the current work we have treated semantic cognition quite abstractly, many other projects have addressed the neural substrate of semantic knowledge through efforts to model particular semantic disorders that arise from different forms of brain damage (Devlin et al. 1998; Farah and McClelland 1991; Gotts and Plaut 2002; Lambon Ralph et al. 2001; Plaut 2002; Rogers et al., forthcoming; Tyler and Moss 2001; Tyler et al. 2000). As yet, there is no unified account for the full variety of different patterns of semantic deficit that have been reported (Rogers and Plaut 2002). Many patients show deficits that appear to be specific to a particular superordinate category (e.g., living things) rather than to a particular information type, but many other patients do not (Garrard, Lambon Ralph, and Hodges 2002). One class of models (Devlin et al. 1998; Gonnerman et al. 1997; Tyler et al. 2000; Tyler and Moss 2001) suggest that apparent category specificity may reflect differences in the pattern of covariation of features in different categories. Another suggestion (Allport 1985; Farah and McClelland 1991; Warrington and Shallice 1984) is that category specificity arises from lesions affecting neurons that represent the type of information most relevant to the affected category, where this type of information is central to the representation of category members. It has been argued that these approaches cannot account for the full range of category-specific cases (Caramazza and Shelton 1998). However, there are several factors that might contribute to category-specific patterns of impairment, that have not yet been fully investigated in this and related frameworks (Rogers and Plaut

2002). In particular, we still lack a full understanding of how representational similarity structure, and coherent covariation of properties across different sensory modalities, might contribute to the patterns of impaired behaviour exhibited by a network under damage for different kinds of objects.

One possibility worthy of further investigation is that some functional specialization in the semantic system might arise in the course of development. Such a suggestion was made by Warrington and McCarthy (1987), building on Warrington's earlier proposal (Warrington 1975) that conceptual differentiation (at an abstract cognitive level) occurs over the course of child development. Possibly, the neural representation of particular types of information is initially quite diffuse, but gradually becomes more strongly topographically organized. As Warrington and McCarthy (1987) suggested, such a process can occur in connectionist networks, and there are now several neural network models, exploiting various different mechanisms, that tend to cause neighboring units to take on related functional specializations (Kohonen 1990; Schyns 1991; Jacobs and Jordan 1992; Plaut 2002). Such models generally start out with little or no spatiotopic organization, and develop more and more specialization and localization in the course of learning. To us this is an interesting possibility, and accords well with the observation that, as a general matter, the consequences of early lesions tend to be less specific than the consequences of lesions later in life (Kolb 1999).

In any case, we suggest that our current abstract model can be brought into line with the neuropsychology of semantic cognition, by placing the input-output units representing different types of information in different brain regions (Rogers et al., forthcoming)—so that units coding for different kinds of movement are located in or near brain regions that represent perceived movement, those coding color are in or near regions mediating color perception, and so on. In addition to these units, however, our theory calls for a set of shared representation units that tie together all of an object's properties across different information types. Such units might lie in the *temporal pole*, which is profoundly affected in semantic dementia (Garrard and Hodges 2000; Hodges, Garrard, and Patterson 1998). Others (Barsalou et al. 2003; Damasio 1989) have emphasized the potential role of this region as a repository of addresses or tags for conceptual representations, but we suggest that the patterns of activation in these areas are themselves "semantic" in two respects. First, their similarity relations capture the semantic similarities among concepts, thereby fostering semantic induction. Second, damage or degeneration in these areas produces a pattern of degradation that reflects this semantic similarity structure. Distinctions between items that are very similar semantically tend to be lost as a result of damage to this system, while distinctions between highly dissimilar objects are maintained (Rogers et al., forthcoming).

Interestingly, the neuroanatomy of the temporal lobes suggests that the principle of convergence we have emphasized as important for the extraction of semantic similarity structure is respected by the brain: the anterior temporal lobe regions are known to receive convergent input from (and send output to) all sensory and motor systems (Gainotti et al. 1995; Gloor 1997). The cortex of the temporal pole has extensive interconnections with all three temporal gyri, which in turn receive projections from earlier sensory processing centers. The anterior part of the inferior temporal gyrus is thought to be the terminus of the ventral visual processing stream; the middle temporal gyrus is generally thought to integrate input from somatosensory, visual, and auditory processing streams; and the superior temporal gyrus as well as the superior temporal sulcus play important roles in auditory perception generally, and speech perception in particular. Both the cortex of the temporal pole and the anterior portion of the inferior temporal gyrus send projections to orbitofrontal and prefrontal cortex as well (Grey and Bannister 1995). The anterior temporal lobes are invariably the regions of greatest atrophy in semantic dementia, a syndrome that affects all domains and modalities of knowledge alike, across many different kinds of tasks and situations. Thus we suggest that the anterior temporal lobe regions encode the convergent representations of objects and contexts that are necessary, under our theory, for the extraction of semantic structure from experience.

As stated above, no complete account of the effects of different types of brain lesions has yet been offered, and the task of providing such an account remains an important challenge for the future. We expect that such an account will encompass many of the principles that have emerged from earlier efforts to model semantic cognition in PDP networks, as well as those arising from our current effort.

Conclusion

It is clear to us that our efforts here are only one step toward the goal of providing an integrative account of human semantic cognition. The issues raised in this chapter are very general ones and we expect they will remain the subject of a great deal of ongoing debate and investigation. The form that a complete theory will ultimately take cannot be fully envisioned at this time. We do believe, however, that the small step represented by this work, together with those taken by Hinton (1981) and Rumelhart (1990), are steps in the right direction, and that, whatever the eventual form of the complete theory, the principles laid out at the beginning of this chapter will be instantiated in it. At the same time, we expect that future work will lead to the discovery of additional principles, not yet conceived, which will help the theory we have laid out here to gradually evolve. Our main hope for this work is that it will contribute to the future efforts of others, thereby serving as a part of the process that will lead us to a fuller understanding of all aspects of semantic cognition.

Appendix A: Simulation Details

Simulations were conducted using the bp++ application from the pdp++ software described in O'Reilly and Munakata 2000, which is documented on the Web at http://psych.colorado.edu/oreilly/PDP++/PDP++.html and may be downloaded from there free of charge. In all simulations, the output units were assigned a fixed, untrainable bias of -2, so that, in the absence of input from the rest of the network, their activation was low. Otherwise, the default objects and settings provided with the bp++ application were used throughout, except where noted below. Following is a summary of the parameterization and methodological details for all simulations described in the book.

Simulations 3.1–3.2

The simulations in chapter 3 employed the model architecture shown in figure 2.2 and the training corpus shown in appendix B, table AB.2. The target values in this corpus were set to 1 for active properties and 0 for inactive properties. Weights were initialized to values from a uniform distribution centered at zero, with a range of -0.9 to 0.9. The learning rate was set to 0.1. The training process was set to use online weight updating, with a permuted presentation of training patterns, so that the model encountered every training pattern once per epoch in random order. No noise, decay, or momentum was employed. The model was trained until all of the output properties were within 0.1 of their target values, usually taking about 3,500 epochs.

To simulate damage in simulation 3.2, random noise was added to the trained weights projecting from *Item* to *Representation* layers, using the AddNoiseToWeights function provided in pdp++. The noise was selected from a Gaussian distribution centered at zero, with variances ranging from 1 to 9, as indicated in the text. On each trial of damage, noise was administered once and all training examples were presented to the network for testing. The weights were then reset to their trained values, and a second trial of damage was initated. Fifty trials at each level of damage were administered, and the results discussed were averaged across these different runs.

Simulations 4.1–7.3

Simulations in chapters 4–7 used the extended-model architecture and training corpus described at the end of chapter 3. The base-model architecture is shown in figure 3.10, which is complete except that it does not depict the output units corresponding to verbal category labels at different levels of specificity, or the corresponding context units (used in chapters 5–7). Training patterns for the extended corpus are presented in appendix B, table AB.3.

All simulations using the extended model and training corpus employed the following parameters and methods, except where noted. The learning rate was set to 0.005 and neither weight decay nor momentum was employed. Bias weights for all output units were fixed at -2. As noted in chapter 4, a small amount of noise was introduced into the activations of all hidden units throughout training. This was accomplished by using the NoisyBpUnitSpec from pdp++ for the hidden units, and configuring these to add noise from a Gaussian distribution centered at 0 with a variance of 0.05. In contrast to the simulations from chapter 3, "soft" targets were used for the training patterns, to prevent frequently occurring items from dominating learning once they had been effectively learned. Thus, properties meant to be active in the output were trained with a target of 0.95, whereas targets meant to be deactivated were trained with a target of 0.05. Finally, weights were updated after every ten pattern presentations, rather than after each presentation, to improve efficiency while approximating pattern-wise updating (which is what we take to be happening in the brain). The model was typically trained for 12,000 epochs, at which point it virtually always succeeded in activating all output properties to within 0.1 of their target values. Where effects of brain damage in semantic dementia are simulated, this was implemented exactly as described above for simulation 3.2. Following is a description of the details specific to particular simulations.

Simulation 4.1

This simulation used two different versions of the general extended-model architecture, one with the usual localist input units, and one with distributed input representations. Both models were trained with a learning rate of 0.01. For the distributed version the localist input units were replaced with a bank of twelve input units, corresponding to seven of the eight *is* properties (excluding only *is living*) and five of the ten *has* properties in the extended training corpus (specifically, *wings*, *legs*, *gills*, *petals*, and *branches*; see appendix B, table AB.3). Each item was then assigned a distributed input representation across these twelve properties, in which properties true of the item were set to 1, and all other properties were set to 0. For example, the distributed representation of *birch* consisted of a pattern of 1s across the input units corresponding to *big*, *white*, and *branches*, and 0s across the other units. In both versions, the model was trained without any explicit category labels (i.e., the *ISA* properties from the extended training corpus were omitted). Training was stopped and the model was tested every 125 epochs, as described in the text.

To derive internal representations of the habituation and test items in our simulation of the infant preference experiment, we used the following procedure. For the distributed version of the model, the patterns shown in figure 4.3 were simply applied across the input units, and the states of the *Representation* units were recorded. In the localist implementation, we used the backprop-to-representation technique as described at the end of this appendix. For each item, error was calculated solely across the property units indicated in figure 4.3, and the algorithm was iterated until the reduction in mean error from the previous iteration fell below a threshold of 0.002. The states of the *Representation* units were then recorded for that item, and the process was repeated for the next item, and so on.

Simulations 5.1–5.6

All simulations in chapter 5 were run using the standard parameters for the extended training corpus described above. The main investigations in this chapter explored effects of frequency and familiarity on learning and processing in the Rumelhart network. Thus, all simulations except 5.3 used the patterns from the extended corpus (appendix B, table AB.3), but varied the frequency with which different patterns occurred during training. To manipulate frequency, the model was trained in a stochastic environment (using the FreqEnv object spec in pdp++), which specifies a probability of occurrence for each pattern within a training epoch. Each pattern was sampled randomly 1,000 times per epoch, so that a pattern occurring with probability 0.03 appeared 30 times an average in a single epoch. For simulation 5.1, the expected frequency with which a given pattern appears in 10,000 trials is shown in table 5.4 in the main text; for simulations 5.2 and 5.3 these frequencies are shown in table 5.6 in the main text; and for simulations 5.4 through 5.6 they are shown in table AB.1 in this appendix. For simulation 5.5, the frequencies shown are for the fish-expert network; to train the bird-expert network, the frequencies shown for fish and birds in table AB.1 were reversed. For simulation 5.6, the frequencies shown are for the network trained with the *is* context most familiar. To train the model with the *can* context most familiar, the frequences shown for the *is* and *can* contexts in table AB.1 were reversed. The rationale for the frequency manipulations in each simulation is presented in the corresponding discussion in the main text.

Simulation 5.3 investigated the effects of varying the attribute structure of the training environment on the model's ability to name at different levels of specificity. In this case, the model was trained on four different sets of patterns, which manipulated different aspects of structure apparent in the extended training corpus from appendix B, table AB.3. The details of how these patterns were manipulated in the different conditions appear in the text.

Simulation 6.1

A model with twenty-four output units was constructed, with an architecture otherwise identical to that shown in figure 3.10. The model was parameterized as described at the beginning of this section. All patterns appeared with equal frequency in the corpus. The model was trained with the patterns shown in figure 6.1 for 18,000 epochs, at which point all target properties were activated above a threshold of 0.7.

Simulation 6.2

The model was parameterized as described at the beginning of this section, and was trained with the extended corpus from appendix B, table AB.3. To find a representation for a novel item with the property *has fur*, the backprop-to-representation procedure was used, as described at the end of this appendix.

Simulation 6.3

Four output units were added to the basic architecture from figure 3.10, corresponding to the properties *is bright*, *is dull*, *is large*, and *is small*. Properties were assigned to the items in the extended training corpus as follows. Among the plants, all trees were large and all flowers were small. The maple, birch, rose, and daisy were bright, whereas the pine, oak, tulip, and sunflower were dull. Among the animals, all birds were bright and all fish were dull. The sparrow, penguin, salmon, and cod were large, whereas the the robin, canary, sunfish, and flounder were small. Note that this assignment is not intended to accurately reflect true properties in the world. Properties were assigned so that brightness but not size is useful for discriminating birds from fish, and size but not brightness is useful for discriminating trees from flowers.

To simulate Macario's (1991) experiment, internal representations were derived for four novel items with the property patterns listed in table 7.1, using the backprop-to-representation technique described at the end of this appendix. Error was propagated only from those properties appearing in table 7.1. The process iterated for each item until the reduction in mean error from the previous iteration fell below a threshold of 0.002, at which point the states of the *Representation* units were recorded to yield the similarities shown in figure 6.7.

Simulations 7.1 and 7.2

Four output units were added to the base-model architecture from figure 3.10, corresponding to the properties *is large*, *is small*, *is bright*, and *is dull* as described above for simulation 6.3. The model was trained just as described in this simulation, and was tested at the points during training indicated in the main text.

To teach the model the novel property *queem* in simulation 7.1, the following procedure was used. A new unit was added to the output layer corresponding to the property *queem*. The weights received by this unit were initialized to random values from a uniform distribution with a mean of zero and a range of −0.9 to 0.9, and the learning rate on these weights was set to 0.01. All other weights in the network were frozen by setting their learning rate to zero. A new environment was created containing a single training pattern, with the new *queem* unit as a target, and inputs corresponding to the pattern being learned. For instance, if the model was being taught that the *maple is queem*, the pattern had the *maple* and *is* units active in the inputs. The model was trained with this single pattern, adjusting only the weights received by the new *queem* unit, until it was activated above a threshold of 0.9. The model was then queried with all items in the extended corpus, using the same context, to see how the property would extend to these items (figure 7.1).

To teach the model novel properties about novel items in simulation 7.2, a combination of the backprop-to-representation technique (see end of this appendix) and the procedure described in the preceding paragraph were used. Properties were assigned to the novel items alpha and beta as described in the text. The representations for alpha and beta were derived using backprop to representation, calculating error across the units corresponding to *skin, legs, large, small, bright,* and *dull*. The process iterated until the mean error reduction from the previous iteration fell below 0.002. Once representations had been discovered for each novel item, the network was taught three new facts about each, just as described above for *queem*. Six new property units were added to the output, corresponding to the novel *ISA, is,* and *has* properties in table 8.1. The weights received by these units were initialized, and all other weights were frozen. The model was then trained to activate the appropriate pattern across these units from the representations it had derived for alpha and beta, in the corresponding relation context. Only the weights received by the novel units were adjusted. Training proceeded until the novel properties were within 0.2 of their targets.

Properties were assigned to the novel item tau as described in the text, and a representation was assigned to tau using backprop to representation from the six novel output properties, as well as the properties corresponding to *skin, legs, large, small, bright,* and *dull*. The process was halted when the mean error reduction from the previous iteration fell below a threshold of 0.002. The activations in table 8.1 were those produced when the representations of alpha, beta, and tau were clamped across *Representation* units, and the network was queried with the contexts indicated.

Simulation 7.3

Three variants of this simulation are reported, all varying the frequency with which items appear in different contexts. All simulations employ the standard parameterization, training methods, and corpus described at the beginning of this section. In variant (a), the model was trained solely with the patterns in the *is* context for the first 500 epochs, and was trained with the full corpus thereafter. In variant (b), training began with patterns in the *is* context 100 times more frequent than those in the other 6 contexts, but these frequencies were gradually adjusted throughout training, so that other contexts were encountered more and more frequently. Specifically, the frequency of the *isa*, *can*, and *has* patterns were increased by one every 10 epochs, so that after 10 epochs these contexts each appeared twice for every 1,000 occurrences of the *is* context; after 20 epochs, they appeared 3 times for every occurrence of the *is context*, and so on. This increase proceeded for 1,000 epochs of learning, at which point all contexts appeared equally frequently through to the end of training. In variant (c), the frequency of each context remained fixed throughout training. However, the model was always required to activate all of an item's *is* properties in the output, regardless of context, in addition to the other properties appropriate in the given context. For example, when probed for an item's properties in the *can* context, the model would activate the item's *is* as well as its *can* properties; when probed for *has* properties, both *is* and *has* properties would be activated, and so on.

Implementation of Backpropagation to Representation

The backpropagation-to-representation technique, described in chapter 2 and used in various places in the book, is a means of allowing a feed-forward network to derive an internal representation of an object when provided with some information about properties of the object that are coded in the network's outputs. In the Rumelhart network, all object attributes are coded by individual output units. Backprop to representation thus allows us to ask of the Rumelhart model, how should an item be represented, given that it has some particular set of attributes?

Conceptually, the technique works as follows. To allow the model to find a representation of a novel item given the predicates *ISA bird* and *is yellow*, we begin by setting inputs to the *Representation* units to zero and activating the *ISA* unit in the *Relation* layer. We propagate activation for all units forward of the *Representation* layer, and calculate the error on just the output units corresponding to *bird* and *yellow*. We then propagate these error signals back to the *Representation* units, without changing any weights, and adjust the activation of these units in the appropriate direction to reduce the error on the *bird* and *yellow* units. At this point we have slightly adjusted the internal representation to accommodate the information that the novel item *ISA bird*, but we have not yet accommodated the information that it *is yellow*, because we have not yet probed the network with the *is* relation. So, maintaining the same pattern of activation across *Representation* units, we next activate the *is* context in the *Relation* layer, and again propagate activation forward. Error is tabulated across both *bird* and *yellow* units and is propagated back to the *Representation* units, where small adjustments are made to their activations. Next we go back to the *ISA* context and make a further adjustment; then again to the *is* context, and so on. With each small adjustment to the activations across *Representation* units, the evolving internal representation comes closer and closer to activating *bird* and *yellow* in the corresponding contexts. The process iterates until the average reduction in error per unit (on just the output units corresponding to the two properties) falls below some threshold, at which point the network has gotten as close as it can to a representation that will simultaneously activate both properties in the appropriate contexts.

The method can be used with any number and combination of output properties. For instance, to derive an internal representation for a novel item that is yellow and green, has feathers and wings, and can grow and sing, we apply the exact same procedure —but with every iteration, the model is now probed with three contexts (*is*, *has*, and *can*); and in each context, error is calculated across all six of the properties. Note that the model very quickly learns to turn off output properties that are inappropriate to a given context (e.g., it turns off all *is*, *isa*, and *has* properties when probed with the *can* relation), so that only those outputs relevant in a given context contribute to how the evolving internal representation changes with each iteration.

Both the forward propagation of activation and the backward propagation of error depend on the states of the intermediating weights, which code the entirety of knowledge in the network. Thus the particular representations the model discovers depend entirely on the configuration of weights, which in turn depend on the network's past training experience.

For all simulations in which it was used, the backprop-to-representation procedure was implemented as follows. Weights throughout the network were frozen. A *novel-item* input unit was added to the network to provide input to the *Representation* layer, and its sending weights were initialized to zero. A new environment was created, with training patterns containing the information from which the representation was to be derived— for instance, if the model was to derive a representation from the properties *ISA bird* and *is yellow*, the new environment would contain two patterns: one with *novel-item* and *ISA* active in the input, and *bird* active as a target; and one with *novel-item is* in the input and *yellow* as a target. Pattern flags in this environment were set so that error accrued solely across the relevant output units (e.g., *bird* and *yellow* in this example). The model was then trained with this environment, making adjustments solely to the weights projecting out from the *novel-item* unit. Since, with the exception of these weights, all weights in the network were frozen, the network's accumulated knowledge remained undisturbed, and served only to determine how activation and errors would propagate through the system.

Changing the weights projecting out from the *novel-item* unit is equivalent to changing the net input of the *Representation* units (see figure 2.3)—hence the adjustment of these weights provides a means of directly changing the net inputs (and activations) of the *Representation* units in response to the backward-propagating error signals. That is, through the adjustment of these weights, the evolution of the model's internal representation could be recorded with each iteration. This provided a convenient means of storing the final representation discovered by the process—once the error reduction at the output fell below threshold, the final representation for the item could be reinstated across *Representation* units at any time, by activating the *novel-item* unit. To determine the stopping criterion, the mean error per unit was recorded with each iteration. The reduction in error was then taken as the difference in error from the current and previous iterations. When this difference fell below threshold, the process was stopped and the network was deemed to have settled on a representation.

Appendix B: Training Patterns

Appendix B.1 Expected frequency with which each pattern appears if sampled 10,000 times in simulations 5.4–5.6

SIMULATION		PINE OAK MAPLE BIRCH	ROSE DAISY TULIP SUNFL	ROBIN CANARY SPARROW PENGUIN	SALMON SUNFISH FLOUNDER COD	CAT MOUSE GOAT PIG	DOG
5.4 (dogs 8× more frequent)	ISA-specific	25.6	25.6	25.6	25.6	205	
	ISA-basic	19.2	19.2	19.2	19.2	76.9	615
	ISA-general	3.21	3.21	1.28	1.28	1.28	10.3
	is	167	167	111	111	37	296
	can	167	167	111	111	37	296
	has	167	167	111	111	37	296
5.4 (dogs 16× more frequent)	ISA-specific	18.2	18.2	18.2	18.2	18.2	291
	ISA-basic	13.6	13.6	13.6	13.6	54.5	873
	ISA-general	2.27	2.27	0.649	0.649	0.649	10.4
	is	167	167	111	111	22.2	355
	can	167	167	111	111	22.2	355
	has	167	167	111	111	22.2	355
5.5 (fish expert, fish names more frequent)	ISA-specific	20.2	20.2	20.2	162	20.2	20.2
	ISA-basic	15.2	15.2	15.2	121	60.6	60.6
	ISA-general	2.52	2.52	0.493	3.94	0.493	0.493
	is	167	167	24.7	198	88.9	88.9
	can	167	167	24.7	198	88.9	88.9
	has	167	167	24.7	198	88.9	88.9
5.5 (fish expert, all names equally frequent)	ISA-specific	62.5	62.5	62.5	62.5	62.5	62.5
	ISA-basic	15.6	15.6	15.6	15.6	62.5	62.5
	ISA-general	7.81	7.81	4.81	4.81	4.81	4.81
	is	167	167	24.7	198	88.9	88.9
	can	167	167	24.7	198	88.9	88.9
	has	167	167	24.7	198	88.9	88.9
5.6 (is context 8× more frequent)	ISA-specific	62.5	62.5	62.5	62.5	62.5	62.5
	ISA-basic	15.6	15.6	15.6	15.6	62.5	62.5
	ISA-general	7.81	7.81	4.81	4.81	4.81	4.81
	is	167	167	24.7	198	88.9	88.9
	can	167	167	24.7	198	88.9	88.9
	has	167	167	24.7	198	88.9	88.9

Appendix B.2 Output patterns for the simulations in chapter 3, incorporating all of the propositions in Quillian's hierarchical model shown in figure 1.2.

CONTEXT	PROPERTY	PINE	OAK	ROSE	DAISY	ROBIN	CANARY	SUNFISH	SALMON
ISA ...	Living thing	1	1	1	1	1	1	1	1
	Plant	1	1	1	1	0	0	0	0
	Animal	0	0	0	0	1	1	1	1
	Tree	1	1	0	0	0	0	0	0
	Flower	0	0	1	1	0	0	0	0
	Bird	0	0	0	0	1	1	0	0
	Fish	0	0	0	0	0	0	1	1
	Pine	1	0	0	0	0	0	0	0
	Oak	0	1	0	0	0	0	0	0
	Rose	0	0	1	0	0	0	0	0
	Daisy	0	0	0	1	0	0	0	0
	Robin	0	0	0	0	1	0	0	0
	Canary	0	0	0	0	0	1	0	0
	Sunfish	0	0	0	0	0	0	1	0
	Salmon	0	0	0	0	0	0	0	1
Is ...	Pretty	0	0	1	1	0	0	0	0
	Big	1	1	0	0	0	0	0	0
	Living	1	1	1	1	1	1	1	1
	Green	1	0	0	0	0	0	0	0
	Red	0	0	1	0	1	0	0	1
	Yellow	0	0	0	1	0	1	1	0
Can ...	Grow	1	1	1	1	1	1	1	1
	Move	0	0	0	0	1	1	1	1
	Swim	0	0	0	0	0	0	1	1
	Fly	0	0	0	0	1	1	0	0
	Sing	0	0	0	0	0	1	0	0
Has ...	Skin	0	0	0	0	1	1	1	1
	Roots	1	1	1	1	0	0	0	0
	Leaves	0	1	1	1	0	0	0	0
	Bark	1	1	0	0	0	0	0	0
	Branch	1	1	0	0	0	0	0	0
	Petals	0	0	1	1	0	0	0	0
	Wings	0	0	0	0	1	1	0	0
	Feathers	0	0	0	0	1	1	0	0
	Gills	0	0	0	0	0	0	1	1
	Scales	0	0	0	0	0	0	1	1

Note: Each row corresponds to a different output property. The first two columns indicate the context in which the property occurs and the name of the property, respectively. The remaining columns indicate the target patterns for the eight concepts in Rumelhart's model. To present a pattern to the network, we activate the *Item* unit corresponding to the particular concept, and one of the four *Context* units. The numbers in the table then indicate the target values for the context in question. For example, if the input is *pine has*, target values for the properties *roots*, *bark*, and *branches* are set to 1, and all other targets are set to 0.

Appendix B.3 Output patterns for the extended training corpus introduced at the end of chapter 3, used for the simulations in chapters 4–7

CONTEXT	PROPERTY	PINE	OAK	MAPLE	BIRCH	ROSE	DAISY	TULIP	SUNFLOWER	ROBIN	CANARY	SPARROW	PENGUIN	SUNFISH	SALMON	FLOUNDER	COD	CAT	DOG	MOUSE	GOAT	PIG
ISA (general)	Plant	1	1	1	1	1	1	1	1	0	0	0	0	0	0	0	0	0	0	0	0	0
	Animal	0	0	0	0	0	0	0	0	1	1	1	1	1	1	1	1	1	1	1	1	1
ISA (basic)	Tree	1	1	1	1	0	0	0	0	0	0	0	0	0	0	0	0	0	0	0	0	0
	Flower	0	0	0	0	1	1	1	1	0	0	0	0	0	0	0	0	0	0	0	0	0
	Bird	0	0	0	0	0	0	0	0	1	1	1	1	0	0	0	0	0	0	0	0	0
	Fish	0	0	0	0	0	0	0	0	0	0	0	0	1	1	1	1	0	0	0	0	0
	Cat	0	0	0	0	0	0	0	0	0	0	0	0	0	0	0	0	1	0	0	0	0
	Dog	0	0	0	0	0	0	0	0	0	0	0	0	0	0	0	0	0	1	0	0	0
	Mouse	0	0	0	0	0	0	0	0	0	0	0	0	0	0	0	0	0	0	1	0	0
	Goat	0	0	0	0	0	0	0	0	0	0	0	0	0	0	0	0	0	0	0	1	0
	Pig	0	0	0	0	0	0	0	0	0	0	0	0	0	0	0	0	0	0	0	0	1
ISA (specific)	Pine	1	0	0	0	0	0	0	0	0	0	0	0	0	0	0	0	0	0	0	0	0
	Oak	0	1	0	0	0	0	0	0	0	0	0	0	0	0	0	0	0	0	0	0	0
	Maple	0	0	1	0	0	0	0	0	0	0	0	0	0	0	0	0	0	0	0	0	0
	Birch	0	0	0	1	0	0	0	0	0	0	0	0	0	0	0	0	0	0	0	0	0
	Rose	0	0	0	0	1	0	0	0	0	0	0	0	0	0	0	0	0	0	0	0	0
	Daisy	0	0	0	0	0	1	0	0	0	0	0	0	0	0	0	0	0	0	0	0	0
	Tulip	0	0	0	0	0	0	1	0	0	0	0	0	0	0	0	0	0	0	0	0	0
	Sunflower	0	0	0	0	0	0	0	1	0	0	0	0	0	0	0	0	0	0	0	0	0
	Robin	0	0	0	0	0	0	0	0	1	0	0	0	0	0	0	0	0	0	0	0	0
	Canary	0	0	0	0	0	0	0	0	0	1	0	0	0	0	0	0	0	0	0	0	0
	Sparrow	0	0	0	0	0	0	0	0	0	0	1	0	0	0	0	0	0	0	0	0	0
	Penguin	0	0	0	0	0	0	0	0	0	0	0	1	0	0	0	0	0	0	0	0	0
	Sunfish	0	0	0	0	0	0	0	0	0	0	0	0	1	0	0	0	0	0	0	0	0
	Salmon	0	0	0	0	0	0	0	0	0	0	0	0	0	1	0	0	0	0	0	0	0
	Flounder	0	0	0	0	0	0	0	0	0	0	0	0	0	0	1	0	0	0	0	0	0
	Cod	0	0	0	0	0	0	0	0	0	0	0	0	0	0	0	1	0	0	0	0	0
Is …	Pretty	0	0	0	0	1	1	1	1	0	1	0	0	0	0	0	0	1	0	0	0	0
	Big	0	1	1	1	0	0	0	1	0	0	0	0	0	1	0	0	0	1	0	1	1
	Living	1	1	1	1	1	1	1	1	1	1	1	1	1	1	1	1	1	1	1	1	1
	Green	1	0	0	0	0	0	0	0	0	0	0	0	0	0	0	0	0	0	0	0	0
	Red	0	0	1	0	1	0	0	0	1	0	0	0	0	1	0	0	0	0	0	0	0
	Yellow	0	0	0	0	0	1	0	1	0	1	0	0	1	0	0	0	0	0	0	0	0
	White	0	0	0	1	0	0	1	0	0	0	0	1	0	0	1	0	0	0	0	0	0
	Twirly	0	0	1	0	0	0	0	0	0	0	0	0	0	0	0	0	0	0	0	0	0

Appendix B.3   (continued)

CONTEXT	PROPERTY	PINE	OAK	MAPLE	BIRCH	ROSE	DAISY	TULIP	SUNFLOWER	ROBIN	CANARY	SPARROW	PENGUIN	SUNFISH	SALMON	FLOUNDER	COD	CAT	DOG	MOUSE	GOAT	PIG
Can …	Grow	1	1	1	1	1	1	1	1	1	1	1	1	1	1	1	1	1	1	1	1	1
	Move	0	0	0	0	0	0	0	0	1	1	1	1	1	1	1	1	1	1	1	1	1
	Swim	0	0	0	0	0	0	0	0	0	0	0	1	1	1	1	1	0	0	0	0	0
	Fly	0	0	0	0	0	0	0	0	1	1	1	0	0	0	0	0	0	0	0	0	0
	Walk	0	0	0	0	0	0	0	0	0	0	0	1	0	0	0	0	1	1	1	1	1
	Sing	0	0	0	0	0	0	0	0	0	1	0	0	0	0	0	0	0	0	0	0	0
Has …	Leaves	0	1	1	1	1	1	1	1	0	0	0	0	0	0	0	0	0	0	0	0	0
	Roots	1	1	1	1	1	1	1	1	0	0	0	0	0	0	0	0	0	0	0	0	0
	Skin	0	0	0	0	0	0	0	0	1	1	1	1	1	1	1	1	1	1	1	1	1
	Legs	0	0	0	0	0	0	0	0	1	1	1	1	0	0	0	0	1	1	1	1	1
	Bark	1	1	1	1	0	0	0	0	0	0	0	0	0	0	0	0	0	0	0	0	0
	Branches	1	1	1	1	0	0	0	0	0	0	0	0	0	0	0	0	0	0	0	0	0
	Petals	0	0	0	0	1	1	1	1	0	0	0	0	0	0	0	0	0	0	0	0	0
	Wings	0	0	0	0	0	0	0	0	1	1	1	1	0	0	0	0	0	0	0	0	0
	Feathers	0	0	0	0	0	0	0	0	1	1	1	1	0	0	0	0	0	0	0	0	0
	Scales	0	0	0	0	0	0	0	0	0	0	0	0	1	1	1	1	0	0	0	0	0
	Gills	0	0	0	0	0	0	0	0	0	0	0	0	1	1	1	1	0	0	0	0	0
	Fur	0	0	0	0	0	0	0	0	0	0	0	0	0	0	0	0	1	1	1	1	0

Note: Targets for a given item and context are indicated by a 1.

Appendix C: Individuating Specific Items in the Input

In chapter 2 we discuss some of the consequences of using localist rather than distributed input representations in the model. In some sense, the use of localist units means that the network is categorizing the individual objects it encounters in its inputs. How does this categorization affect the behavior of the model? Is this categorization necessary for the model to work? To address these issues, we conducted a simulation to examine what happens in a model that uses a separate input unit to represent each of several unique instances of some category, which do not differ in their observed properties (e.g., five individual cats). How might the network behave under these circumstances?

The simulations presented in chapter 3 suggest an answer to this question: distinct concepts with similar sets of output properties receive similar internal representations when the network is trained. Thus, when two instances are associated with identical output properties, we might expect them to receive near-identical internal representations. That is, the network's learned representations for a given set of localist inputs will only differ to the extent that the sets of properties true of the individual items differ.

To illustrate this, we trained a model with patterns based on the extended training corpus displayed in appendix B, table AB.3. However, instead of using a single input unit for every dog and another for every cat, we employed five dog input units, meant to represent five individual dogs (for our convenience, we give them the names Lassie, Laddie, Snoopy, Benji, and Spot), and five cat input units representing five individual cats (Mimi, Fifi, Kiki, Lili, and Boots). For each cat, the network was required to activate the same set of properties in the output (the properties of the cat listed

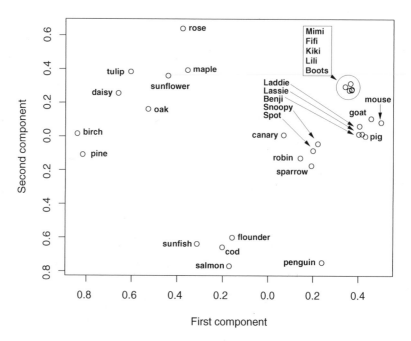

Figure AC.1   MDS plot of the final learned internal representations for the model trained with five individual cat and dog inputs. The cats, undifferentiated in the output, receive essentially the same internal representation. The dogs, which differed slightly in their output properties, are similar to one another, but are better differentiated. The two dogs that did not differ in their output properties (Laddie and Lassie) receive near-identical internal representations.

in appendix B). The dogs shared most properties in the output; however, the basic *dog* pattern in appendix B was altered slightly for each, so every individual dog had at least one property that distinguished it from each of the other dogs, with the exception of Lassie and Laddie, who had identical attributes.

We trained the network with these ten dogs and cats mixed in with all the other items from the extended training corpus. Training proceeded just as described in appendix A for the localist version of simulation 4.1. The model was not trained to produce names for any of the items. In this simulation, each individual dog and cat appeared one-fifth as often as the other input items. In total, then, the five dogs together appeared as often as (for example) the single pine tree.

Figure AC.1 shows the similarity across learned internal representations for all items in the simulation, compressed to two dimensions. The network learned near-identical representations for all five cat items. The five dog items, while similar to one another, are better differentiated. Laddie and Lassie, who have identical output attributes, are represented as almost identical.

The simulation shows that distinct items with the same set of output properties will be assigned near-identical internal representations in the network. Thus the use of localist inputs to "group together" different instances of a specific concept such as *cat* or *pig* is not in and of itself responsible for the model's ability to capture the structure of a semantic domain in its internal representations. The network will treat as identical all items that have identical sets of attributes in the output, and so it does not matter whether we use one or many localist units to differentiate individuals in the input. So long as the individuals are not differentiated in the output, they will remain undifferentiated in the internal representations, in either case. Of course, whenever individual items differ at all in their attributes, there must be some difference in the input if the network is to be able to assign distinct representations.

Notes

Chapter 1

1. Following Quillian (1968) and Hinton (1981), we use the term *ISA* to differentiate the class-inclusion predicate (meaning *belongs to category X*, as in the statement "a canary is a bird") from the predicate *is* (*meaning has the property X*, as in the statement "a canary is yellow").

Chapter 2

1. Technically, the δ terms correspond to the partial derivative of the error with respect to the net input to each unit, and the adjustments are made to a variable that specifies its value, which is initialized to 0. The activations of the units are derived from these values by applying the logistic activation function shown in figure 2.3.

Chapter 3

1. We tried several different threshold values, and the qualitative pattern of results was not substantially affected.

Chapter 4

1. Scholars of philosophy and other students of Quine (1960) might observe that it is not a trivial matter for the child to determine what is being named when a name is given, and the argument can be extended to noting that it is not at all clear what particular aspects of a situation are the ones that support the appropriate predictions of outcomes that might be expected to arise from it. Attentional foregrounding and characteristics of perceptual systems can influence these processes. Elsewhere we have argued as well that gradual learning in connectionist networks can sort out ambiguities that arise in individual cases (St. John and McClelland 1990). For example, a naive listener may not know what aspects of an event are picked out by the words "cat" and "dog" in a sentence like "The dog is chasing the cat," but over many other sentence-event pairs (e.g., events described with the sentences "The dog is chewing the bone," "The cat is drinking the milk," and so on), some of these ambiguities will naturally sort themselves out.

Chapter 5

1. To get the actual probabilities, simply divide these numbers by 10,000.

Chapter 6

1. Billman uses the term *value systematicity* to describe what we have been calling *coherent covariation*, but the terms are roughly synonymous.

2. Of particular interest here is the fact that children attribute to the echidna a property that it does not appear to have. A second interesting issue is why they choose to mention the property *feet* when asked how they know the object can move by itself—a choice that seems to indicate knowledge about a special causal relationship between having feet and self-initiated movement. We will return to this issue in chapter 8.

Chapter 8

1. It may perhaps be useful to note that the learning envisioned here does not depend on explicit correction of overt errors. Rather, learning occurs through the mismatch between the implicit predictions generated in the network and subsequent events observed in the environment. For example in Elman 1990, the experience used in training consists of a stream of words—as each word is presented, the network uses it both to correct its predictions from past words and to generate a prediction for the following word.

2. In work not yet published, Thompson and McClelland have carried out a series of simulations illustrating the account of the blicket detector findings described here and on the next two pages. The simulations also capture the finding (Schulz and Gopnik, forthcoming) that prior experience can bias initial expectations about the causal efficacy of a particular action (e.g., taking to a person should be more likely to affect the person's behavior than pressing a button), but these expectations can then be revised with subsequent input (e.g., a child observes that pressing a button actually influences a person's behavior, but talking to the person does not).

3. On other trials of the experiment, children were asked to say whether a pictured object was an animal or whether it was alive, and also gave explanations on these trials. The breakdown of explanation types includes explanations of these other types of judgments, and so it is difficult to know the exact frequencies with which different explanation types were used on up/down trials, but it is clear that these three types were often used on up/down trials.

Chapter 9

1. We should note that an initial pressure to generalize broadly can benefit the semantic system, which must extract common structure across different items and events, but such a pressure would not benefit other systems, such as the episodic memory system, which must maintain distinct representations for different events regardless of their similarity. Thus our suggestion that the initial weight configuration gives rise to similar representa-

tions for all items and events is meant to apply to the neocortical knowledge system that has been the focus of our investigation—other systems may conform to different initial constraints.

2. It may be worth noting that some, but not all, of the properties seen in the Rumelhart network also arise in localist networks that make use of bidirectional propagation of activation (Page 2000). For example, the "Jets and Sharks" model proposed by McClelland (1981) exhibited generalization and sensitivity to coherent covariation of properties. This model had localist "item" units for each of several individuals, along with separate pools of units for each of several different types of attributes (age, education, gang membership, occupation, and name), as well as bidirectional excitatory connections between the various units in each pool. When the name of an individual is activated, the corresponding item unit also becomes active and passes its activity to the other known properties. These units in turn feed back to activate the item units for individuals known to share the same properties, and these item units return their acitivity back to the property level— supporting or filling in properties shared among the set of similar individuals, and weakening properties of the probed individual that are not shared. While this model does exhibit a form of generalization, it would by no means capture all of the properties of the Rumelhart model. For one thing, there is no progressive differentiation of concepts in this model; if anything, as additional items are stored in the network, the retrieval of the particular properties of a given individual will become more and more problematic.

3. The technique is similar to a procedure used by Miikkulainen and Dyer (1987) to assign semantic representations to words, but in their application the representation was discovered by applying very small changes over many presentations of each word, rather than using a single experience to assign an unfamiliar object a representation.

References

Aha, D. W., and Goldstone, R. 1990. Learning attribute relevance in context in instance-based learning algorithms. In M. Piatelli-Palmarini, ed., *Proceedings of the Twelfth Annual Conference of the Cognitive Science Society*, 141–148. Hillsdale, NJ: Erlbaum.

Ahn, W. 1998. Why are different features central for natural kinds and artifacts?: The role of causal status in determining feature centrality. *Cognition, 69*, 135–178.

Ahn, W., Gelman, S., Amsterlaw, J. A., Hohenstein, J., and Kalish, C. W. 2000. Causal status effect in children's categorization. *Cognition, 76*, B35–B43.

Ahn, W., and Kalish, C. W. 2000. The role of mechanism beliefs in causal reasoning. In F. C. Keil and R. A. Wilson, eds., *Explanation and cognition*. Cambridge, MA: MIT Press.

Ahn, W., Kalish, C. W., Medin, D. L., and Gelman, S. 1995. The role of covariation versus mechanism information in causal attribution. *Cognition, 54*, 299–352.

Ahn, W., Marsh, J. K., and Luhmann, C. C. 2002. Effect of theory-based feature correlations on typicality judgments. *Memory and Cognition, 30*(1), 107–118.

Allport, D. A. 1985. Distributed memory, modular systems and dysphasia. In S. K. Newman and R. Epstein, eds., *Current perspectives in dysphasia*, 207–244. Edinburgh: Churchill Livingstone.

Altmann, G. T. M., and Dienes, Z. 1999. Rule learning by seven-month-old infants and neural networks. *Science, 284*, 875. (With reply by G. Marcus.)

Alvarez, P., and Squire, L. R. 1994. Memory consolidation and the medial temporal lobe: A simple network model. *Proceedings of the National Academy of Sciences, USA, 91*, 7041–7045.

Anderson, C. A., and Lindsay, J. J. 1998. The development, perseverance, and change of naive theories. *Social Cognition, 16*(1), 8–30.

Anderson, J. R. 1983. *The Architecture of Cognition*. Cambridge, MA: Harvard University Press.

Anderson, J. R. 1990. *The Adaptive Character of Thought*. Hillsdale, NJ: Erlbaum.

Anderson, J. R. 1991. The adaptive nature of human categorization. *Psychological Review, 98*(3), 409–426.

Anderson, J. R., and Fincham, J. M. 1996. Categorization and sensitivity to correlation. *Journal of Experimental Psychology: Learning, Memory, and Cognition, 22*(2), 259–277.

Anderson, J. R., and Matessa, M. 1992. Explorations of an incremental, Bayesian algorithm for categorization. *Machine Learning, 9*, 275–308.

Anglin, J. W. 1977. *Word, Object, and Conceptual Development*. New York: Norton.

Asch, S. 1952. *Social Psychology*. New York: Prentice-Hall.

Bailey, P. J., and Squire, L. R. 2002. Medial temporal lobe amnesia: Gradual acquisition of factual information by non-declarative memory. *Journal of Neuroscience, 22*, 5741–5748.

Baillargeon, R. 1995. *Physical Reasoning in Infancy*. Cambridge, MA: MIT Press.

Barsalou, L., Simmons, W., Barbey, A., and Wilson, C. D. 2003. Grounding conceptual knowledge in modality-specific systems. *Trends in Cognitive Sciences*, *7*(2), 84–91.

Battig, W. F., and Montague, W. E. 1969. Category norms for verbal items in 56 categories: A replication and extension of the Connecticut category norms. *Journal of Experimental Psychology*, *80*, 1–46.

Bauer, P., and Mandler, J. 1989. Taxonomies and triads: Conceptual organization in one- to two-year-olds. *Cognitive Psychology*, *21*, 156–184.

Becker, S., Moscovitch, M., Behrmann, M., and Joordens, S. 1997. Long-term semantic priming: A computational account and empirical evidence. *Journal of Experimental Psychology: Learning, Memory, and Cognition*, *23*, 1059–1082.

Behl-Chada, G. 1996. Basic-level and superordinate-like categorical representations in infancy. *Cognition*, *60*, 105–141.

Berlin, B. 1972. Speculations on the growth of ethnobotanical nomenclature. *Language in Society*(1), 51–86.

Bertenthal, B. 1993. Infants' perception of biomechanical motions: Intrinsic image and knowledge-based constraints. In C. Grandrud, ed., *Visual Perception and Cognition in Infancy*, 175–214. Hillsdale, NJ: Erlbaum.

Besner, D., Twilley, L., McCann, R. S., and Seergobin, K. 1990. On the connection between connectionism and data: Are a few words necessary? *Psychological Review*, *97*(3), 432–446.

Billman, D., and Knutson, J. 1996. Unsupervised concept learning and value systematicity: A complex whole aids learning the parts. *Journal of Experimental Psychology: Learning, Memory, and Cognition*, *22*, 458–475.

Bloom, P. 2000. *How Children Learn the Meanings of Words*. Cambridge, MA: MIT Press.

Boster, J. S., and Johnson, J. C. 1989. Form or function: A comparison of expert and novice judgments of similarity among fish. *American Anthropologist*, *91*, 866–889.

Boyd, R. 1986. *Natural kinds, homeostasis, and the limits of essentialism*. Unpublished manuscript.

Brown, R. 1958. How shall a thing be called? *Psychological Review*, *65*, 14–21.

Brown, R. 1973. *A First Language*. Cambridge, MA: Harvard University Press.

Burgess, C., and Lund, K. 1997. Modeling parsing constraints with high-dimensional context space. *Language and Cognitive Processes*, *12*(2), 177–210.

Caramazza, A., and Shelton, J. R. 1998. Domain-specific knowledge systems in the brain: The animate-inanimate distinction. *Journal of Cognitive Neuroscience*, *10*(1), 1–34.

Carey, S. 1985. *Conceptual Change in Childhood*. Cambridge, MA: MIT Press.

Carey, S. 2000. The origin of concepts. *Cognition and Development*, *1*, 37–42.

Carey, S., and Bartlett, E. 1978. Acquiring a single new word. *Papers and Reports on Child Language Development*, *15*, 17–29.

Carey, S., and Gelman, R. 1991. *The Epigenesis of Mind: Essays on Biology and Cognition*. Hillsdale, NJ: Erlbaum.

Carey, S., and Spelke, E. 1994. Domain-specific knowledge and conceptual change. In L. A. Hirschfeld and S. Gelman, eds., *Mapping the Mind: Domain Specificity in Cognition and Culture*, 169–200. New York: Cambridge University Press.

Carey, S., and Spelke, E. 1996. Science and core knowledge. *Philosophy of Science*, *63*, 515–533.

Chapman, K. L., and Mervis, C. B. 1989. Patterns of object-name extension in production. *Journal of Child Language*, *16*(3), 561–571.

Chapman, L. J. 1967. Illusory correlation in observational report. *Journal of Verbal Learning and Verbal Behavior, 6*, 151–155.

Chomsky, N. 1980. Rules and representations. *Behavioral and Brain Sciences, 3*, 1–61.

Chomsky, N. 1985. *Knowledge of Language: Its Nature, Origin, and Use.* New York: Praeger.

Clark, E. V. 1973. What's in a word? On the child's acquisition of semantics in his first language. In T. E. Moore, ed., *Cognitive Development and the Acquisition of Language.* New York: Academic Press.

Cleeremans, A., Servan-Schreiber, D., and McClelland, J. L. 1989. Finite state automata and simple recurrent networks. *Neural Computation, 1*, 372–381.

Cohen, J. D., and Servan-Schreiber, D. 1992. Context, cortex, and dopamine: A connectionist approach to behavior and biology in schizophrenia. *Psychological Review, 99*(1), 45–77.

Cohen, L. B., Chaput, H. H., and Cashon, C. H. 2002. A constructivist model of infant cognition. *Cognitive Development, 17*, 1323–1343.

Cohen, L. B., Rundell, L. J., Spellman, B. A., and Cashon, C. H. 1999. Infants' perception of causal chains. *Psychological Science, 10*, 412–418.

Coley, J. D., Medin, D. L., and Atran, S. 1997. Does rank have its privilege? Inductive inferences within folkbiological taxonomies. *Cognition, 64*, 73–112.

Collins, A. M., and Loftus, E. F. 1975. A spreading-activation theory of semantic processing. *Psychological Review, 82*, 407–428.

Collins, A. M., and Quillian, M. R. 1969. Retrieval time from semantic memory. *Journal of Verbal Learning and Verbal Behavior, 8*, 240–247.

Colunga, E., and Smith, L. B. 2002. *A connectionist account of the object-substance distinction in early noun learning.* Unpublished manuscript.

Conrad, C. 1972. Cognitive economy in semantic memory. *Journal of Experimental Psychology, 92*(2), 149–154.

Cree, G., McRae, K., and McNorgan, C. 1999. An attractor model of lexical conceptual processing: Simulating semantic priming. *Cognitive Science, 23*(4), 371–414.

Damasio, A. R. 1989. The brain binds entities and events by multiregional activation from convergence zones. *Neural Computation, 1*, 123–132.

Danks, D. 2003. Equilibria of the Rescorla-Wagner model. *Journal of Mathematical Psychology, 47*, 109–121.

Devlin, J. T., Gonnerman, L. M., Andersen, E. S., and Seidenberg, M. S. 1998. Category-specific semantic deficits in focal and widespread brain damage: A computational account. *Journal of Cognitive Neuroscience, 10*(1), 77–94.

Eimas, P. D., and Quinn, P. C. 1994. Studies on the formation of perceptually based basic-level categories in young infants. *Child-Development, 65*(3), 903–917.

Elman, J. L. 1990. Finding structure in time. *Cognitive Science, 14*, 179–211.

Elman, J. L. 1991. Distributed representations, simple recurrent networks, and grammatical structure. *Machine Learning, 7*, 194–220.

Elman, J. L., Bates, E. A., Johnson, M. H., Karmiloff-Smith, A., Parisi, D., and Plunkett, K. 1996. *Rethinking Innateness: A Connectionist Perspective on Development.* Cambridge, MA: MIT Press.

Farah, M., and McClelland, J. L. 1991. A computational model of semantic memory impairment: Modality-specificity and emergent category-specificity. *Journal of Experimental Psychology: General, 120*, 339–357.

Fodor, J. 2000. *The Mind Doesn't Work that Way: The Scope and Limits of Computational Psychology.* Boston, MA: MIT Press/Bradford Books.

Fodor, J. A. 1983. *Modularity of Mind: An Essay on Faculty Psychology*. Cambridge, MA: MIT Press.

Fodor, J. A., and Pylyshyn, Z. W. 1988. Connectionism and cognitive architecture: A critical analysis. *Cognition, 28*, 3–71.

Gainotti, G., Silveri, M. C., Daniele, A., and Giustoli, L. 1995. Neuroanatomical correlates of category-specific semantic disorders: A critical survey. *Memory, 3*(3/4), 247–264.

Garcia, J., Ervin, F. R., and Koelling, R. A. 1966. Learning with prolonged delay of reinforcement. *Psychonomic Science, 5*, 121–122.

Garcia, J., and Koelling, R. A. 1966. Relation of cue to consequence in avoidance learning. *Psychonomic Science, 4*(3), 123–124.

Garrard, P., and Hodges, J. R. 2000. Semantic dementia: Clinical, radiological, and pathological perspectives. *Journal of Neurology, 247*, 409–422.

Garrard, P., Lambon Ralph, M., and Hodges, J. R. 2002. Semantic dementia: A category-specific paradox. In E. M. Forde and G. W. Humphreys, eds., *Category Specificity in Brain and Mind*, 149–179. Hove, East Sussex, U.K.: Psychology Press.

Gelman, R. 1990. First principles organize attention to and learning about relevant data: Number and the animate/inanimate distinction as examples. *Cognitive Science, 14*, 79–106.

Gelman, R., and Williams, E. M. 1998. Enabling constraints for cognitive development and learning: A domain-specific epigenetic theory. In D. Kuhn and R. Siegler, eds., *Handbook of Child Psychology, Volume 2: Cognition, Perception and Development*, 5th ed., 575–630. New York: Wiley.

Gelman, S., and Coley, J. D. 1990. The importance of knowing a dodo is a bird: Categories and inferences in 2-year-old children. *Developmental Psychology, 26*, 796–804.

Gelman, S. A., and Kremer, K. E. 1991. Understanding natural cause: Children's explanations of how objects and their properties originate. *Child Development, 62*, 396–414.

Gelman, S. A., and Markman, E. M. 1986. Categories and induction in young children. *Cognition, 23*, 183–209.

Gelman, S. A., and Wellman, H. M. 1991. Insides and essences: Early understandings of the nonobvious. *Cognition, 38*, 213–244.

Gergely, G., Nadasdy, Z., Csibra, G., and Biro, S. 1995. Taking the intentional stance at 12 months of age. *Cognition, 56*, 165–193.

Gloor, P. 1997. *The Temporal Lobe and Limbic System*. New York: Oxford University Press.

Glymour, C. 2001. *The Mind's Arrows: Bayes Nets and Graphical Causal Models in Psychology*. Cambridge, MA: MIT Press.

Gonnerman, L. M., Andersen, E. S., Devlin, J. T., Kempler, D., and Seidenberg, M. S. 1997. Double dissociation of semantic categories in Alzheimer's disease. *Brain and Language, 57*, 254–279.

Goodman, N. 1954. *Fact, Fiction, and Forecast*. London: Athelone Press.

Gopnik, A. 2001. Scientist in the crib. Paper presented at the 2001 meeting of the American Association for the Advancement of Science, San Francisco, CA.

Gopnik, A., Glymour, C., Sobel, D. M., Schulz, L. E., Schulz, T., and Danks, D. Forthcoming. A theory of causal learning in children: Causal maps and Bayes nets. *Psychological Review*.

Gopnik, A., and Meltzoff, A. N. 1997. *Words, Thoughts, and Theories*. Cambridge, MA: MIT Press.

Gopnik, A., and Sobel, D. M. 2000. Detecting blickets: How young children use information about novel causal powers in categorization and induction. *Child Development*, *71*(5), 1205–1222.

Gopnik, A., and Wellman, H. M. 1994. The theory theory. In L. A. Hirschfeld and S. A. Gelman, eds., *Mapping the Mind: Domain Specificity in Cognition and Culture*, 257–293. New York: Cambridge University Press.

Gotts, S., and Plaut, D. C. 2002. The impact of synaptic depression following brain damage: A connectionist account of "access/refractory" and "degraded-store" semantic impairments. *Cognitive, Affective and Behavioral Neuroscience*, *2*, 187–213.

Graham, K., Simons, J., Pratt, K., Patterson, K., and Hodges, J. 2000. Insights from semantic dementia on the relationship between episodic and semantic memory. *Neuropsychologia*, 313–324.

Graham, K. S., and Hodges, J. R. 1997. Differentiating the roles of the hippocampal complex and the neocortex in long-term memory storage: Evidence from the study of semantic dementia. *Neuropsychology*, *11*(1), 77–89.

Grey, H., and Bannister, L. H. 1995. *Grey's Anatomy*. 38th ed. Edinburgh: Churchill Livingstone.

Hampton, J. 1993. Prototype models of concept representation. In I. Van Mechelen, J. A. Hampton, R. S. Michalski, and P. Theuns, eds., *Categories and Concepts: Theoretical Views and Inductive Data Analysis*, 64–83. London: Academic Press.

Hampton, J. 1997. Psychological representation of concepts. In M. A. Conway and S. E. Gathercole, eds., *Cognitive models of memory*, 81–110. Hove, East Sussex, U.K.: Psychology Press.

Heit, E. 1998. A Bayesian analysis of some forms of inductive reasoning. In M. Oaksford and N. Chater, eds., *Rational Models of Cognition*, 248–274. Oxford: Oxford University Press.

Heit, E. 2000. Properties of inductive reasoning. *Psychonomic Bulletin and Review*, *7*, 569–592.

Hertz, J., Krogh, A., and Palmer, R. G. 1991. *Introduction to the Theory of Neural Computation*. Reading, MA: Addison-Wesley.

Hinton, G. E. 1981. Implementing semantic networks in parallel hardware. In G. E. Hinton and J. A. Anderson, eds., *Parallel Models of Associative Memory*, 161–187. Hillsdale, NJ: Erlbaum.

Hinton, G. E. 1986. Learning distributed representations of concepts. In *Proceedings of the Eighth Annual Conference of the Cognitive Science Society*, 1–12. Hillsdale, NJ: Erlbaum.

Hinton, G. E. 1989. Learning distributed representations of concepts. In R. G. M. Morris, ed., *Parallel distributed processing: Implications for psychology and neurobiology*, 46–61. Oxford: Clarendon Press.

Hinton, G., and Anderson, J. 1981. *Parallel Models of Associative Memory*. Hillsdale, N.J.: Lawrence Erlbaum Associates.

Hinton, G. E., McClelland, J. L., and Rumelhart, D. E. 1986. Distributed representations. In D. E. Rumelhart, J. L. McClelland, and the PDP Research Group, eds., *Parallel Distributed Processing: Explorations in the Microstructure of Cognition*, vol. 1, 77–109. Cambridge, MA: MIT Press.

Hinton, G. E., and Sejnowski, T. J. 1986. Learning and relearning in Boltzmann machines. In D. E. Rumelhart and J. L. McClelland, eds., *Parallel Distributed Processing: Explorations in the Microstructure of Cognition*, vol. 1, 282–317. Cambridge, MA: MIT Press.

Hodges, J. R., Garrard, P., and Patterson, K. 1998. Semantic dementia and Pick complex. In A. Kertesz and D. Munoz, eds., *Pick's Disease and Pick Complex*, 83–104. New York: Wiley Liss.

Hodges, J. R., Graham, N., and Patterson, K. 1995. Charting the progression in semantic dementia: Implications for the organisation of semantic memory. *Memory*, *3*, 463–495.

Hodges, J. R., and Patterson, K. 1995. Is semantic memory consistently impaired early in the course of Alzheimer's disease? Neuroanatomical and diagnostic implications. *Neuropsychologia*, *33*(4), 441–459.

Hummel, J. E., and Holyoak, K. J. 1997. Distributed representations of structure: A theory of analogical access and mapping. *Psychological Review*, *104*(3), 427–466.

Inhelder, B., and Piaget, J. 1958. *The Growth of Logical Thinking from Childhood to Adolescence*. New York: Basic Books.

Jacobs, R. A., and Jordan, M. I. 1992. Computational consequences of a bias toward short connections. *Journal of Cognitive Neuroscience*, *4*(4), 323–336.

Joanisse, M. F., and Seidenberg, M. S. 1999. Impairments in verb morphology after brain injury: A connectionist model. *Proceedings of the National Academy of Science, USA*, *96*, 7592–7597.

Johnson, K. E., and Mervis, C. B. 1997. Effects of varying levels of expertise on the basic level of categorization. *Journal of Experimental Psychology: General*, *126*(3), 248–277.

Jolicoeur, P., Gluck, M., and Kosslyn, S. 1984. Pictures and names: Making the connection. *Cognitive Psychology*, *19*, 31–53.

Jones, S. S., Smith, L. B., and Landau, B. 1991. Object properties and knowledge in early lexical learning. *Child Development*, *62*(3), 499–516.

Kaplan, A. S., and Murphy, G. 2000. Category learning with minimal prior knowledge. *Journal of Experimental Psychology: Learning, Memory and Cognition*, *26*(4), 829–846.

Katz, J. 1972. *Semantic Theory*. New York: Harper and Row.

Keil, F. 1979. *Semantic and Conceptual Development: An Ontological Perspective*. Cambridge, MA: Harvard University Press.

Keil, F. 1989. *Concepts, Kinds, and Cognitive Development*. Cambridge, MA: MIT Press.

Keil, F. 1991. The emergence of theoretical beliefs as constraints on concepts. In S. Carey and R. Gelman, eds., *The Epigenesis of Mind: Essays on Biology and Cognition*, 237–256. Hillsdale, NJ: Erlbaum.

Keil, F. 1994. The birth and nurturance of concepts by domains: The origins of concepts of living things. In L. A. Hirschfeld and S. A. Gelman, eds., *Mapping the Mind: Domain Specificity in Cognition and Culture*, 234–254. New York: Cambridge University Press.

Keil, F. Forthcoming. Grasping the causal structure of the world: The ends and beginnings of science in cognitive development. In L. Gershkoff-Stowe and D. Rakison, eds., *Building object categories in developmental time*, vol. 32. Mahwah, NJ: Erlbaum.

Keil, F., Carter Smith, W., Simons, D. J., and Levin, D. T. 1998. Two dogmas of conceptual empiricism: Implications for hybrid models of the structure of knowledge. *Cognition*, *65*(2–3), 103–135.

Keil, F. C., and Wilson, R. A., eds. 2000. *Explanation and Cognition*. Cambridge, MA: MIT Press.

Kellenbach, M., Brett, M., and Patterson, K. 2001. Large, colorful or noisy? Attribute- and modality-specific activations during retrieval of perceptual attribute knowledge. *Cognitive, Affective and Behavioral Neuroscience, 1*(3), 207–221.

Kersten, A. W., and Billman, R. 1997. Event category learning. *Journal of Experimental Psychology: Learning, Memory and Cognition, 23*(2), 638–658.

Knudsen, E. 1983. Early auditory experience aligns the auditory map of space in the optic tectum of the barn owl. *Science, 222*, 939–942.

Kohonen, T. 1990. The self-organizing map. *Proceedings of the IEEE, 78*, 1464–1480.

Kolb, B. 1999. Synaptic plasticity and the organization of behavior after early and late brain injury. *Canadian Journal of Experimental Psychology, 53*, 62–76.

Kruschke, J. K. 1992. ALCOVE: An exemplar-based connectionist model of category learning. *Psychological Review, 99*(1), 22–44.

Kucera, H., and Francis, W. N. 1967. *Computational Analysis of Present-Day American English*. Providence, RI: Brown University Press.

Lakoff, G. 1987. *Women, Fire, and Dangerous Things: What Categories Reveal about the Mind*. Chicago: University of Chicago Press.

Lambon Ralph, M. A., McClelland, J., Patterson, K., Galton, C. J., and Hodges, J. 2001. No right to speak? The relationship between object naming and semantic impairment: Neuropsychological evidence and a computational model. *Journal of Cognitive Neuroscience, 13*, 341–356.

Landauer, T. K., and Dumais, S. T. 1997. A solution to Plato's problem: The latent semantic analysis theory of acquisition, induction, and representation of knowledge. *Psychological Review, 104*(2), 211–240.

Leslie, A. M. 1984. Spatiotemporal continuity and the perception of causality in infants. *Perception, 13*, 287–305.

Leslie, A. M. 1995. A theory of agency. In D. Sperber, D. Premack, and A. J. Premack, eds., *Causal cognition*, 121–141. Oxford: Clarendon Press.

Leslie, A. M., and Keeble, S. 1987. Do six-month-olds perceive causality? *Cognition, 25*, 265–288.

Levelt, W. J. M. 1989. *Speaking: From Intention to Articulation*. Cambridge, MA: MIT Press.

Lin, E. L., and Murphy, G. 1997. Effects of background knowledge on object categorization and part detection. *Journal of Experimental Psychology: Human Perception and Performance, 23*(4), 1153–1169.

Linsker, R. 1986. From basic network principles to neural architecture, I: Emergence of spatial-opponent cells. *Proceedings of the National Academy of Sciences, USA, 83*, 7508–7512.

Lopez, A., Atran, S., Coley, J. D., Medin, D., and Smith, E. E. 1997. The tree of life: Universal and cultural features of folkbiological taxonomies and inductions. *Cognitive Psychology, 32*, 251–295.

Macario, J. F. 1991. Young children's use of color in classification: Foods and canonically colored objects. *Cognitive Development, 6*, 17–46.

MacDonald, M. C., Pearlmutter, N. J., and Seidenberg, M. S. 1994. The lexical nature of syntactic ambiguity resolution. *Psychological Review, 101*(4), 676–703.

MacKay, D. J. 1992. A practical Bayesian framework for backpropagation networks. *Neural Computation, 4*, 448–472.

MacWhinney, B. 1994. *The Childes Project: Tools for Analyzing Talk*. 2nd ed. Hillsdale, NJ: Erlbaum.

Maier, N. R. F. 1931. Reasoning in humans, II: The solution of a problem and its appearance in consciousness. *Journal of Comparative Psychology*, *12*, 181–194.

Malt, B. C., and Smith, E. E. 1984. Correlated properties in natural categories. *Journal of Verbal Learning and Verbal Behavior*, *23*, 250–269.

Mandler, J. M. 1988. How to build a baby: On the development of an accessible representational system. *Cognitive Development*, *3*, 113–136.

Mandler, J. M. 1990. From perception to conception. In P. van Geert and L. Mos, eds., *Developmental Psychology*. New York: Plenum.

Mandler, J. M. 1992. How to build a baby II: Conceptual primitives. *Psychological Review*, *99*(4), 587–604.

Mandler, J. M. 1997. Representation. In D. Kuhn and R. Siegler, eds., *Cognition, Perception, and Language*, vol. 2, *Handbook of Child Psychology*, 5th ed., 255–308. New York: Wiley.

Mandler, J. M. 2000a. Perceptual and conceptual processes in infancy. *Journal of Cognition and Development*, *1*, 3–36.

Mandler, J. M. 2000b. What global-before-basic trend? Commentary on perceptually based approaches to early categorization. *Infancy*, *1*(1), 99–110.

Mandler, J. M. 2002. On the foundations of the semantic system. In E. M. Forde and G. Humphreys, eds., *Category specificity in mind and brain*, 315–340. Hove, East Sussex, U.K.: Psychology Press.

Mandler, J. M., and Bauer, P. J. 1988. The cradle of categorization: Is the basic level basic? *Cognitive Development*, *3*, 247–264.

Mandler, J. M., Bauer, P. J., and McDonough, L. 1991. Separating the sheep from the goats: Differentiating global categories. *Cognitive Psychology*, *23*, 263–298.

Mandler, J. M., and McDonough, L. 1993. Concept formation in infancy. *Cognitive Development*, *8*, 291–318.

Mandler, J. M., and McDonough, L. 1996. Drinking and driving don't mix: Inductive generalization in infancy. *Cognition*, *59*, 307–355.

Marcus, G. F. 2001. *The Algebraic Mind*. Cambridge, MA: MIT Press.

Mareschal, D. 2000. Infant object knowledge: Current trends and controversies. *Trends in Cognitive Science*, *4*, 408–416.

Mareschal, D., French, R. M., and Quinn, P. C. 2000. A connectionist account of asymmetric category learning in early infancy. *Developmental Psychology*, *36*(5), 635–645.

Mareschal, D., Plunkett, K., and Harris, P. 1999. A computational and neuropsychological account of object-oriented behaviours in infancy. *Developmental Science*, *2*(3), 306–317.

Marr, D. 1969. A theory of cerebellar cortex. *Journal of Physiology (London)*, *202*, 437–470.

Marr, D. 1971. Simple memory: A theory for archicortex. *Philosophical Transactions of the Royal Society of London*, *262*(series B), 23–81.

Marr, D. 1976. Early processing of visual information. *Proceedings of the Royal Society of London, Series B—Biological Sciences*, *275*, 483–524.

Marr, D. 1982. *Vision*. New York: Freeman.

Martin, A., and Chao, L. L. 2001. Semantic memory in the brain: Structure and processes. *Current Opinion in Neurobiology*, *11*, 194–201.

Martin, A., Haxby, J. V., Lalonde, F. M., Wiggs, C. L., and Ungerleider, L. G. 1995. Discrete cortical regions associated with knowledge of color and knowledge of action. *Science*, *270*, 102–105.

Massey, C. M., and Gelman, R. 1988. Preschooler's ability to decide whether a photographed unfamiliar object can move by itself. *Developmental Psychology, 24*(3), 307–317.

McClelland, J. L. 1981. Retrieving general and specific information from stored knowledge of specifics. In *Proceedings of the Third Annual Conference of the Cognitive Science Society,* Berkeley, CA, 170–172.

McClelland, J. L. 1989. Parallel distributed processing: Implications for cognition and development. In R. G. M. Morris, ed., *Parallel Distributed Processing: Implications for Psychology and Neurobiology,* 8–45. New York: Oxford University Press.

McClelland, J. L. 1991. Stochastic interactive activation and the effect of context on perception. *Cognitive Psychology, 23,* 1–44.

McClelland, J. L. 1993. Toward a theory of information processing in graded, random, and interactive networks. In D. E. Meyer and S. Kornblum, eds., *Attention and Performance XIV: Synergies in Experimental Psychology, Artificial Intelligence, and Cognitive Neuroscience,* 655–688. Cambridge, MA: MIT Press.

McClelland, J. L. 1994a. The interaction of nature and nurture in development: A parallel distributed processing perspective. In P. Bertelson, P. Eelen, and G. D'Ydewalle, eds., *International Perspectives on Psychological Science, Volume 1: Leading Themes,* 57–88. Hillsdale, NJ: Erlbaum.

McClelland, J. L. 1994b. Learning the general but not the specific. *Current Biology, 4,* 357–358.

McClelland, J. L. 1995. A connectionist perspective on knowledge and development. In T. J. Simon and G. S. Halford, eds., *Developing Cognitive Competence: New Approaches to Process Modeling,* 157–204. Hillsdale, NJ: Erlbaum.

McClelland, J. L. 1998. Connectionist models and Bayesian inference. In M. Oaksford and N. Chater, eds., *Rational Models of Cognition,* 21–53. Oxford: Oxford University Press.

McClelland, J. L., and Chappell, M. 1998. Familiarity breeds differentiation: A subjective-likelihood approach to the effects of experience in recognition memory. *Psychological Review, 105,* 724–760.

McClelland, J. L., McNaughton, B. L., and O'Reilly, R. C. 1995. Why there are complementary learning systems in the hippocampus and neocortex: Insights from the successes and failures of connectionist models of learning and memory. *Psychological Review, 102,* 419–457.

McClelland, J. L., and Rumelhart, D. E. 1985. Distributed memory and the representation of general and specific information. *Journal of Experimental Psychology: General, 114,* 159–188.

McClelland, J. L., and Rumelhart, D. E. 1988. *Explorations in Parallel Distributed Processing: A Handbook of Models, Programs, and Exercises.* Cambridge, MA: MIT Press.

McClelland, J. L., and Seidenberg, M. S. 1995. *The basis of human language: Rules or connections?* Unpublished manuscript.

McClelland, J. L., St. John, M. F., and Taraban, R. 1989. Sentence comprehension: A parallel distibuted processing approach. *Language and Cognitive Processes, 4,* 287–335.

McCloskey, M. 1991. Networks and theories: The place of connectionism in cognitive science. *Psychological Science, 2*(6), 387–395.

McCloskey, M., and Cohen, N. J. 1989. Catastrophic interference in connectionist networks: The sequential learning problem. In G. H. Bower, ed., *The Psychology of Learning and Motivation,* vol. 24, 109–165. New York: Academic Press.

McCloskey, M., and Glucksberg, S. 1979. Decision processes in verifying category membership statements: Implications for models of semantic memory. *Cognitive Psychology*, *11*, 1037.

McNaughton, B. L., and Morris, R. G. M. 1987. Hippocampal synaptic enhancement and information storage within a distributed memory system. *Trends in Neurosciences*, *10*, 408–415.

McRae, K., and Cree, G. 2002. Factors underlying category-specific deficits. In E. M. E. Forde and G. Humphreys, eds., *Category specificity in brain and mind*. Hove, East Sussex, U.K.: Psychology Press.

McRae, K., De Sa, V., and Seidenberg, M. 1997. On the nature and scope of featural representations of word meaning. *Journal of Experimental Psychology: General*, *126*(2), 99–130.

Medin, D. L., Lynch, E. B., and Coley, J. D. 1997. Categorization and reasoning among tree experts: Do all roads lead to Rome? *Cognitive Psychology*, *32*, 49–96.

Medin, D. L., and Shaffer, M. M. 1978. Context theory of classification learning. *Psychological Review*, *85*, 207–238.

Mervis, C. B. 1984. Early lexical development: The contributions of mother and child. In C. Sophian, ed., *Origins of Cognitive Skills: The Eighteenth Carnegie Symposium on Cognition*, 339–370. Hillsdale, NJ: Erlbaum.

Mervis, C. B. 1987a. Acquisition of a lexicon. *Contemporary Educational Psychology*, *8*(3), 210–236.

Mervis, C. B. 1987b. Child basic object categories and early lexical development. In U. Neisser, ed., *Concepts and Conceptual Development: Ecological and Intellectual Factors in Categorization*. Cambridge: Cambridge University Press.

Mervis, C. B., Catlin, J., and Rosch, E. 1976. Relationships among goodness-of-example, category norms, and word frequency. *Bulletin of the Psychonomic Society*, *7*(3), 283–284.

Mervis, C. B., and Mervis, C. A. 1982. Leopards are kitty-cats: Object labeling by mothers for their thirteen-month-olds. *Child Development*, *53*(1), 267–273.

Mervis, C. B., and Rosch, E. 1981. Categorization of natural objects. *Annual Review of Psychology*, *32*, 89–115.

Michotte, A. 1963. *The Perception of Causality*. New York: Basic Books.

Miikkulainen, R. 1993. *Subsymbolic Natural Language Processing: An Integrated Model of Scripts, Lexicon, and Memory*. Cambridge, MA: MIT Press.

Miikkulainen, R. 1996. Subsymbolic case-role analysis of sentences with embedded clauses. *Cognitive Science*, *20*(1), 47–74.

Miikkulainen, R., and Dyer, M. G. 1987. *Building Distributed Representations Without Microfeatures*. Technical Report No. UCLA-AI-87-17. Los Angeles: Department of Computer Science, UCLA.

Miikkulainen, R., and Dyer, M. G. 1991. Natural language processing with modular PDP networks and distributed lexicon. *Cognitive Science*, *15*, 343–399.

Miller, K. D., Keller, J. B., and Stryker, M. P. 1989. Ocular dominance column development: Analysis and simulation. *Science*, *245*, 605–615.

Minsky, M., and Papert, S. 1969. *Perceptrons: An Introduction to Computational Geometry*. Cambridge, MA: MIT Press.

Moss, H. E., Tyler, L. K., and Devlin, J. T. 2002. The emergence of category-specific deficits in a distributed semantic system. In E. M. E. Forde and G. W. Humphreys, eds., *Category Specificity in Brain and Mind*, 115–148. Hove, East Sussex, U.K.: Psychology Press.

Moss, H. E., Tyler, L. K., Durrant-Peatfield, M., and Bunn, E. M. 1998. Two eyes of a see-through: Impaired and intact semantic knowledge in a case of selective deficit for living things. *Neurocase: Case Studies in Neuropsychology, Neuropsychiatry, and Behavioural Neurology, 4*, 291–310.

Movellan, J., and McClelland, J. L. 2001. The Morton-Massaro law of information integration: Implications for models of perception. *Psychological Review, 108*, 113–148.

Munakata, Y. 1997. Infant perseveration and implications for object permanence theories: A PDP model. *Developmental Science, 1*, 161–184.

Munakata, Y., and McClelland, J. L. 2003. Connectionist models of development. *Developmental Science, 6*, 413–429.

Munakata, Y., McClelland, J. L., Johnson, M. H., and Siegler, R. 1997. Rethinking infant knowledge: Toward an adaptive process accout of successes and failures in object permanence tasks. *Psychological Review, 104*, 686–713.

Murphy, G. L. 2000. Explanatory concepts. In F. Keil and R. A. Wilson, eds., *Explanation and Cognition*, 361–392. Cambridge, MA: MIT Press.

Murphy, G. L. 2002. *The Big Book of Concepts*. Cambridge, MA: MIT Press.

Murphy, G. L., and Allopenna, P. D. 1994. The locus of knowledge effects in concept learning. *Journal of Experimental Psychology: Learning, Memory and Cognition, 20*(4), 904–919.

Murphy, G. L., and Brownell, H. H. 1985. Category differentiation in object recognition: Typicality constraints on the basic category advantage. *Journal of Experimental Psychology: Learning, Memory, and Cognition, 11*(1), 70–84.

Murphy, G. L., and Kaplan, A. S. 2000. Feature distribution and background knowledge in category learning. *Quarterly Journal of Experimental Psychology: Human Experimental Psychology, 53A*(4), 962–982.

Murphy, G. L., and Lassaline, M. E. 1997. Hierarchical structure in concepts and the basic level of categorization. In K. Lamberts and D. Shanks, eds., *Knowledge, Concepts and Categories*, 93–132. Hove, East Sussex, U.K.: Psychology Press.

Murphy, G. L., and Medin, D. L. 1985. The role of theories in conceptual coherence. *Psychological Review, 92*, 289–316.

Newell, A. 1990. *Unified Theories of Cognition*. Cambridge, MA: MIT Press.

Nisbett, R. E., and Wilson, T. D. 1977. Telling more than we can know: Verbal reports on mental processes. *Psychological Review, 84*(3), 231–259.

Nosofsky, R. M. 1986. Attention, similiarity and the identification-categorization relationship. *Journal of Experimental Psychology: Learning, Memory, and Cognition, 115*(1), 39–57.

Oaksford, M., and Chater, N. 1994. A rational analysis of the selection task as optimal data selection. *Psychological Review, 101*, 608–631.

Oaksford, M., and Chater, N. 1996. Rational explanation of the selection task. *Psychological Review, 103*, 381–391.

Oaksford, M., and Chater, N., eds. 1998. *Rational Models of Cognition*. Oxford: Oxford University Press.

O'Reilly, R. 1996. *The LEABRA model of neural Interactions and Learning in the Neocortex*. Unpublished doctoral dissertation, Department of Psychology, Carnegie Mellon University, Pittsburgh, PA.

O'Reilly, R. C., Dawson, C. K., and McClelland, J. L. 1995. *The PDP++ Software*. (Carnegie Mellon University, Pittsburgh, PA, 15213. Updated version maintained by Randall C. O'Reilly available from http://psych.colorado.edu/oreilly/PDP++/PDP++.html.)

O'Reilly, R., and Munakata, Y. 2000. *Computational Explorations in Cognitive Neuroscience*. Cambridge, MA: MIT Press.

Ortony, A., Vondruska, R. J., Foss, M. A., and Jones, L. E. 1985. Salience, similes, and the asymmetry of similarity. *Journal of Memory and Language, 24*, 569–594.

Page, M. 2000. Connectionist modeling in psychology: A localist manifesto. *Behavioral and Brain Sciences, 23*(4), 443–512.

Palmer, C. F., Jones, R. K., Hennessy, B. L., Unze, M. G., and Pick, A. D. 1989. How is a trumpet known? The "basic object level" concept and the perception of musical instruments. *American Journal of Psychology, 102*, 17–37.

Patterson, K., Graham, N., and Hodges, J. R. 1994a. The impact of semantic memory loss on phonological representations. *Journal of Cognitive Neuroscience, 6*(1), 57–69.

Patterson, K., Graham, N., and Hodges, J. R. 1994b. Reading in Alzheimer's type dementia: A preserved ability? *Neuropsychology, 8*(3), 395–412.

Patterson, K., and Hodges, J. R. 1992. Deterioration of word meaning: Implications for reading. *Neuropsychologia, 30*(12), 1025–1040.

Pauen, S. 2002a. Evidence for knowledge-based category discrimination in infancy. *Child Development, 73*(4), 1016.

Pauen, S. 2002b. The global-to-basic shift in infants' categorical thinking: First evidence from a longitudinal study. *International Journal of Behavioural Development, 26*(6), 492–499.

Pearl, J. 1988. *Probabilistic Reasoning in Intelligent Systems*. San Mateo, CA: Morgan Kaufmann.

Pearl, J. 2000. *Causality*. New York: Oxford University Press.

Piaget, J. 1930. *The Child's Conception of Physical Causality*. New York: Harcourt Brace.

Pinker, S. 1991. Rules of language. *Science, 253*, 530.

Pinker, S., and Ullman, M. T. 2002. The past and future of the past tense. *Trends in Cognitive Sciences, 6*, 456–463.

Plaut, D. C. 1997. Structure and function in the lexical system: Insights from distributed models of naming and lexical decision. *Language and Cognitive Processes, 12*, 767–808.

Plaut, D. C. 1999. Systematicity and specialization in semantics. In D. Heinke, G. W. Humphreys, and A. Olson, eds., *Connectionist Models in Cognitive Neuroscience: Proceedings of the Fifth Annual Neural Computation and Psychology Workshop*. New York: Springer.

Plaut, D. C. 2002. Graded modality-specific specialization in semantics: A computational account of optic aphasia. *Cognitive Neuropsychology, 19*(7), 603–639.

Plaut, D. C., and Booth, J. R. 2000. Individual and developmental differences in semantic priming: Empirical and computational support for a single-mechanism account of lexical processing. *Psychological Review, 107*(4), 786–823.

Plaut, D. C., McClelland, J. L., and Seidenberg, M. S. 1995. Reading exception words and pseudowords: Are two routes really necessary? In J. P. Levy, D. Bairaktaris, J. A. Bullinaria, and P. Cairns, eds., *Connectionist Models of Memory and Language*, 145–159. London: UCL Press.

Plaut, D. C., McClelland, J. L., Seidenberg, M. S., and Patterson, K. E. 1996. Understanding normal and impaired word reading: Computational principles in quasi-regular domains. *Psychological Review, 103*, 56–115.

Plaut, D. C., and Shallice, T. 1993a. Deep dyslexia: A case study of connectionist neuropsychology. *Cognitive Neuropsychology, 10*(5), 377–500.

Plaut, D. C., and Shallice, T. 1993b. Perseverative and semantic influences on visual object naming errors in optic aphasia: A connectionist account. *Journal of Cognitive Neuroscience*, *5*(1), 89–117.

Plunkett, K., and Sinha, C. 1992. Connectionism and developmental theory. *British Journal of Developmental Psychology*, *10*(3), 209–254.

Quillian, M. R. 1968. Semantic memory. In M. Minsky, ed., *Semantic information processing*, 227–270. Cambridge, MA: MIT Press.

Quine, W. V. O. 1960. *Word and Object*. Cambridge, MA: MIT Press.

Quinn, P., and Eimas, P. 1997. Perceptual organization and categorization in young infants. In C. Rovee-Collier and L. P. Lipsitt, eds., *Advances in Infancy Research*, vol. 11. Norwood, NJ: Ablex.

Quinn, P., and Eimas, P. 2000. The emergence of category representations during infancy: Are separate perceptual and conceptual processes really required? *Journal of Cognition and Development*, *1*, 55–61.

Quinn, P., Eimas, P., and Rosenkrantz, S. 1991. Evidence for representations of perceptually similar natural categories by 3-month-old and 4-month-old infants. *Perception*, *22*, 463–475.

Quinn, P. C. 2002. Early categorization: A new synthesis. In U. Goswami, ed., *Blackwell Handbook of Childhood Cognitive Development*, 84–101. Oxford: Blackwell.

Quinn, P. C., and Johnson, M. H. 1997. The emergence of perceptual category representations in young infants: A connectionist analysis. *Journal of Experimental Child Psychology*, *66*, 236–263.

Quinn, P. C., and Johnson, M. H. 2000. Global-before-basic object categorization in connectionist networks and 2-month-old infants. *Infancy*, *1*, 31–46.

Rakison, D. 2003. Parts, categorization, and the animate-inanimate distinction in infancy. In L. M. Oakes and D. H. Rakison, eds., *Early Concept and Category Development: Making Sense of the Blooming, Buzzing Confusion*, 159–192. New York: Oxford University Press.

Rakison, D., and Butterworth, B. 1998a. Infant attention to object structure in early categorization. *Developmental Psychology*, *34*(6), 1310–1325.

Rakison, D., and Butterworth, B. 1998b. Infants' use of parts in early categorization. *Developmental Psychology*, *34*(1), 49–62.

Rakison, D., and Cohen, L. B. 1999. Infants' use of functional parts in basic-like categorization. *Developmental Science*, *2*, 423–432.

Rakison, D., and Oakes, L. M., eds. 2003. *Early Category and Concept Development: Making Sense of the Blooming, Buzzing Confusion*. New York: Oxford University Press.

Rakison, D., and Poulin-Dubois, D. 2001. The developmental origin of the animate-inanimate distinction. *Psychological Bulletin*, *127*, 209–228.

Reber, A. S. 1969. Transfer of syntactic structure in synthetic languages. *Journal of Experimental Psychology*, *81*, 115–119.

Rehder, B., and Ross, B. H. 2001. Abstract coherent categories. *Journal of Experimental Psychology: Learning, Memory, and Cognition*, 1261–1275.

Rips, L. J., Shoben, E. J., and Smith, E. E. 1973. Semantic distance and the verification of semantic relations. *Journal of Verbal Learning and Verbal Behavior*, *12*, 1–20.

Rogers, T. T., and Griffin, R. 2001. *Goal attribution without goal representation: A connectionist approach to infants' early understanding of intentional actions*. Unpublished manuscript.

Rogers, T. T., Lambon Ralph, M., Garrard, P., Bozeat, S., McClelland, J. L., Hodges, J. R., and Patterson, K. Forthcoming. *The structure and deterioration of semantic memory: A computational and neuropsychological investigation. Psychological Review.*

Rogers, T. T., and Plaut, D. C. 2002. Connectionist perspectives on category specific deficits. In E. Forde and G. Humphreys, eds., *Category Specificity in Mind and Brain*, 251–289. Hove, East Sussex, U.K.: Psychology Press.

Rohde, D. L. T. 2002. *A connectionist model of sentence comprehension and production.* Unpublished doctoral dissertation, Computer Science Department, Carnegie Mellon University, Pittsburgh. (Available as Technical Report CMU-CS-02-105.)

Rohde, D. L. T., and Plaut, D. C. 1999. Language acquisition in the absence of explicit negative evidence: How important is starting small? *Cognition, 72*(1), 67–109.

Rolls, E. T. 1990. Principles underlying the representation and storage of information in neuronal networks in the primate hippocampus and cerebral cortex. In S. F. Zornetzer, J. L. Davis, and C. Lau, eds., *An Introduction to Neural and Electronic Networks*, 73–90. San Diego, CA: Academic Press.

Rolls, E. T. 2000. The orbitofrontal cortex and reward. *Cerebral Cortex, 10*, 284–294.

Rosch, E. 1975. Cognitive representations of semantic categories. *Journal of Experimental Psychology: General, 104*, 192–233.

Rosch, E. 1978. Principles of categorization. In E. Rosch and B. Lloyd, eds., *Cognition and Categorization*, 27–48. Hillsdale, NJ: Erlbaum.

Rosch, E., and Mervis, C. B. 1975. Family resemblances: Studies in the internal structure of categories. *Cognitive Psychology, 7*, 573–605.

Rosch, E., Mervis, C. B., Gray, W., Johnson, D., and Boyes-Braem, P. 1976. Basic objects in natural categories. *Cognitive Psychology, 8*, 382–439.

Rosch, E., Simpson, C., and Miller, R. 1976. Structural bases of typicality effects. *Journal of Experimental Psychology: Human Perception and Performance, 2*, 491–502.

Rumelhart, D. E. 1990. Brain style computation: Learning and generalization. In S. F. Zornetzer, J. L. Davis, and C. Lau, eds., *An Introduction to Neural and Electronic Networks*, 405–420. San Diego, CA: Academic Press.

Rumelhart, D. E., Durbin, R., Golden, R., and Chauvin, Y. 1995. Backpropagation: The basic theory. In Y. Chauvin and D. E. Rumelhart, eds., *Back-propagation: Theory, Architectures, and Applications*, 1–34. Hillsdale, NJ: Erlbaum.

Rumelhart, D. E., Hinton, G. E., and Williams, R. J. 1986a. Learning internal representations by error propagation. In D. E. Rumelhart, J. L. McClelland, and the PDP Research Group, eds., *Parallel Distributed Processing: Explorations in the Microstructure of Cognition*, vol. 1, 318–362. Cambridge, MA: MIT Press.

Rumelhart, D. E., McClelland, J. L., and the PDP Research Group. 1986b. *Parallel Distributed Processing: Explorations in the Microstructure of Cognition, Volume 1: Foundations.* Cambridge, MA: MIT Press.

Rumelhart, D. E., Smolensky, P., McClelland, J. L., and Hinton, G. E. 1986c. Schemata and sequential thought processes in PDP models. In J. L. McClelland, D. E. Rumelhart, and the PDP research group, eds., *Parallel Distributed Processing: Explorations in the Microstructure of Cognition*, vol. 2, 7–57. Cambridge, MA: MIT Press.

Rumelhart, D. E., and Todd, P. M. 1993. Learning and connectionist representations. In D. E. Meyer and S. Kornblum, eds., *Attention and Performance XIV: Synergies in Experimental Psychology, Artificial Intelligence, and Cognitive Neuroscience*, 3–30. Cambridge, MA: MIT Press.

Shulz, L. E., and Gopnik, A. Forthcoming. Causal learning across domains. *Developmental Psychology.*

Schyns, P. G. 1991. A modular neural network model of concept acquisition. *Cognitive Science, 15*, 461–508.

Seidenberg, M. S., and McClelland, J. L. 1989. A distributed, developmental model of word recognition and naming. *Psychological Review, 96*, 523–568.

Sejnowski, T. J., and Rosenberg, C. R. 1987. Parallel networks that learn to pronounce English text. *Complex Systems, 1*, 145–168.

Servan-Schreiber, D., Cleeremans, A., and McClelland, J. L. 1991. Graded state machines: The representation of temporal contingencies in simple recurrent networks. *Machine Learning, 7*, 161–193.

Shiffrin, R. M., and Steyvers, M. 1997. A model of recognition memory: REM—Retrieving effectively from memory. *Psychonomic Bulletin and Review, 4*, 145–166.

Shultz, T. R., Mareschal, D., and Schmidt, W. C. 1994. Modeling cognitive development of balance scale phenomena. *Machine Learning, 16*, 57–86.

Siegler, R. S. 1976. Three aspects of cognitive development. *Cognitive Psychology, 8*(4), 481–520.

Siegler, R. S. 1997. *Emerging Minds: The Process of Change in Children's Thinking.* New York: Oxford University Press.

Siegler, R. S., and Klahr, D. 1982. When do children learn? The relationship between existing knowledge and the acquisition of new knolwedge. In R. Glaser, ed., *Advances in Instructional Psychology*, vol. 2, 121–211. Hillsdale, NJ: Erlbaum.

Siegler, R. S., and Stern, E. 1998. Conscious and unconscious strategy discoveries: A microgenetic analysis. *Journal of Experimental Psychology: General, 127*(4), 377–397.

Sloman, S. A., and Rips, L. J., eds. 1998. *Similarity and Symbols in Human Thinking.* Cambridge, MA: MIT Press.

Sloutsky, V. M. 2003. The role of similarity in the development of categorization. *Trends in Cognitive Sciences, 7*(6), 246–251.

Smith, E. E., and Medin, D. L. 1981. *Categories and Concepts.* Cambridge, MA: Harvard University Press.

Smith, E. E., Shoben, E. J., and Rips, L. J. 1974. Structure and process in semantic memory: A featural model for semantic decision. *Psychological Review, 81*, 214–241.

Smolensky, P. 1986. Information processing in dynamical systems: Foundations of harmony theory. In D. E. Rumelhart and J. L. McClelland, eds., *Parallel Distributed Processing: Explorations in the Microstructure of Cognition*, vol. 1, 194–281. Cambridge, MA: MIT Press.

Snodgrass, J. G., and Vanderwart, M. 1980. A standardized set of 260 pictures: Norms for name agreement, image agreement, familiarity, and visual complexity. *Journal of Experimental Psychology: Learning, Memory, and Cognition, 6*, 174–215.

Snowden, J. S., Goulding, P. J., and Neary, D. 1989. Semantic dementia: A form of circumscribed temporal atrophy. *Behavioural Neurology, 2*, 167–182.

Sobel, D. M., Tenenbaum, J., and Gopnik, A. 2002. *Causal learning from indirect evidence in young children: Children use rational inference, not simply associations.* Unpublished manuscript.

Spelke, E. S., Breinlinger, K., Macomber, J., and Jacobson, K. 1992. Origins of knowledge. *Psychological Review, 99*(4), 605–632.

Spirtes, P., Glymour, C., and Scheines, R. 2001. *Causation, prediction, and search.* 2nd ed. Springer Lecture Notes in Statistics. Cambridge, MA: MIT Press.

Springer, K., and Keil, F. 1991. Early differentiation of causal mechanisms appropriate to biological and nonbiological kinds. *Child Development, 62*, 767–781.

Squire, L. R. 1992. Memory and the hippocampus: A synthesis from findings with rats, monkeys, and humans. *Psychological Review, 99*, 195–231.

Squire, L. R., Cohen, N. J., and Nadel, L. 1984. The medial temporal region and memory consolidation: A new hypothesis. In H. Weingartner and E. Parker, eds., *Memory Consolidation*, 185–210. Hillsdale, NJ: Erlbaum.

St. John, M. F. 1992. The Story Gestalt: A model of knowledge-intensive processes in text comprehension. *Cognitive Science, 16*, 271–306.

St. John, M. F., and McClelland, J. L. 1990. Learning and applying contextual constraints in sentence comprehension. *Artificial Intelligence, 46*, 217–257.

Sutton, R. S. 1988. Learning to predict by the method of temporal diferences. *Machine Learning, 3*, 9–44.

Tanaka, J., and Taylor, M. 1991. Object categories and expertise: Is the basic level in the eye of the beholder? *Cognitive Psychology, 23*, 457–482.

Tomasello, M. 1999. Having intentions, understanding intentions, and understanding communicative intentions. In P. D. Zelazo and J. W. Astington, eds., *Developing Theories of Intention: Social Understanding and Self-Control*, 63–75. Mahwah, NJ: Erlbaum.

Tyler, L., Moss, H. E., Durrant-Peatfield, M. R., and Levy, J. P. 2000. Conceptual structure and the structure of concepts: A distributed account of category-specific deficits. *Brain and Language, 75*(2), 195–231.

Tyler, L. K., and Moss, H. E. 2001. Towards a distributed account of conceptual knowledge. *Trends in Cognitive Sciences, 5*(6), 244–252.

Warrington, E. K. 1975. Selective impairment of semantic memory. *Quarterly Journal of Experimental Psychology, 27*, 635–657.

Warrington, E. K., and McCarthy, R. 1987. Categories of knowledge: Further fractionation and an attempted integration. *Brain, 110*, 1273–1296.

Warrington, E. K., and Shallice, T. 1984. Category specific semantic impairments. *Brain, 107*, 829–854.

White, H. 1989. Learning in artificial neural networks: A statistical perspective. *Neural Computation, 1*, 425–464.

Williams, R. J., and Zipser, D. 1989. A learning algorithm for continually running fully recurrent neural networks. *Neural Computation, 1*, 270–280.

Wilson, R. A., and Keil, F. C. 2000. The shadows and shallows of explanation. In F. C. Keil and R. A. Wilson, eds., *Explanation and Cognition*, 87–114. Cambridge, MA: MIT Press.

Wittgenstein, L. 1953. *Philosophical Investigations*. Oxford: Blackwell.

Younger, B., and Fearing, D. 2000. A global-to-basic trend in early categorization: Evidence from a dual-category habituation task. *Infancy, 1*, 47–58.

Zeki, S. M. 1978. Functional specialization in the visual cortex of the rhesus monkey. *Nature, 274*, 423.

Index